Dr. Avani Maniar
Dr. Shivani Mehta

A Study on Silver Workers Residing in Vadodara City

Anchor Academic Publishing

Maniar, Avani, Mehta, Shivani: A Study on Silver Workers Residing in Vadodara City, Hamburg, Anchor Academic Publishing 2017

Buch-ISBN: 978-3-96067-111-4
PDF-eBook-ISBN: 978-3-96067-611-9
Druck/Herstellung: Anchor Academic Publishing, Hamburg, 2017

Bibliografische Information der Deutschen Nationalbibliothek:
Die Deutsche Nationalbibliothek verzeichnet diese Publikation in der Deutschen Nationalbibliografie; detaillierte bibliografische Daten sind im Internet über http://dnb.d-nb.de abrufbar.

Bibliographical Information of the German National Library:
The German National Library lists this publication in the German National Bibliography. Detailed bibliographic data can be found at: http://dnb.d-nb.de

All rights reserved. This publication may not be reproduced, stored in a retrieval system or transmitted, in any form or by any means, electronic, mechanical, photocopying, recording or otherwise, without the prior permission of the publishers.

Das Werk einschließlich aller seiner Teile ist urheberrechtlich geschützt. Jede Verwertung außerhalb der Grenzen des Urheberrechtsgesetzes ist ohne Zustimmung des Verlages unzulässig und strafbar. Dies gilt insbesondere für Vervielfältigungen, Übersetzungen, Mikroverfilmungen und die Einspeicherung und Bearbeitung in elektronischen Systemen.

Die Wiedergabe von Gebrauchsnamen, Handelsnamen, Warenbezeichnungen usw. in diesem Werk berechtigt auch ohne besondere Kennzeichnung nicht zu der Annahme, dass solche Namen im Sinne der Warenzeichen- und Markenschutz-Gesetzgebung als frei zu betrachten wären und daher von jedermann benutzt werden dürften.

Die Informationen in diesem Werk wurden mit Sorgfalt erarbeitet. Dennoch können Fehler nicht vollständig ausgeschlossen werden und die Diplomica Verlag GmbH, die Autoren oder Übersetzer übernehmen keine juristische Verantwortung oder irgendeine Haftung für evtl. verbliebene fehlerhafte Angaben und deren Folgen.

Alle Rechte vorbehalten

© Anchor Academic Publishing, Imprint der Diplomica Verlag GmbH
Hermannstal 119k, 22119 Hamburg
http://www.diplomica-verlag.de, Hamburg 2017
Printed in Germany

Acknowledgements

First and foremost I would like to express my sincere gratitude and thanks to my guide Dr. Avani Maniar for her continuous support, for her patience, inspiration, and immense encouragement. It has been an honour to be her first Ph.D. student. I appreciate all her contributions of time, ideas, to make my Ph.D. experience productive and stimulating. The joy and enthusiasm she has for research was contagious and motivational for me, even during tough times in the Ph.D. pursuit. She has routinely gone beyond her duties to fire fight my worries, concerns, and anxieties, and have worked to instil great confidence in both myself and my work.

Most importantly, I owe a lot to my parents, Mr. Rajul .B. Mehta and Roma .R. Mehta who encouraged, helped and supported me endlessly at every stage of my personal and academic life, and longed to see this achievement come true. Special thanks to my mother for standing by me like my shadow and accompanying me at the time of data collection and for being with me in each and every stage of my PhD. Without their support it would not have been possible for me to accomplish my research.

Sincere thanks are extended to Prof. Rameshwari Pandya, Head, Department of Extension and Communication, Faculty of Family and Community Sciences, The Maharaja Sayajirao University of Vadodara for her valuable suggestions, advice, constructive criticism at the time of validation of the tool and various stages of the study.

I show extensive gratitude to all of the silver workers who warmly contributed their stories, histories, and experiences. Without this willingness to share, the research would not have even been possible in the same vein. I also want to express my appreciation for cooperation to all the business houses, banks, corporate, firms, and who have supported and obliged me by providing required details during data collection.

I would like to extend great thanks to Mr. Harendra Parmar for helping in statistical analysis of the data, from Psychology Department, Faculty of Education and

Psychology. The Maharaja Sayajirao University of Baroda, Vadodara for helping in statistical analysis of the data.

I am really grateful to Dr. Jitesh Parikh for generously offering time for the grammatical checking of my thesis.

I would like to extend special thanks to my friends and fellow mate Ms. Dhara Bhatt and Ms. Leena Chauhan, for the stimulating discussions, their constant support various capacities towards completing this study and for all the fun we have had. I specially thank Ms. Sarika Patel for her support during data analysis phase.

- **Ms. Shivani Mehta**

Abstract

The present study was aimed to assess the reason of silver workers to work after retirement and also to assess the employer's attitude towards the employment of such silver workers who wants to work after retirement.

The study was explorative and analytical in nature. Population of the study comprised of elderly residing State who were working after retirement and the employers who recruit retired elderly in their organizations, firms, corporate, banks, and business houses. The sample consisted of 300 elderly and 50 employers residing in Vadodara City of Gujarat State

Primary data for the study was collected through questionnaire and personal interviews. Analysis of the study was using different statistical measures like mean, percentage, t-test, f-test, correlation, standard deviation, intensity indices, range and coefficient of correlation.

The study was set to investigate the reasons, factors that influence elderly to work after retirement, problems they face due to work and workplace, perceptions about old age, and satisfaction while working after retirement. It also focused on acquiring the suggestions that elderly workers wanted to give for the betterment of work sector, policies framing for retired people, change that they would like to in societies' attitudes towards them. In relation to the employers study aimed at investigating the attitudes of employers towards recruiting elderly after they retire, advantages and disadvantages of recruiting them

Many stereotypes and prejudices related to the employment of elderly persons that employers usually exhibit to avoid employing them find no justification today and cannot be taken as valid arguments. Primarily, the demand for manual work has decreased, which suits elderly workers to a large extent. Similarly, due to the advances in medicine and better life conditions, the physical and mental health of elderly population have improved, which enable them to be able to work longer hours than it was possible in the past. Besides, the living style has completely changed in the last two decades. All this has led to a situation that even those who count as the richest and who can safely retire, wish to continue to work and feel useful to themselves, to their families and to their society. The poor ones are forced to work even after they have formally retired because their pensions are small and often insufficient to allow a decent life.

The elderly are keen on redefining retirement. Instead of surfing and mountain-biking, the elderly will prefer spend at least part of retirement not in leisure but working. It may be sometimes for money or, out of necessity, or sometimes for no money but just because it is personally rewarding. Not long ago, many employers appeared to be askance at elderly workers. They thought that elderly workers lacked the spirit and imagination that youthful cohorts can display. But now the times are changing. The motives of elderly people to go out to work may differ; however, what is common to all of these people is that they want to be actively working as long as they are able to work.

It appears that population ageing is one of the most important and challenging issues in this millennium. It may infer that in this country, the ageing process has been largely influenced by socio-economic development of society. However, the problems call for serious thinking on a part that the government and civil society can play. In this context, the present research would like to find the reasons of silvers workers for working after retirement.

CONTENTS

Acknowledgements

Abstract

List of Tables

List of Figures

Sr. No.	Contents	Page No.
1.	***INTRODUCTION***	1-52

    1.1 Demography of Elderly Population

    1.2 Elderly Defined

    1.3 Elderly and Retirement

    1.4 Work after Retirement amongst Elderly

    1.5 Reasons of Working after Retirement

    1.6 Perceptions about Retirement

    1.7 Influence of Work on Elderly

    1.8 Problems faced by Elderly at Workplace

    1.9 Satisfaction at Workplace

    1.10 Employers Attitude towards Recruiting Elderly after Retirement

    1.11 Statement of the Problem

    1.12 Research Questions

    1.13 Justification

    1.13.1 Justification of the Subject of the Study

    1.13.2 Justification of the Sample of the Study

    1.13.3 Significance of the Study in the Department of Extension and Communication

    1.13.4 Justification of the Variables

1.14 Objectives of the Study

1.15 Null Hypothesis of the Study

1.16 Delimitation of the Study

1.17 Assumptions of the Study

1.18 Operational Definitions of Silver Workers and Employers

2. *REVIEW OF LITERATURE* 53-82

2.1 Studies Related to Reasons of Silver Workers to Work after Retirement

2.2 Studies related to Employment Status of Silver Workers

2.3 Studies related to Factors Influencing Silver Workers to Work beyond Retirement Age

2.4 Studies related to Employers Perspectives towards recruiting Silver Workers

2.5 Studies related to Perceptions of Silver Workers related to Retirement

2.6 Studies related to Problems faced by Silver Workers

3. *METHODOLOGY* 83-117

(A) Methodology for Quantitative Data

(B) Methodology for Qualitative Data

3.1 Pilot Study

3.1.1 Findings of the Pilot Study

3.1.2 Conclusion of the Pilot Study

3.2 Population of the Study

3.3 Sampling Unit

3.4 Sampling Frame

3.5 Sample Size and Selection Procedure of the Sample (Silver Workers and Employers)

3.5.1 Sample Size for Qualitative Data

3.6 Construction of Research Tool

3.6.1 Description of Research tools used for Silver Workers

3.6.1.1 Section 1 Profile of Silver Workers

3.6.1.2 Section 2 Reasons of Working after Retirement and Perceptions about Retirement

3.6.1.3 Section 3 Influence of Work on Silver Workers

3.6.1.4 Section 4 Problems faced by Silver Workers at Workplace

3.6.1.5 Section 5 Satisfaction at Workplace

3.6.1.6 Suggestions

3.6.2 Description of Research tool Used for Employers

3.6.2.1 Research tool used for Data Collection of Employers

3.7 Validity of Research Tools

3.8 Reliability of Research Tools

3.9 Pre-Testing of Research Tools

3.10 Procedure of Data Collection

3.11 Scoring and Categorization of the Data of Silver Workers

3.11.1 Categorization of Variables

3.11.2 Reasons to Work after Retirement

3.11.3 Perception about Retirement

3.11.4 Influence of Work on Silver Workers

3.11.5 Problems faced by Silver Workers at Workplace

3.11.6 Satisfaction at Workplace

3.12 Scoring categorization of Data of Employers

3.12.1 Qualities of recruiting Silver Workers

3.12.2 Advantages of recruiting Silver Workers

3.12.3 Disadvantages of recruiting Silver Workers

3.12.4 Influential Factors in recruiting Silver Workers

3.13 Statistical Analysis of the Data

3.14 Sampling Unit

3.15 Sampling Frame

3.16 Sample Size

3.17 Process of Conducting In-depth Interviews

3.18 Analysis of the Interviewed Data

4.   *FINDINGS and DISCUSSION*   118-358

Part – 1 Silver Workers   120-326

A)   *Findings and Discussion of the Quantitative Data*   120-288

4.1 Profile of the Selected Silver Workers

4.1.1 Details about Family

4.1.2 Silver Worker and their Present Occupation

4.1.3 Work History

4.1.4 Health Status

4.2 Overall and Aspects Wise Reasons of Silver Workers to Work after Retirement

4.3 Differences in the Reasons of Silver Workers to Work after Retirement in Relation to the Selected Variables

4.4 Item Wise Findings regarding Reasons Prompting Silver Workers to Work after Retirement

4.5 Perceptions of Silver Workers about Retirement

4.6 Item wise Findings of the Perceptions of Silver Workers about their Retirement

4.7 Preparation of Retirement

4.8 Influence of Work on Silver Workers

4.9 Differences in the Overall Influence of Work on Silver Workers in relation to the Selected Variables

4.10 Item Wise Findings of the Influence of Work on Silver Workers

4.11 Problems Confronted by Silver Workers due to Work and Workplace

4.12 Differences in the Problems Confronted by the Silver Workers due to work and Workplace in relation to the Selected Variables

4.13	Item Wise Findings of the Problems Confronted by the Silver Workers due to work and Workplace	
4.14	Satisfaction of the Silver Workers related to Work and Workplace	
4.15	Differences in the Satisfaction of Silver Workers related to Work and Workplace in relation to the Selected Variables	
4.16	Item wise Findings of the Satisfaction of Silver Workers related to Work and Workplace	
4.17	Suggestion by the Silver Workers	

B) Findings and Discussion of the Qualitative Data 289-326

- 4.18 Profile of the Selected Silver Workers
- 4.19 Interviews Conducted with Selected Silver Workers

Part – 2 Employers 327-358

- 4.20 Profile of the Employers
- 4.21 Details about the Employees
- 4.22 Item wise Findings Regarding Influential Factors in Deciding the Time to Retire
- 4.23 Item Wise Findings in view of the Qualities Considered by the Employers While Recruiting Silver Workers
- 4.24 Item Wise Findings Regarding Advantages of the Employers while Recruiting Silver Worker
- 4.25 Item Wise Findings Regarding Disadvantages Considered by Employers in Recruiting Silver Workers.

5. **SUMMARY** 359-386

Cited literature

Bibliography

Webliography

Appendices

Sr. No.	List of Tables	Page No.
1.	Description of Research Tools of the Silver Workers	92
2.	Content and Number of Statements under each Aspect.	95
3.	Content and Number of Statements under each Aspect.	96
4.	Description of Research Tools of the Employers	98
5.	Categorization of Independent Variables for Silver Workers	102
6.	Categorization of Dependent Variables for Silver Workers	103
7.	Plan for Statistical Analysis of the Data of Silver Workers	114
8.	Plan for Statistical Analysis of the Data of Employers	116
9.	Percentage Distribution of the Silver Workers According to their Background Information	123
10.	Percentage Distribution of the Silver Workers According to their Native State	127
11.	Percentage Distribution of the Silver Workers According to the Type of House they Possess	128
12.	Percentage Distribution of the Silver Workers According to the Type of Vehicle they Own and Drive.	129
13.	Percentage Distribution of the Silver Workers According to their Purpose of Driving	130
14.	Percentage Distribution of the Silver Workers According to their Participation in Number of Leisure time Activities	131
15.	Percentage Distribution of the Silver Workers According to their Participation in Specific Leisure time Activities	132
16.	Percentage Distribution of the Silver Workers According to their Type of Family	141
17.	Percentage Distribution of the Silver Workers According to their Relation between Type of Family and Marital Status	142
18.	Percentage Distribution of the Silver Workers According to their Size of Family	143

Sr. No.	List of Tables	Page No.
19.	Percentage Distribution of Silver Workers According to the Educational Qualification of their Spouse (Husband/Wife)	144
20.	Percentage Distribution of Silver Workers According to the Occupational Status 145 of their Spouse (Husband/wife)	145
21.	Percentage Distribution of Silver Workers According to the Sex of their Children and their Marital Status	146
22.	Percentage Distribution of Silver Workers According to the Occupational Status of their Sons, Daughters and Daughters-in-Law	147
23.	Percentage Distribution of the Silver Workers According to their Sources of Family Income per Month	147
24.	Percentage Distribution of the Silver Workers According to the Gap of time between the year of Retirement and the year of Joining Present Job	157
25.	Percentage Distribution of the Silver Workers According to Organization they are working in after Retirement	159
26.	Percentage Distribution of the Silver Workers According to their Employment Status	160
27.	Percentage Distribution of the Silver Workers According to the Type of Organization	161
28.	Percentage Distribution of the Silver Workers According to the Type of Work they are doing	162
29.	Percentage Distribution of the Silver Workers According to their Present Designation	162
30.	Percentage Distribution of the Silver Workers According to Their Type of Designation	163
31.	Percentage Distribution of the Silver Workers According to their Present Salary and Type of Salary	164

Sr. No.	List of Tables	Page No.
32.	Percentage Distribution of the Silver Workers According to Duties Performed by them Prior to Retirement and in their Present Job	165
33.	Percentage Distribution of the Silver Workers According to the Type of Duties Performed as the part of Present Job	166
34.	Percentage Distribution of the Silver Workers According to their Working Hours Per Day	167
35.	Percentage Distribution of the Silver Workers According to the Distance of their Workplace	167
36.	Percentage Distribution of the Silver Workers According to the People who helped them in getting Present Job/Work	168
37.	Overall Intensity Indices and Percentage wise Distribution of the Silver Workers According to the Problems they faced in Searching Jobs after Retirement	169
38.	Percentage Distribution of the Silver Workers According to Procuring the Present Job	171
39.	Percentage Distribution of the Silver Workers According to Social Security Benefits that they receive from their Present Job	172
40.	Percentage Distribution of the Silver Workers According to their Reasons for Working on the Present Job	173
41.	Percentage Distribution of the Silver Workers According to their Expectations to Work after Retirement	174
42.	Percentage Distribution of the Silver Workers According to Work they expected to do after Retirement	174
43.	Percentage Distribution of the Silver Workers According to the Lacunas noticed in the Present Job as compared to the Previous Jobs before Retirement	175
44.	Percentage Distribution of the Silver Workers According to Passion for the Present Work	176
45.	Percentage Distribution of the Silver Workers According to the Current Retirement Benefits Received	177

Sr. No.	List of Tables	Page No.
46.	Percentage Distribution of the Silver Workers According Importance of their Present Work	177
47.	Percentage Distribution of the Silver Workers According to Age they think appropriate for their Second Retirement (age when they will be financially able to Retire from full/part time Work for pay)	178
48.	Percentage Distribution of the Silver Workers According to the Extent of Appreciation they receive for the Present Work	179
49.	Percentage Distribution of the Silver Workers According to the Extent they fulfil the Demands of Present Work	180
50.	Percentage Distribution of the Silver Workers According to their Past Designation	193
51.	Percentage Distribution of Silver Workers according to Work Experience Pre- Retirement	194
52.	Percentage Distribution of the Silver Workers According to their Past Salary	194
53.	Percentage Distribution of the Silver Workers According to their Type of Salary	195
54.	Percentage Distribution of the Silver Workers According to their Employment Status	196
55.	Percentage Distribution of the Silver Workers According to the Type of Work	196
56.	Percentage Distribution of the Silver Workers According to the Type of Organizations	197
57.	Percentage Distribution of the Silver Workers According Importance of their Work in Past	197
58.	Percentage Distribution of the Silver Workers According to their Health Status	203
59.	Overall Extent Aspects and Percentage wise distribution of the Reasons of the Silver Workers to Work after Retirement	206
60.	Overall Extent of the Reasons of the Silver Workers to Work after Retirement in Relation to the Selected Variables	207

Sr. No.	List of Tables	Page No.
61.	Extent of Social and Familial Reasons of Silver Workers to Work after Retirement in Relation to the Selected Variables	209
62.	Extent of Financial Reasons of Silver Workers to Work after Retirement in Relation to the Selected Variables	211
63.	Extent of Personal Reasons of Silver Workers to Work after Retirement in Relation to the Selected Variables	213
64.	Extent of Work Related Reasons of Silver Workers to Work after Retirement in Relation to the Selected Variables	215
65.	t-Ratio Showing the Difference in the Reasons of Silver Workers to Work after retirement in Relation to their Age	217
66.	Analysis of Variance (ANOVA) Indicating Reasons of Silver Workers to Work after Retirement in Relation to their Educational Qualification	218
67.	t- Ratio Showing the Difference in the Reasons of Silver Workers to Work after retirement in Relation to their Educational Qualification	218
68.	Analysis of Variance (ANOVA) Showing Difference between Reasons of Silver Workers to Work after Retirement in Relation to their Last Designation	220
69.	Ratio Showing the Difference in the Reasons of Silver Workers to Work after retirement in Relation to their Educational Qualification	221
70.	Analysis of Variance (ANOVA) Showing Difference between Reasons of Silver Workers to Work after Retirement in Relation to their Health Status	222
71.	t-Ratio Showing the Difference in the Reasons of Silver Workers to Work after retirement in Relation to their Health Status	222
72.	Analysis of Variance (ANOVA) Showing Difference in Reasons of Silver Workers to Work after Retirement in Relation to their Type of Family	223

Sr. No.	List of Tables	Page No.
73.	Intensity Indices Showing Reasons to a great extent of the Silver Workers to Work after Retirement	225
74.	Item Wise Intensity Indices showing the Social and Familial Reasons of Silver Workers to Work after Retirement	226
75.	Item Wise Intensity Indices showing the Financial Reasons of Silver Workers to Work after Retirement	228
76.	Item Wise Intensity Indices showing the Personal Reasons of the Silver Workers to Work after Retirement	229
77.	Item Wise Intensity Indices showing the Work related Reasons of Silver Workers to Work after Retirement	231
78.	Percentages wise Distribution of Overall Perceptions of the Silver about Retirement	235
79.	Percentage Distribution of the Silver Workers According to the Considerations in Deciding the Time to Retire	235
80.	Percentage Distribution of the Silver Workers According to their Preparation for Retirement	236
81.	Percentage Distribution of the Silver Workers According to Personnel's primarily responsible for preparing the Workers for Retirement	237
82.	Percentage Distribution of the Silver Workers According to the Circumstances that they thought could be the Reasons for the Inadequate Retirement Savings of their Fellow Workers	237
83.	Item Wise Intensity Indices showing the Favourable Perceptions of Silver Workers about Retirement	239
84.	Item Wise Intensity Indices showing the Unfavourable Perceptions of Silver Workers about Retirement	241
85.	Percentage Distribution of the Silver Workers According to their Stages of Planning Finance	244
86.	Percentage Distribution of the Silver Workers According to the Specific Age when they started to Plan for Finance	244

Sr. No.	List of Tables	Page No.
87.	Overall Intensity Indices and Percentage Wise Distribution of the Silver Workers According to the Stages of Life that they enjoyed the most	245
88.	Percentage Distribution of the Silver Workers According to the Need of money During Retirement Age	246
89.	Percentage Distribution of the Silver Workers According to the Purpose to Need Money during the Retirement Age	247
90.	Percentage Distribution of the Silver Workers According to the Preparedness to Spend More Money during Retirement	249
91.	Percentages Wise Distribution of Overall Influence of Work on Silver Workers	252
92.	Extent of Influence of Work on the Silver Workers in Relation to the Selected Variables	252
93.	t-Ratio Showing the Difference in the Influence of Work on Silver Workers in Relation to Age	253
94.	t-Ratio Showing the Difference in the Influence on Silver Workers in Relation to their Type of Work	254
95.	Analysis of Variance (ANOVA) Showing Difference in Influence of work on Silver Workers in Relation to their Present Designations	255
96.	Analysis of Variance (ANOVA) Showing Difference in Influence of Work on the Silver Workers in Relation to their Health Status	255
97.	Item Wise Intensity Indices Showing Influence of Work on Silver Workers	256
98.	Percentage Distribution of the Silver Workers according to the Problems they confronted due to Work and Workplace	260
99.	Percentage Distribution of the Silver Workers According to the Problems confronted due to Work and Workplace in Relation to the Selected Variables	261
100.	Percentage Distribution of the Silver Workers According to the Treatment received at Workplaces	263

Sr. No.	List of Tables	Page No.
101.	t-Ratio Showing the Difference in the Problems Confronted by Silver Workers due to Work and Work Place in Relation to their Age	264
102.	Analysis of Variance (ANOVA) Showing Difference between Problems Confronted by Silver Workers due to Work and Workplace in Relation to their Educational Qualification	265
103.	t-Ratio Showing the Difference in the Problems Confronted by Silver Workers due to Work and Workplace in Relation to their Educational Qualification	265
104.	Analysis of Variance (ANOVA) Showing Difference between Problems Confronted by Silver Workers due to Work and Workplace in Relation to their Present Salary	266
105.	t-Ratio Showing the Difference in the Problems Confronted by Silver Workers due to Work and Workplace in Relation to their Present Salary	267
106.	Analysis of Variance (ANOVA) Showing Difference between Problems Confronted by Silver Workers due to Work and Workplace in Relation to their Health Status	268
107.	Analysis of Variance (ANOVA) Showing Difference between the Problems Confronted by Silver Workers due to Work and Workplace in Relation to their Present Designation	268
108.	t-Ratio Showing the Difference in the Problems Confronted by Silver Workers due to Work and Workplace in Relation to their Perceptions about Retirement	269
109.	Item Wise Intensity Indices Showing the Problems Confronted by the Silver Workers due to Work and Workplace	270
110.	Item Wise Intensity Indices Showing the Problems Confronted by the Silver Workers at Workplaces due to Self	272
111.	Percentage Distribution of the Silver Workers according to their Satisfaction related to Work and Workplace	273

Sr. No.	List of Tables	Page No.
112.	Percentage Distribution of the Silver Workers According to their Satisfaction related to Work and Workplace in Relation to the Selected Variables	274
113.	Percentage Distribution of what the Silver Workers thought about an Ideal Age of Retirement	275
114.	t-Ratio Showing the Difference in the Overall Satisfaction related to Work and Workplace of Silver Workers in Relation to their Type of Work	277
115.	Analysis of Variance (ANOVA) Showing Difference in Overall Satisfaction related to Work and Workplace on Silver Workers in Relation to Present Salary	278
116.	t-Ratio Showing the Difference in the Overall Satisfaction of Silver Workers related to Work and Workplace in Relation to their Present Salary	278
117.	Analysis of Variance (ANOVA) Showing Difference in Overall Satisfaction of the silver workers related to Work and Workplace in Relation to their Present Designation	279
118.	t-Ratio Showing the Difference in the Overall Satisfaction of Silver Workers related to Work and Workplace in Relation to their Present Designation	279
119.	Item Wise Intensity Indices Showing the Satisfaction of Silver Workers related to their Work and Workplace	281
120.	Percentage Distribution of the Silver Workers according to their Suggestions for Specific Personnel Policy for Elderly Employees	283
121.	Percentage Distribution of the Silver Workers According to the Need for Action Concerning Engagement of Elder Employees	284
122.	Percentage Distribution of the Silver Workers Suggestions for the Important Services for Elder Employees	285
123.	Percentage Distribution According to the Facilities that Employer can Provide to the Silver Workers	286

Sr. No.	List of Tables	Page No.
124.	Percentage Distribution of the Silver Workers interviewed according to their Background Information	293
125.	Percentage Distribution of the Employers According to their Designations	329
126.	Percentage Distribution of the Employers According to their Age	330
127.	Percentage Distribution of the Employers According to their Experience in the organisation/company/institution/corporate/firm	330
128.	Percentage Distribution of the Employers According to the Type of Organizations	331
129.	Percentage Distribution of the Employers According to the Finance Resource that they Resort for the Organizations	332
130.	Percentage Distribution According to the Age of Retirement Prescribed at the organizations	333
131.	Percentage Distribution of the Employers According to Number of the Silver Workers working in their Organisations	334
132.	Percentage Distribution of the Employers According to Increase in Number of Elderly Workers in the Organizations	334
133.	Percentage Distribution of the Employers According to Increase in Number of Elderly Workers in the Organizations	335
134.	Percentage Distribution of the Employers According to their Roles in the Organisations	336
135.	Percentage Distribution of the Employers According to Reasons Organisations for not Retaining retired Silver Workers after Retirement	337
136.	Percentage Distribution of the Employers According to the Best Age to Contribute to the Organizations	338
137.	Percentage Distribution of the Employers According to their Opinions regarding Formal Policies/Programmes for Recruitment of Employees who are Approaching Retirement Age	339

Sr. No.	List of Tables	Page No.
138.	Percentage Distribution of the Employers Concerned about Loss of Valuable Knowledge faced by the Company/Organization	340
139.	Overall Intensity Indices Showing the Influential Factors in Deciding Time to Retire	342
140.	Overall Intensity Indices Showing the Qualities Considered by Employer Expect while Employing Silver Workers	344
141.	Overall Intensity Indices showing the Advantages of the Employers while recruiting Silver Workers	346
142.	Overall Intensity Indices showing the Disadvantages if the Employers in Recruiting Silver Workers	348

ILLUSTRATIONS

Figure No.	List of Figures	Page No.
1.	Global Population by Age Group	3
2.	Percentage of People Aged 60 and Over in the Labour Force	15
3.	Percentage of Labour Force Participation by People 65 and Older by Region	17
4.	Overview of the Study	84
5.	Percentage Distribution of the Silver Workers according to their Age	134
6.	Percentage Distribution of the Silver Workers according to their Sex	134
7.	Percentage Distribution of the Silver Workers according to their Marital Status	135
8.	Percentage Distribution of the Silver Workers according to their Educational Qualification	135
9.	Percentage Distribution of the Silver Workers according to their Religion	136
10.	Percentage Distribution of the Silver Workers according to their Caste	136
11.	Percentage Distribution of the Silver Workers according to their Native Place	137
12.	Percentage Distribution of the Silver Workers according to their Type of House	137
13.	Percentage Distribution of the Silver Workers according to Vehicle they Own	138
14.	Percentage Distribution of Silver Workers according to the Type of Vehicle they Own	138
15.	Percentage Distribution of Silver Workers according to the Type of Vehicle they Drive	139
16.	Percentage Distribution of Silver Workers according to their Purpose of Driving	139
17.	Percentage Distribution of Silver Workers according to their Leisure Time Activities	140
18.	Percentage Distribution of the Silver Workers according to their Type of Family	150

Figure No.	List of Figures	Page No.
19.	Percentage Distribution of the Silver Workers according to their Marital Status	150
20.	Percentage Distribution of the Silver Workers according to their Size of Family	151
21.	Percentage Distribution of the silver workers according to the Educational Qualification of Spouse (Husband)	151
22.	Percentage Distribution of the Silver Workers according to the Educational Qualification of Spouse (Wife)	152
23.	Percentage Distribution of the Silver Worker's according to the Occupational Status of Spouse (Husband)	152
24.	Percentage Distribution of the Silver Worker's according to the Occupational Status of Spouse (Wife)	153
25.	Percentage Distribution of the Silver Workers according to the Marital Status of the Son	153
26.	Percentage Distribution of the Silver Worker according to the Marital Status of Daughter	154
27.	Percentage Distribution of the Silver Workers according to the Occupational Status of the Son	154
28.	Percentage Distribution of the Silver Workers according to the Occupational Status of the Daughters	155
29.	Percentage Distribution of the Silver Workers according to the Occupational Status of the Occupational Status of Daughter in Law	155
30.	Percentage Distribution of the Silver Workers according their Sources of Income	156
31.	Percentage Distribution of the Silver Workers according to the Gap between Retirement Year and Year of Joining Present Job	181
32.	Percentage Wise Distribution of the Silver Workers According to Organization they are working in after Retirement	181
33.	Percentage Distribution of the Silver Workers according to the Employment Status	182

Figure No.	List of Figures	Page No.
34.	Percentage Distribution of the Silver Workers according to the Type of Organization	182
35.	Percentage Distribution of the Silver Workers according to the Type of Work	183
36.	Percentage Distribution of the Silver Workers according to the Present Designation	183
37.	Percentage Distribution of the Silver Workers according to the Type of Designation	184
38.	Percentage Distribution of the Silver Workers according to the Present Salary	184
39.	Percentage Distribution of the Silver Workers according to the Type of Salary	185
40.	Percentage Distribution of the Silver Workers according to the Duties Performed before Retirement	185
41.	Percentage Distribution of the Silver Workers according to the Type of Duties Performed in Present Job	186
42.	Percentage Distribution of the Silver Workers according to the Type of Duties Performed as Part of Present Job Wise	186
43.	Percentage Distribution of the Silver Workers according to the Working Hours	187
44.	Percentage Distribution of the Silver Workers according to the Distance of Work	187
45.	Percentage Distribution of the Silver Workers according to the Persons who helped in Getting Present Job	188
46.	Procuring present job Wise Percentage Distribution of the Silver Workers	188
47.	Percentage Distribution of the Silver Workers according to the Social Security Benefits	189
48.	Reasons of Working on Present Job Wise Percentage Distribution of the Silver Workers	189
49.	Percentage Distribution of the Silver Workers according to the Expectations to Work after Retirement	190

Figure No.	List of Figures	Page No.
50.	Percentage Distribution of the Silver Workers according to the work they expected to do after Retirement	190
51.	Percentage Distribution of the Silver Workers according to the Lacunas in the Present Job as Compared to the Previous jobs before Retirement	191
52.	Percentage Distribution of the Silver Workers according to the Retirement Benefits	191
53.	Percentage Distribution of the Silver Workers according to the Importance of Present work	192
54.	Percentage Distribution of the Silver Workers according to the Age of Re-retirement	192
55.	Percentage Distribution of the Silver Workers according to the Past Designation	199
56.	Percentage Distribution of the Silver Workers according to the Work Experience of Pre –Retirement	199
57.	Percentage Distribution of the Silver Workers according to their Past Salary	200
58.	Percentage Distribution of the Silver Workers according to the Type of Salary	200
59.	Percentage Distribution of the Silver Workers according to the Employment Status	201
60.	Percentage Distribution of the Silver Workers according to the Type of Work Wise	201
61.	Percentage Distribution of the Silver Workers according to the Type of Organization	202
62.	Percentage Distribution of the Silver Workers according to the Work in Past	202
63.	Percentage Distribution of the Silver Workers according to their Health Status	203

CHAPTER -1
INTRODUCTION

1.1 Demography of Elderly Population

The world is growing older. Longevity should be a matter for congratulations since long life expectancy is regarded as an indicator to a successful society and an effective health care system (World Health Organization2000).An ageless world is not a myth anymore. Age is getting invisible as we move from longetivity to super longetivity.

According to Gaminiratne (2004) "Population Ageing, Elderly Welfare and Extending Retirement Cover: The Case Study of Srilanka" Population ageing is a process no longer confined to industrialized countries. Many developing countries are now also experiencing ageing of their populations – reflected by the rising share of the elderly in the total population. Not only are developing countries ageing, they are ageing at a much faster rate and at a much earlier stage of economic development, thus placing them at a greater disadvantage in terms of their ability to respond to ageing developments. The availability of domestic resources, for example, to finance ageing pressures on public finances and public services are likely to be more limited. In addition, the political time frame available to formulate and implement appropriate policy responses will be shorter. Developing countries are confronting ageing pressures at a time when social security coverage is still limited to a minority of the better-off elderly population, and when the systems of protection which have supported the elderly in the past are gradually eroding.

Across the world, countries are experiencing population ageing. The growth rate of the elderly population is more rapid in developing countries like India than developed countries. Apart from demographic transitions, socio-economic and political changes together with increased individualism have altered living conditions of the elderly.

Today, the elderly demand that society should not only ensure independence and participation, but also provide care, fulfilment and dignity. Limited understanding of factors influencing their quality of life is largely responsible for the elderly being denied a dignified existence. After all, the last stage of life holds as much potential for growth and development as earlier stages. The diversity among the elderly and varied inter-related influencing aspects from their environment need significant consideration of researchers and policy planners.

According to the Report on the Status of Elderly in selected States of India 2011, by United Nations Population Fund (UNFPA) a major demographic issue for India in the 21st century is population ageing, with wide implications for economy and society in general. With the rapid changes in demographic indicators over the last few decades, it is certain that India will move from being a young country to an old country over the next few decades. Presently, India has around 90 million elderly and by 2050, the number is expected to increase to 315 million, constituting 20 percent of the total population. The analysis found that around three-fourths of the elderly live in rural areas, of which 48 percent are women and 55 percent of them are widows. Nearly 70 percent of rural elderly are dependent on others, and their health problems increase with age. In addition to problems of illiteracy, unemployment, widowhood and disabilities, older women in India also face life-long gender based discrimination, resulting in differential patterns of ageing of men and women.

The Global Report on Ageing in the 21st Century (2012) reinforces the observations made in India that there is multiple discrimination experienced by elderly persons, particularly elderly women, including in access to jobs and health care, subjection to abuse, denial of the right to own and inherit property, and lack of basic minimum income and social security (UNFPA and Help Age International, 2012).

Further, the majority of the people at 60+ in India are socially backward and economically poor. In addition, there is also extreme heterogeneity in the demographic transition across states, resulting in vast differences in the demographic scenario across social, economic and spatial groups. For instance, the state of Kerala which had 11 percent of the elderly population in 2001 is expected to have 18 per cent by the year 2026, with an absolute number of around seven million elderly. On the other hand, Uttar Pradesh in 2001 had only six percent and will have around 10 per cent elderly population in 2026. Though the proportion of the elderly population in Uttar Pradesh is smaller than in Kerala, the absolute number of elderly in Uttar Pradesh is expected to be thrice that of Kerala as mentioned in the Report on the

Status of Elderly in selected States of India 2011, by United Nations Population Fund (UNFPA) .Thus, adding life to the years that have been added to life is a significant challenge. Yet, ageing is not to be viewed from a problem perspective; its potential must be recognised and realised.

The demographic transition has altered age structure of the population where sizeable proportion in the population of elderly persons becoming the norm today. Decline in fertility rate, decline in mortality rate, improvement in child survival and increased life expectancy signify development. These are the trends towards which the world is progressing today. These are desired transitions. But these transitions are not devoid of challenges. One significant challenge is the change in demographic composition. The number of elderly in the world is set to increase significantly and rapidly.

The elderly population in India is the second largest in the world, next only to China. This population, which was 77 million according to the 2001 census (7.5% of the total population), is projected by the UN to increase to 137 million by 2021. Three-fourth of the elderly population live in rural areas. Their annual growth rate is higher (3%) as compared to the growth rate of the total population (1.9%). Population projections show that by 2050, the elderly population in India will surpass the population of children below 14 years.

Figure 1: Global Population by Age Group

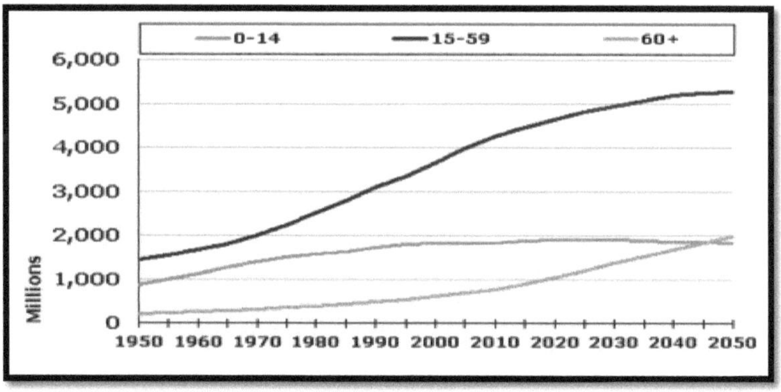

Source: World Population Prospects: the 2006 revision population database.

- Globally, the number of people over 80 is growing at 4 percent per annum, whereas the population as a whole is growing at 1 percent per annum. 3.5 million People will be over 100 years old by 2050. Over half will live in Asia.
- The 21st century will witness a gradual transition to an ageing society the world over. The process which first started in low fertility western societies and in Japan is now spreading to the developing countries of Asia, Africa and Latin America.
- Countries like China and India will not only be at the forefront in terms of absolute number of total population, but also in terms of absolute number of the elderly (60+) population.
- Is the country ready to embrace this transition? Do we have adequate and appropriate elderly care systems in place in the context of changing socio-economic conditions? What is the plight of the elderly among the poor? Are there options to set the poor on the trajectory of graceful ageing?
- In brief, the long-term impact of decline in fertility and reduction in the size of family will lead to a decrease in the population of children (0-14 years), which in turn will push up the population in the working age group.
- Looking to these data, it is obvious that elderly would require special attention and care. It is said that a person starts aging one he/she is out of work place. The "retirement period" is considered as dangerous for the health of individual.
- Old age is commonly associated with retirement, illness and dependency. Most government jobs have set the retirement age at 60. This has tuned many urban minds to think that working life beyond 60 is incidental. However the truth speaks to the contrary.
- About 70 percent of the elderly in India work. They work like rest of the adults. The number of elderly that work in rural areas is more than their counterparts in urban areas.
- Even at the age of 80 and above there are about 35 percent elderly working. Most of the elderly workforce is engaged as cultivators and agricultural laborers.
- Elderly are also engaged in trade and commerce, non-household industry, household industry, sense of lowered self-esteem and loss of control. Living with children determines the physical and psychological well being of the elderly to some extent. But complete dependence takes away the degree of autonomy in the

economic and social decision making. Therefore the elderly want to work for as long as they wish.
- Experiential studies indicate that health is closely connected to active life. Activity drives away isolation and boredom to a large extent. Among the poor gainful employment of the elderly brings in economic security.
- Currently in India the opportunities for the elderly to work are less compared to their willingness and ability to work. This has to change. They should get opportunities to work as long as they wish in productive jobs without being forced into retirement.
- This work should their current abilities. Fortunately, many of these abilities are in demand. When designing poverty reduction/livelihoods programs it is very important to make the elderly part of the designing and planning process.
- The active-elderly can be prepared for graceful ageing to make the transition as smooth as possible. Attention can be paid towards improving the livelihoods and income levels of these groups so they have decent reserves to take care of themselves in times of need.

The primary reason for such demographic ageing is improved Medicare in all its aspects. Due to the phenomenal advances in medical and biological sciences, infant mortality has been substantially reduced. The general healthcare of the population has improved. People have become, over the years, nutrition and health conscious. There has been a general increase in the overall standard of living. What are the likely effects of people living longer on the society and country at large? An immediate impression that grips everyone is that the ageing population might become a burden to the concerned country and the world at large.

The reduction in fertility level, reinforced by steady increase in the life expectancy has produced fundamental changes in the age structure of the population, which in turn leads to the aging population. India had the second largest number of elderly (60+) in the world as of 2001. The analysis of historical patterns of mortality and fertility decline in India indicates that the process of population aging intensified only in the 1990's. The older population of India, which was 56.7 million in 1991, is 76 million in 2001 and is expected to grow to 137 million by 2021. Today India is home to one out of every ten eldely of the world. Both the absolute and relative size of the population of the elderly in India will gain in strength in future.

1.2 Elderly Defined

The use of words 'elderly',' older persons' and 'senior citizens' in both popular and scholarly works gives an impression that they make a homogeneous group. But, in fact, there prevails great deal of variation between and among these various categories of old people. The concept of an old age varies between societies and it has undergone great deal of change in diverse context. Population ageing is a multidimensional phenomenon and, as such, it is difficult to provide its clear definition. Some would wonder whether an old age is a problem in India in the first place or it is one of those unwanted legacies inherited from the West. In fact, the discussion demands to clarify. What constitutes old age? Is it an age at which employees retire? or is it only a mental process?. Does it pose a challenge that organs do not co-operate and the body becomes inhabits number of diseases or it is viewed as an opportunity to take up a renewed vigour and cultivate hobbies or interests for which he/she had little time earlier in life.

Gorman, (2000) defines "The ageing process is of course a biological reality which has its own dynamic, largely beyond human control. However, it is also subject to the constructions by which each society makes sense of old age. In the developed world, chronological time plays a paramount role. The age of 60 or 65, roughly equivalent to retirement ages in most developed countries is said to be the beginning of old age. In many parts of the developing world, chronological time has little or no importance in the meaning of old age. Other socially constructed meanings of age are more significant such as the roles assigned to older people; in some cases it is the loss of roles accompanying physical decline which is significant in defining old age. Thus, in contrast to the chronological milestones which mark life stages in the developed world, old age in many developing countries is seen to begin at the point when active contribution is no longer possible."Although there are commonly used definitions of old age, there is no general agreement on the age at which a person becomes old. The common use of a calendar age to mark the threshold of old age assumes equivalence with biological age, yet at the same time, it is generally accepted that these two are not necessarily synonymous.

Different writers have viewed ageing in different contexts as the outcome of biological, demographic, sociological, physiological or other processes. Hermanova, (1988) views "Ageing in its demographic sense is not the same as the biological process of ageing which is dynamic and continuous. Chronological age does not measure psychological age".

According to Talib (April, 2000), every society marks the biographical trajectory of its members into recognized scenes of a play. Each scene represents different roles and narrations, varying colours and costumes. As individuals graduate from one scene to another, they acquire newer identities and relations in the structure and dynamics of the play. The imagery of drama is somewhat restrictive if deployed to understand life. While a play has clear cut scenes, actual life has several replays of the same drama enacted simultaneously. The final, the middle and the early scenes of a play coexist in actual life; it is their inter-relation, which makes a scene or a group of actors' problematic. The last scene in life has invariably been understood either segmentally or integrally. In a segmental view, old age is set apart, constructed through stereotypes and discriminated against, simply because those enacting the last scene are considered worn out and removed from the central concerns of active, healthy and productive life".

Since the present study proposes to conduct study on silver workers in India , based specifically in the city of Vadodara, it would be interesting to know how the Indian concept of old age was originated and implemented in the context of societies in India. Majority of the Indians population consist of people with Indian way of living. Irrespective of caste or creed, they mostly follow the system of 'ashrams' or stages of life and the caste system. However, deterioration has occurred in the spirit of systems which has originally based on division of work in human life of society. Accordingly, human life is presumed to be of 100 years which is divided into four stages or ashrams according to an age. 'Brahmacharya ashrama' from birth to 25th year, second is 'Grihasthashrama' , from 26th year to 50 years and third is 'Vanaprastha ashrama', from 51st year to 75th year and fourth is 'Sanayastashrama' , from 76th year to 100th year. Of these four stages, the later two stages relate to old age like , say from 50 years to 60 years as early –old age- age or young-old age, from 60 years to 70 years as middle –old-age and 70 years and above as old age.

The silver workers that are referred in the present study fall in a range of 60 years and above.

In the Indian context, a person beyond 50 years is supposed to be relived from family responsibilities entrusting all powers and duties to their grown-up sons and daughters. They are supposed to lead almost a retired life under the care of their families. In case of financially strong family, things go smoothly. But with families undergoing financial constraints, things are bit difficult to manage and its effect surfaces in attitude and behaviour of younger members to elders. Eventually, growing apathy and neglect of elders in families forces the elderly to decide to work even after retirement.

Ageing is measured in many ways. To a nonprofessional an elderly means a person who lives longer. Ageing refers to the process of growing older or the effect of age i.e. the deterioration in psychological capabilities.

Considering the facts first—7 percent of India's population is elderly today. The definition of elderly as given by World Health Organization (WHO) and other agencies determines an old age at sixty years. But interestingly, now the agencies divide the elderly population into 3 age groups

1. YOUNG-OLD-AGED---60 to 70 years old
2. MIDDLE-OLD- AGED—70 to 80 years.
3. OLD-OLD- AGED---- above 80 years.

An old age is a part of life cycle about which there are numerous myths and stereotypes. They present an overstatement of commonly held beliefs; the old age is portrayed in reference to dependent individuals .It is characterized by a lack of social autonomy. It carries a sense of being unloved and neglected by both their immediate family and friends, and posing a threat to the living standard of younger age groups by proving a "burden" that consumes without producing anything. These negative notions cause decline a status of old people in society. Stereotyping is judging, reacting to, or treating another person on the basis of one's perception of the group to which that person belongs or in which they have been placed. The terms old or older describe a group of people to which certain characteristics are assigned. They may include positive traits such as experience, good judgment, strong work ethic, and a commitment to quality. In a more negative vein, older workers have been characterized as lacking flexibility, resentful to new technology, unwilling or unable to learn new skills, and unable to compromise or adapt to new conditions. Viewing in the context of work sector, as Lord and Farrington, (2006) state that "many people attribute high absenteeism, and high job turnover to the older population due to the stereotype of a physically and mentally declining individual". So there prevail variety of observations as regarded to elderly and retirement. They may be explained in view of establishing the basic theme of the resent research.

1.3 Elderly and Retirement

"Retirement kills more people than hard work ever did."- Malcolm S. Forbes

Given the trend of population aging in the country, the elderly population faces a number of problems and adjusts to them in varying degrees. These problems range from absence of ensured and sufficient income to support themselves and their dependents after retirement to ill health, absence of social security, loss of social role and recognition and to the non-availability of opportunities for creative use of free time. The needs and problems of the elderly vary significantly according to their age, socio-economic status, health, living status and other such background characteristics.

Retirement refers to an ongoing period in life that traditionally has been considered to begin at the point of withdrawal from working life. Retirement is a social concept implemented primarily during the past 100 years due to changes in life expectancies and population demographics. Increase in life expectancies over the past century has produced both challenges and opportunities during the retirement phase of life. It continually calls for increased attention and resources. The arrival of the elderly generation arriving at an retirement age has enormous implications for population demographics, workforce, and a host of social and economic issues. A dramatic trend toward early retirement, coupled with increased life expectancy, ensures a growing focus on issues related to retirement.

For individual retiree, this retirement period of life holds remarkable potential and risk as well. The usual definitions of retirement imply withdrawal from the workforce and from remaining years of life. Operationally, retirement has been conceived in a variety of ways:

a) A well-deserved rest as a reward for years of work
b) A means of maintaining an effective work force
c) A period of transition to old age
d) A distinct period of human development
e) A period for postretirement careers
f) A period of adjustment to loss of work identity.

Perhaps all of these concepts are applicable across to or within particular cases. Developing of a general theory or model for retirement has been difficult for several reasons. For example, the number of factors that influence the nature and quality of experience of retirement are substantial. Further, there is no real standard to determine the beginning of retirement. Some workers choose to retire early and some choose not to retire at all, some others are forced to retirement; whereas some retire partially; and some even return to work after retirement. Viewing retirement in socio economic economical context "Age-based retirement arbitrarily severs productive persons from their livelihood, squanders their talents, scars their health, strains an already overburdened social security system, and drives many elderly people into poverty and despair. Ageism is as odious as racism and sexism."

The word "Retirement" implies by its very nature letting go, dropping or giving up. Some people legitimately wish to spend their later years relaxing. It may be true but, according to studies carried out at Harvard University and Johns Hopkins University, a vast majority of retired people list boredom as their complaints. Turning sixty? Time to sit back and relax? But it would not be a case anymore. In fact life begins at sixty! There is lot to do in life after sixty. Age is just a number of years for growing number of elderly citizens. The population after age 60 is smart and not at all the 'sathya gaya' types as made out in the past. Living life of dignity, self sufficient, at ease in parties, not to content with babysitting of their grand kids. It makes a true face of aged. Ageing is now fashion and not even negativity about life. "Life ki Second Innings Back foot pe nahi front foot pe khelni chahiye". This is a mantra for the sixty plus and it has fascinated many elders who do not want to retire.

Retirement is an occupational transition. It is therefore considered important in the field of occupational therapy. Life after so-called "retirement" is defined in India as an age after sixty years. The question arises, are these elderly helpless as made out? The reply is not at all. Retirement is not an end. It is the beginning. It is a phase in which an old chapter closes and a person moves forward to live a new chapter in life to face another. People can do many things after retirement. Gone are the days when the post retirement plans did not extend beyond undertaking regular pilgrimages and live happily in company of grandchildren .In recent years the concept of retirement, mostly in the metros and towns, has almost become defunct. An idea of "Second Innings" is now more acceptable and appropriate terms its claimants are living it up every moment.

The manner in which people leave the work force does not always translate simply into "retirement" in a customary sense. About one-third and one-half of people who leave their full-time career jobs move into, what can be described "bridge jobs"- these jobs are full-time or part-time paying jobs. As Quinn (2002, 2003) explains, other than those in which they spent the better part of their working years and that presumably "bridge" the transition from work to retirement. Still others leave the work force entirely for a while and return later on. Prisuta (2004) explains what is more, as many as half of current retirees left the work force earlier than they planned or had wanted to, most often because of poor health or adverse economic events, such as plant closings, layoffs, or downsizing . Several specific factors may interact to influence individuals' experience of retirement. These factors include finance, health and medical care, relationship, housing, existential issues, security, and satisfaction with career.

Retirement can lead to a sense of social isolation. Especially when work relationships are just primary or retirement involves a geographical movement. Social support systems are critical to most people. A need for social support also changes across years of retirement. It requires some significant planning and adjustment. It is generally thought advisable to start discussing retirement issues and plans with friends and family much before the time to retire actually approaches. Access to family or others relatives who can play supportive role in retirement is a key dimension of satisfaction. Consequently, everyone ought to be involved in the planning process. Certain kind of support, with financial matters for example, may be best handled through professionals approach. From the perspective of generating supportive atmosphere, retirees also need to make plans to contribute to the support of the significant others (e.g., spouse, children, and siblings). The retiree can do it by sharing responsibilities with these individuals.

There is substantial increase in number of retirees who wish to return to work, at least part-time. It reflects shifting financial demands. Some others however may choose to return to work for a variety of reasons other than financial. For instance, they may see work as an opportunity to help others; to meet achievement/productivity needs; to stay engaged cognitively and socially; to share knowledge, skills, or experiences; or to gain the intrinsic rewards associated with engagement in work. Any of these objectives can also be satisfied by doing volunteer work as well. Objectives for any work or activities have to be thoughtfully planned. Retirees who wish to return to work ought to consider both the reason for assuming work responsibility and their specific expectations regarding the work.

It is very normal for retirees to have with a lifetime of experience and getting more of free time to reflect on the meaning of life. The reality of mortality increases with age. Retirement can serve a great opportunity, not only to reflect on purpose of life issues, accomplishments, and failures, but also to develop and project a vision of the future. Sharing the reflections of retirement with younger generations, staying engaged with social and religious institutions and activities, and engaging in service to others are all easily accessible ways to enhance meaning and value of life in retirement. They can be realized with, these skills, abilities, and motives that were set up and nurtured in the earlier phase of life.

At any age a person can do new things, learn new skills, and be more active with the community. Many countries have witnessed major changes in the work and retirement patterns of their older citizens during the last 3 decades (Jacobs, Kohli and Rein, 1991). In developed countries, until the 1950's retirement from the workforce was an event that occurred almost exclusively at a regulated age, with little possibility of receiving a pension prior to that age (Tracy, 1979). Since then, countries have adopted a wide range of approaches to provide old age security, to old age persons. As a result, different potential routes have emerged to benefit for persons who make the transition from labour force participation to retirement. Changes in view of part-time work, unemployment, disability pensions, and early retirement have hastened withdrawal from the labour force, and increased an average number of years that an individual spends outside formal economic activities (Torrey, 1982).

The American Association of Retired Persons received 36,000 responses to a working life survey, covering 375 job titles from workers age 50 and who had returned to the workplace after an initial period of retirement (Bird 1994). The three most frequently cited reasons for returning to work include those of financial need, liking to work, and keeping busy. However, closer examination of the data revealed that "financial need" would refer to money to help the children as well as to meet basic needs. "Liking to work" would include feeling of being successful, enjoying excitement of the workplace, and contributing. Further the reasons of "Keeping busy" would mean working with a spouse, staying healthy, and fulfilling a social need. Reasons cited for remaining or returning to the workplace expressed the social meaning of work. Ginsberg (1983) viewed that work provides income, status, and personal achievement; structures time; and provides opportunities to explore interpersonal relationships. In the study by Stein, Rocco, and Goldenetz (2000), older workers who remain in workplaces or return to workplace were mentioned as not planning wisely. A need to contribute, expecting appreciation from others, and desire to create something would form reasons for not retiring from the workplace. Work is something more than mere earning livelihood; it is a way to life. When people live longer, what mechanisms are available to them to remain active and productive in employment and other gainful activities? How much unemployment and poverty are there among elderly? Are they covered under existing social security schemes and/or do they own financial assets and property? Are they assured of income through pension and retirement benefits? Is there any special social security provisions for elderly? What are the policy responses? This study aims to finds out answers to such questions.

1.4 Work after Retirement amongst Elderly

In the view of the elderly work, it is said,
"The race is over, but the work never is done
while the power to work remains...
it cannot be, while you still live.
For to live is to function;
that is all there is in living."

These thoughts may reflect a perspective of current older generation about work.

Age is identified as a fundamental organising principle of modern society. One of the areas of our lives that are structured with reference to age is employment. In particular, a practice of withdrawing from the labour force resulting into retirement is age related. Retirement can thus be socially constructed phenomenon. Yet it has more the economies of the organised labour markets than with preferences and abilities of older people to participate in paid employment

Old age is commonly associated with retirement and illness and dependency are its by-products. Most government jobs have an age of retirement set at sixty years. This conveys to many in urban societies that working life beyond sixty years is just incidental. However, the truth speaks about the contrary. About seventy percent of the elderly in India are to be working, they work like other workers. The society needs to recognize strengths of the old and empower them rather than adopting a paternalistic attitude to cause devastating impact on self –esteem of the elderly citizens. According to AARP study (2007), 'Old age' calls for much more personal and individualistic definition like: A 60-year-old may be known as 'old,' while an 85-year-old remains youthful. What works in it is not longevity of life in years, but spirit of living that sees no age. Therefore, people, especially in the West, now see retirement as a time of reinvention and a new chapter in life. People in more affluent societies want to carry on working even in retirement.

Figure 2: Percentage of People Aged 60 and Over in the Labour Force

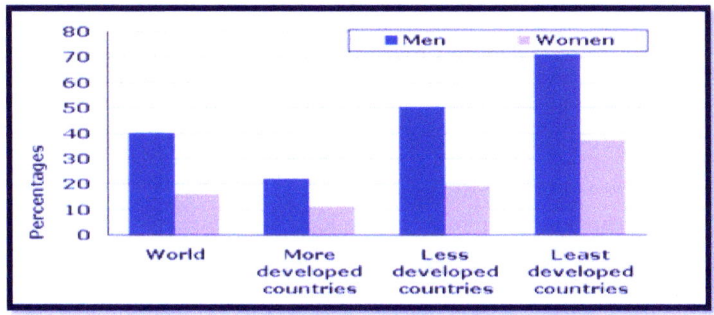

Source: World Population Prospects: the 2006 revision population database.

The above figure reflects that in least developed country more number of persons ageing 60 and beyond, both men and women, were engaged in labour force as compared to those in less developed countries. However, those in more developed countries remain lower than world statistics. In more recent times, a line between working full-time a.nd not working has blurred. Many elderly persons prefer partial retirement or they look to find for other ways of raising income after they leave full-time employment. The AARP (2002) survey has found that 70 percent of mature workers plan to work into what they view as their retirement years. Updating the 2002 survey, the survey "Staying Ahead of the Curve 2007: The AARP Work and Career Study" reports that 27 percent of the 45-75 year olds questioned admit about a need for money as a reason to continue to work, while 21 percent attributed their decision to work in retirement to the reason that they enjoy working.

The study further reports that 51 of those interviewed said they plan to work part-time in retirement, while 29 percent of them do not have any plan to work. Another 11 percent of the respondents even plan to start their own business or work for themselves and 6 percent plan to work full-time. The final report includes a section called "Blueprint for Change" that focuses on creative policies adopted by progressive employers. These creative practices include among other things flexible work schedules and work arrangements, competitive health and other benefits, restructuring jobs or workplaces to accommodate employees' unique needs related to later life, recharging late-career workers with updated training, and utilizing knowledge retention strategies. There has been growing emphasis on lifestyle and consumption in retirement rather than on idleness and leisure. It is supported with a new rhetoric that emphasizes that 'retirees' have worked hard and they deserve their time in the sun. This kind of reformulation of retirement seems to be driven in part by cultural changes arising from social transformations of persons in sixties in which the elderly generation gave a new legitimacy and cachet to youthfulness. The elderly fascination for youth culture leads them to denial about own ageing, and redefine old age and retirement. The elderly who create the cult of youth are now confronted with the unreality of the sixties to refrain 'Hope I die before I get old'. Nonetheless, elderly seem determined to prolong their adolescence and resist the future (Mackay 1997). In keeping with their ability to rewrite the rules, it seems that the elderly can live up to lament simply by redefining what is 'old' with slogans like '50 is the new 40'etc. Redefinition of old age is further supported by the government campaigns like 'Positive Ageing'. It emphasizes that retirement is an active time to call for social and cultural involvement. It may also further contribute to the perception that retirement is just the next lifestyle phase. Such new understanding of retirement is echoed in the demos study. Many older persons work for economic reasons, but as an old age increases the ratio of older persons who work for economic reasons decreases, while the ratio of those who work for health increases.

It has been observed over the world that if more people avail enjoys opportunities for dignified work earlier in life, (properly remunerated, in adequate environments, protected against the hazards) the more they would be able to reach old age able to participate in the workforce in old age by it, the whole society would benefit. In all parts of the world, there is an increasing recognition of a need to support active and productive contribution by older people in the form of formal work, informal work, and unpaid activities at home or in voluntary occupations. Volunteering need not be an isolated activity. Instead, it is a reflection of an underlying quality of social connectedness. It may manifest itself in many ways like through work for social life, formal community service, informal helping, secular civic engagement, or faith-based good works. Social connectedness is also strongly associated with health and welfare of individuals in a community, which is a necessary precondition for engaging in community service (Berkman et al. 2000; Fried et al. 2004; Rowe and Kahn 1997). A critical question, then, arises in relation to the elderly's potential as a community resource about an extent to which they will embrace and enhance quality of social connectedness. This is where the real promise of improving the quality of community life lies. It is played out through a variety of mechanisms, formal and informal, structured and unstructured, organized and unorganized

In developed countries, the potential gain of older people encouraged to work longer is not being fully realized. But when unemployment is high, there is often a tendency to see reduced number of older workers as a way to create more jobs for younger people. However, experience shows early retirement to free up new jobs for the unemployed has not been an effective solution (OECD, 1998).In less developed countries, older people are by necessity more likely to remain

Figure 3: Percentage of Labour Force Participation by People 65 and Older, by Region

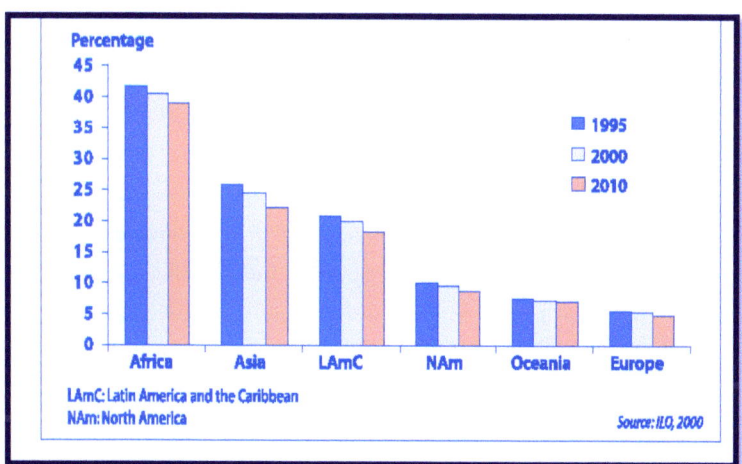

economically active into old age (see Figure 3). However, industrialization, adoption of new technologies and labour market mobility threaten much of the traditional work of older people, particularly in rural areas. Development projects need to ensure that older people are eligible for credit schemes and full participation in income- generating work opportunities.

Study after study disproves stereotypes about old people. Older workers can indeed learn new processes and technologies. They are no less efficient or productive; they are less absent than younger workers. They are less likely to shift jobs for a new career, and are no more inflexible about full-time and overtime than any other worker. The world of the aged may appear to be ugly and undesirable and young may reject them. Young people with vigour and strength forget that one day they will find themselves in the same shoes. It is just same life that we all have. Why cannot we build a world of love to shelter all, irrespective of age? Why cannot life begin after retirement, rather than end? .This can be possible only if the society will understand the importance of the elderly. It is important that society understands that retirement of a person does not mean end of his/her capabilities and potentials of the person. They still have capacity to work. It is the responsibility of the society to encourage them to work and live their life with dignity and respect so that they do not have to depend on their family for their daily requirements. This will definitely facilitate understanding and adjustment necessary for the old and the young to appreciate mutual problems and create harmony, love and respect for each other.

The problem to promote an idea of "Active Elderly" amongst society is a challenge pose by the age related stereotypes about elderly that they are weak, they have health related problems, and they are stubborn and slow. These preconceived stereotypes occupy minds of people to be resentful to employ elderly, or associate them with work. It is not enough; they also lead to misconceptions about the elderly that keep them away from work. There is a need to develop a bridge between the elderly and other segment of society. Society needs to listen to problems of the elderly and the elderly as well should learn about the expectations that society keeps from them. There is an urgent need to bridge this gap and build alternative bridges of productive interaction between two to far alien generations. Some solution has to be sought to put an end to a situation like two aliens locked in the same cell denying communicating with each other and share ideas and concern about life.

1.5 Reasons of Working after Retirement

"Retirement at sixty-five is ridiculous. When I was sixty-five, I still had pimples."
George Burns

"Age is only a number, a cipher for the records. A man can't retire his experience. He must use it. Experience achieves more with less energy and time."
Bernard Mannes Baruch

The above quotations express spirit of youthfulness among elderly persons who are still zealous to work more and be active to contribute. There are various reasons for employment of older persons. They work mainly to earn their living, but it is also noticed that even if they do not need money, they do not retire from their jobs. This is because they want to work for self-satisfaction, for friendly relations with colleagues and also for realization of their social participation.

To some extent, older workers remain in the workplace because they are healthier, cognitively able and want to remain engaged in work. In view of the study on older workers, Rix (1990) observed that many elderly workers continue to work at peak efficiency and that there is virtually much more variation within age groups than among age groups. Cognitive performance and personality have little effect on workers output except in the most physically demanding tasks. Farr, Tesluk and klein (1998) find in their study that there is no consistent relationship between an age and performance across settings. Some more observations among faculties like in the sciences, an age had a slight negative relationship to publicity productivity (Levin and Stephan 1989).Some studies indicate stronger negative relationship between an age and work performance for non-professional and low-level clerical jobs than for higher-level craft service and professional jobs. (Avolio, Waldman and Mc Daniel 1990; Waldman and Avolio 1993)

According to the study conducted by AARP titles "Staying Ahead of the Curve 2003: The AARP Working in Retirement". It is observed that more than three in four pre-retirees (77- 87 percent) who plan to work in retirement indicate that their desire to stay mentally and physically active and to remain productive and useful are among the major factors causing them to consider work in retirement work. In contrast, no more than two in three (54-66 percent) indicate that the need for health benefits or the needing money are among the major factors influencing their decision to work.

However, when the respondents were asked to indicate only one major factor for their decision to work in retirement, it became clear that the need for money is the most common primary motivator. Specifically, when they were asked to choose only one major influence to their decision to work, respondents were more likely to cite the need for money (22 percent) than any other factor. The second to importance of money is a need for health benefits (17 percent) .It is followed closely by a desire to remain mentally active (15 percent) and a desire to remain productive or useful (14 percent).

Numerous AARP reports present evidence that older workers form an active segment of the workforce (AARP 2004).One evidence indicate that 1,200 elderly and almost 80 percent of the respondents were found to be planning to work in some capacity during their retirement years(AARP 2005).The following factors impacted older workers for decision making.

- Inadequate retirement savings
- Stagnating pension coverage and other benefits reduced to extent to many workers with little or no pension protection and inadequate health benefits
- Changes and reduction in eligibility for full social security benefits
- Higher education levels educated workers are more likely to stay in labour force
- Increased life expectancy and improved health status
- Labour shortages that may prompt employers to implement programme and polices to attract and retain older workers

Although it appears that pre-retirees would expect that retirement work will avail them to provide a variety of nonfinancial benefits as well as financial benefits, the fact remains that a need for money is the most frequently cited as "one major factor" for working in retirement .It suggests that a sizable portion of these workers would choose to spend their retirement years outside of the workforce if they felt them financially secure doing so. Not surprisingly as compared to workers who do not plan to work in retirement, those who plan to continue working in retirement are more likely to have lower household family incomes.

Retirement from economic activities need not mean retirement from non-economic activities. Some retired persons live alone in later years and some participate in a variety of non economic activities like community work, hobbies, religious groups, and the like. Smooth and satisfied retirement would mean smooth transition from economic activities to such personal and social kind of activities.

Ageing and changes in work force may prompt us to re-examine and revalue meaning and necessity of work for older workers. An ageing work force might influence cultures and values at workplaces in ways may that change our notions of meaning and necessity of work. A workplace that blends training opportunities, flexible employment patterns, and policies supportive to needs of ageing work force becomes a workplace that value elderly workers as capable, productive, and knowledgeable workers. Elderly workers will need organizational and social supports to encourage the extension of the work life (Bailey and Hansson 1995).

Discovering meaning of work in the lives of elderly workers would provide is fertile ground to adult educators. They might explore more of learning-teaching approaches that would prove more effective to provide career guidance to older adults making while transition to part-time work, returning from periods of retirement, or thinking about leaving the work force. Flexible schedules, job sharing, reduced loads, and seasonal employment can be redefined in the context of a changing and ageing work force. Notions of full-time, part-time and career are applied usually to workers of the age between 18-65–may need to be re-examined in a light of employees who wish to work beyond even eighth decades of life. Elderly workers possess rich source of experience, accumulated knowledge, and wisdom. The quality and sensitivity reflected in an institution's program for counselling, training, retraining, and preparing elderly workers transition of life and career might indicate way by which organizations can recruit and retain their valued and productive workers

1.6 Perceptions about Retirement

Aging is judged by different criterion in different societies. The transition to old age is identified with several factors such as chronological age, ill health, retirement, physical/mental deterioration, and death of spouse. Studies reveal that changes in social role (widowhood, grandparenthood, retirement) and physical health dominate the definition of age identity. At the same time, studies also reveal that, like other age group, some aged separate illness or disability from aging. While they feel their health has deteriorated because of aging, their personality continues to remain the same. Thus, self-image remains unaltered, as the subjective image of age is not changed.

For many of us, it can be unpleasant to grow older. Our society and culture value youth, and being old is sometimes treated like a disease that has no cure. Of course, it's a reality that all of us have to face at some point, so aging is a huge topic of study for sociologists. Among other things, they observe patterns of social activity and identify the challenges we all face as we age. The larger challenge that has been identified is retirement.

Retirement may seem like something to strive for - a goal - not a challenge to face. It's nice to imagine not having to go to work every day, travelling and living a life of leisure. However, retirement like this doesn't happen too often anymore. In our current economy, more and more individuals have no choice but to work well past the age of 65. The harsh reality is that most of those who cannot work - and even some of those who can - live in or close to poverty.

Money aside, another part of the challenge of retirement is adjusting to retired life. Work provides us not only with income but also with social interaction and a sense of purpose. So, our job is often an important part of our identity. When it ends, it's common to struggle with the loss of that identity.

Retirement is a fluid concept because it connotes different things and is fraught with different experiences for different people. While some individuals perceive it positively and anticipate it with nostalgia others dread its eventuality with great anxiety. Thus, it could be said that it is not a homogenous experience for everyone.

Retirement is a time of significant transition as far as the use of time is concerned. However, the importance of retirement is made more glaring by the fact that the retired person is made to face some challenges because of his/her new status (as a retired person). It has been noted that retirement is a stressful experience to many because of its associated life decision change in the matter of life arrangement generally. It has been postulated by Elezua (1998) that the moment retirement comes knocking on the door (of an employee) it enters with challenges and expectations.

Retirement has been defined as a state of being withdrawn from business, public life or active service. According to the Industrial Training Fund, Centre for Excellence (2004), retirement is a real transition. In the views of Kemps and Buttle (1979) in Ubangba and Akinyemi (2004), retirement is a transfer from one way of life to another; they note that many people suffer from retirement shock such as a sense of deprivation during the early period of their retirement. In the opinion of Olusakin (1999), retirement involves a lot of changes in values, monetary involvements and social aspects of life. Olusakin further noted that for some retirees, it leads to termination of a pattern of life and a transition to a new one. However, Billings (2004) described retirement as the transition from first adulthood to second adulthood which is often a jarring and unsettling experience. It follows from these descriptions/definitions of retirement that a retired person or retiree is any person who performs no gainful employment during a given year or any person who is receiving a retirement pension benefit and any person not employed full time, all year round after his/her disengagement from a previous work schedule. It is deducible; therefore, that retirement implies a transition from active working life at youthful age with adequate financial capability to less rigorous work schedule or lack of any tangible work schedule at old age.

Retirement usually entails changes to economic circumstances. The loss of paid employment may lead to lower life satisfaction due to financial insecurity and a lower standard of living. On the other hand, for people with substantial financial resources these factors may not be of concern, while for others moving from unemployment to retirement may entail greater financial security if eligible for the aged pension or superannuation funds.

The negative effect of retirement due to financial insecurity may be particularly marked if the retirement is involuntary. Research has found that control over the timing of retirement may be important to higher levels of wellbeing (Quine et al., 2007; Sharpley and Layton, 1998; Szinovacz, 2003; Schulz and Heckhausan, 1997; Mirowsky and Ross, 1989; Herzog et al., 1998; Heckhausan and Schulz, 1995; Seeman and Lewis, 1995).

There are many social circumstances which may change at retirement. The end of working life may be associated with the loss of a role fundamental to personal identity and social status. This can result in disengagement from society due to the loss of social support and networks. Retirees may also experience low motivation and boredom if they are unable to replace the lost role with new activities (Pinquart and Schindler, 2007: 442).

1.7 Influence of Work on Elderly

One of the most influencing factors is decision-making in the work /retirement transition that will be influenced by the degree of control which individuals have over key events affecting their lives. Researchers contrast those with total choice and control to those with virtually no choice at all. Between these extremes will be a variety of circumstances and experiences, these influencing the extent to which work and retirement pathways are open to individual control. Social class appears as a significant variable, with those from manual occupations much less able to make meaningful choices about whether or not to extend work or take flexible retirement.

The context for decision-making is likely to be important. Organisational factors are likely to influence decision-making in the move from work to retirement. Family circumstances may be relevant for some, notably for those with responsibilities for caring for a spouse or parent. Women in their 50s have been identified as a 'pivot' generation, juggling care as well as work roles. Decisions about work and retirement must also be located in the wider social networks within which personal ties are embedded.

Retiring early or late may be normative among a group of colleagues within a particular occupational setting. Personal relationships are themselves likely to influence work and retirement options, notably in respect of the timing of decisions made by couples about leaving or staying on at work.

Retirement decisions are directly related to labour force, and especially elderly labour force participation. Major factors affecting elderly participation include education, working spouse or spousal labour force supply, health, personal properties and family debt, financial status of the family, marital status, number of children and fertility rate.

According to the discussed arguments, postponing or advancing retirement which happens in response to different factors, causes a change in the rate of participation from the elderly and the participation of all labour force in the labour market. There may be people who are still active in the labour market even after retiring and receiving pension. Although there is a close relationship between retirement and getting out of the market in developed countries, as the retirement pension they receive is not enough to support their family.

Therefore, any factor relating to retirement and retirement decisions has a direct effect on labour force participation, though outflow of labour force from the market and lack of labour force participation in the labour market may be a more general and comprehensive concept than retirement. In other words, factors that influence labour force participation and retirement decisions can also affect retired people's decision to return to the labour market.

1.8 Problems faced by Elderly at Workplace

Retiring from paid work may be different from the transition to retirement while unemployed. Many people transition to retirement from unemployment due to the large proportion of unemployed people (ABS, 2010). Older people may have difficulties in finding work because of employer preference or because of rapid changes in technology.

What problems do elderly employees face in the workplace?

Reduced employment opportunities: Those who are returning to the workforce or making a career change later in life find it harder to maintain salary and benefit levels comparable to their previous employment, because fewer options are available.

Decreased training participation: When compared to younger workers, elderly are less likely to participate in workplace training activities (35 hours per year for younger workers versus 9 hours per year for elderly).11 Contributing factors to this disparity potentially originate from perceptions of both employers and employees that prolonged tenure means greater level of workplace knowledge or lack of interest. Employees also may feel diminished support from management to participate in training opportunities.

Increased discrimination: Employer anxiety around salary and benefit costs have driven some to avoid interviewing and hiring elderly, even though evidence suggests it would not cut workplace productivity or earnings to employ them.

More challenging workplace conditions: When the need arises for elderly to care for aging family members or slowly transition out of the workplace, they may be confronted with inflexible work hours. Flexible work conditions, such as unconventional work schedules or the ability to telecommute, are important for employers to consider when employing elderly.

Salary expectations: Salary expectations also can be a major obstacle for older workers, many of whom made high incomes because of their experience level and length of time at their former company.

1.9 Satisfaction at Workplace

For many life events, people can be expected to experience a common reaction. For example, getting a job could be expected to be associated with an increase in life satisfaction for a period of time. Life events such as unemployment, ill health or bereavement are typically accompanied by low levels of life satisfaction (Carroll, 2007; Cole et al., 2009). The effect of retirement on life satisfaction differs for a range of reasons, depending on the individual circumstances surrounding the retirement transition. The associated change may be negative or positive, or there may be no change at all.

Previous studies generally found that job satisfaction is not only associated with salary but also with achievement, personal growth or relationship with others (Robbins, 2001). For the situational predictors, none of the occupational characteristics predicted life satisfaction, while all measured characteristics experienced by individuals during post retirement activity predicted work satisfaction. This is largely consistent with the Job Characteristics Model (Hackman and Oldham, 1975) with the important addition that opportunities to pass on knowledge (generativity opportunities) are also important in post-retirement work, which corresponds to findings on work motives at older ages (e.g., Calo, 2005; Grube and Hertel, 2008; Loi and Shultz, 2007). But the main part of the variance in work satisfaction is explained by opportunities to fulfill one's own achievement goals, perceived appreciation, and autonomy. This might suggest that persons who engage in unpaid post-retirement activities live in a different 'work world' than older employees still embedded in traditional work settings.

According to the study conducted by Over half of employees say job satisfaction is more important than salary in ensuring they are happy at work, a survey has revealed.

Job satisfaction was the most important factor for 56% of UK workers in securing happiness in the workplace, in contrast to just over a third (36%) who ranked pay above all else, according to the findings from Capital One. Furthermore, more than six in ten (62%) workers are happy in their current role, with one in five (19%) going so far as to say they love it.

Happiness in work was also noticably higher among older employees, with 67% of those aged over 55 saying they loved their job. Job satisfaction appeared a primary motivator in ensuring happiness at work for older employees, with 61% of those aged over 55 "Good employers recognise that their staff are their best asset and invest in creating positive working environments, empowering through trusted leadership and offering secondary benefits that support employees work life, well-being and interest. Creating an environment for success boosts morale, innovation and productivity."

1.10 Employers Attitude towards Recruiting Elderly after Retirement

Despite the lack of consensus regarding the point at which a worker officially becomes an "older worker," there is no debate that elderly face a number of challenges in the workforce, some of which are due to common perceptions of elderly—whether they are accurate or not. Studies of employer attitudes toward elderly workers consistently find that elderly are perceived to have a number of positive characteristics such as a good work ethic, acquired knowledge and experience, loyalty to the company, dependability, a commitment to quality, and productivity

Employment at older ages, however, depends not only on the willingness and ability of elderly to work but also on employers' willingness to hire and retain them. In surveys, employers usually say they value elderly' experience, maturity and work ethic, but often express concern about their relatively high salaries and benefit costs. One-quarter of employers in a 2006 survey said they were reluctant to hire elderly. Furthermore, some employers appear to discriminate against elderly. For companies happy to employ elderly, studies have shown that employers can reduce the barriers to working at older ages by offering phased retirement opportunities and reduced and flexible hours.

Many stereotypes and prejudices related to the employment of elderly persons that employers usually exhibit to avoid employing them find no justification today and cannot be taken as valid arguments. Primarily, the demand for manual work has decreased, which suits elderly to a large extent. Similarly, due to the advances in medicine and better life conditions, the physical and mental health of elderly population have improved, which enable them to be able to work longer hours than it was possible in the past. Besides, the living style has completely changed in the last two decades. All this has led to a situation that even those who count as the richest and who can safely retire, wish to continue to work and feel useful to themselves, to their families and to their society. The poor ones are forced to work even after they have formally retired because their pensions are small and often insufficient to allow a decent life. There is also a category of people that were laid off due to the crisis, who cannot exercise their right to retirement and hence want to find a new job. The motives of elderly people to go out to work may differ; however, what is common to all of these people is that they want to be actively working as long as they are able to work. Some wish to try new jobs and start up their own firms. Here they encounter numerous barriers of different forms.

One stereotype is that older people are less physically active and less mentally prepared to answer the demands of their jobs than the younger age groups. These attitudes cannot be fully accepted given that the health (both mental and physical) of elderly people is much better nowadays than it used to be in the past. Hence, they represent a valid potential in terms of labour force, skills and experience that societies need to put to productive use. Experience with "active aging" shows that older people, when integrated into the society, lead a better quality life, live longer and stay healthier. A conclusion can be drawn that integration and participation in employment are closely connected with the concept of social cohesion, a vital constituent of a healthy society. This can be achieved through a more substantial support the society should provide for this category of population in terms of encouraging them to be economically active as long as they choose or are able to be. The lack of policy that will regulate these issues leaves elderly people to live their lives in poverty instead of recognizing their active economic and social contributions. It is in this view that we can rightfully conclude that aging is a natural process, and that healthy elderly people are an important resource for their families, their communities, as well as for the economies of their countries.

Since there are elderly workers active on the labour market, organizations may benefit by employing elderly workers with intrinsic work values, since these elderly workers are more willing to invest in their work and relationship with the organization (Bal and Kooij, 2011).

In view of this reality, the present research seeks to conduct an enquiry into economical, social and psychological undercurrents in the reality today that prompt elderly decide to work even after they retire from their first employment. Does it turn out to be a kind of compulsion or because of familial responsibilities on their part or they wanted to do it out of their willingness or passion for work, or some other kind of considerations? The present research focuses on these issues to review the decisions of elderly to work after retirement. Popularly these workers are termed as "Silver Workers". The focus is laid on silver workers in the city of Vadodara to conduct a sample study on the related issues at large. Emerges from the responses and reflections of the silver workers against the questions asked to them. As a result we can obtain perspective on the silver workers decision to work after retirement.

1.11 Statement of the Problem

Keeping in view above discussion a study entitled "A Study on Silver Workers Residing in Vadodara City was undertaken"

1.12 Research Questions

There are questions concerning to the elderly and their decision to work in retirement. They reflect on variety of issues related to them. So they need an in-depth inquiry. The present research proposes to dwell on the following questions and analyse their implication in the interest of projecting the reality about silver workers and focus on some pertinent reasons, influencing factors, perceptions about retirement and problems puzzling and troubling them. In the light of the above, discussion, the following questions need to be responded by assessing

Q-1 How many elderly get success in seeking job after retirement?

Q-2 Do the companies welcome them as silver workers?

Q-3 Do they respect their work experience?

Q-4 Are they paid what they deserve? Or are they exploited?

Q-5 Are they treated in the way same as young colleague in a unit?

Q-6 Are they given any extra benefits for being in their third stage of life?

Q-7 Are elderly happy and satisfied with the type of job they do after their retirement?

To seek answers to these questions it was proposed to take up "A study on Silver Workers residing in Vadodara City"

1.13 Justification

1.13.1 JUSTIFICATION OF THE SUBJECT OF THE STUDY

The subject of working and caring has gained much attention in the last decades. However the research carried out in the field is mostly concentrated on childcare and mothers of young children. Only recently, a subject of caring for an elderly and its impact on employment and individual choice gets serious attention. Such sudden growth in interest for the elderly care cannot be accidental. We live in a time when the elderly generations are increasingly growing into a big cohort and the younger generation is constantly shrinking to minority causing care deficit.

The elderly are keen on redefining retirement. Instead of surfing and mountain-biking, the elderly will prefer spend at least part of retirement not in leisure but working. It may be sometimes for money or, out of necessity, or sometimes for no money but just because it is personally rewarding. Not long ago, many employers appeared to be askance at elderly workers. They thought that elderly workers lacked the spirit and imagination that youthful cohorts can display. But now the times are changing.

With respect to living arrangement and gender significant variations in morbidity exist among the elderly. Elderly population has become a challenge for many developing countries because their socio-economic development does not keep pace with rapid increase of the ageing population. Many nations are not adequately equipped with the social and economic potentiality to facilitate their elderly people to lead a dignified healthy life (Kalache A and Keller I, 2000). Healthy elders are a resource to their families, communities, countries and economies (WHO, 2002). But for many elderly with no savings, lack of old age economical security, poor health, no economic support from their children and little help from their children, friends and communities, the old age is not a phase of life worthy of looking forward to (UNFPA, 2002).

In a country like as India, in which no universal social security exists, people tend to work as long as they can (Irudaya Rajan,2005).In India ,there are several mechanism of social safety nets for vulnerable groups in the form of the gratuity, provident funds and social insurance programmes. The coverage of these schemes is restricted to 12 percent of elderly engaged at work mostly in the organized sector. The remaining 88 percent of elderly are engaged at work in unorganized sectors. They may have an access, though to limited extent to social assistance, social insurance, employer's liability and social allowance. In order to address limited coverage of these schemes, in view of ensuring fiscal viability, new initiative are undertaken, including the pension reforms. The increased life expectancy and improved health status of older people allow them to work after retirement. As soon as a person retires, he does not necessarily become old, inactive or non-contributory. His / her capacity to contribute to society is not reduced and hence, an opportunity to continue working should be allowed to the elderly.

Opening the doors to welcome elderly would prove very beneficial to organizations in time when a talent crunch is faced. Elderly can help in transmitting knowledge within the organization to benefit younger workers. Abundance of experience and wisdom that the aged possess cannot be gained from books or friends or can never be downloaded from the websites. The elderly who possess enough experience and maturity to cope with problems in life can help to enhance productivity by alleviating problems that a company confronts in its day to day functioning.

In order to remain active, the elderly have to find out adequate the possible work in which they can engage themselves. It may be part time or some kind of social work or of counselling about education. At such a stage in life a person should become a participant in life instead remaining a mere spectator. It will help them to remain economically independent. In addition, by utilizing of their time in constructive activities they can review enthusiasm and interest in life. One elderly person from Vadodara city shared his experience of retirement. He said "I am killing my time every day. I play with my grandchildren, help my wife in household chores, watch television and read newspapers. But I always feel that I must utilize my time by sharing my expertise with others. I must contribute to the society". This expression reflects that an elderly person would not be satisfied with normal household duty and hobbies as pastime activities. Along with them he would rather be aspirant to find out ways to share his/her knowledge and experience, benefit younger generation and, in that way, to impart valuable contribution into making of a new better work for generations to come.

Life expectancy has reportedly increased over the past few decades. With the elderly population in a country is increasing both in terms of absolute numbers in proportion of the total population; yet, traditional family norms and values to support the elderly are eroding gradually. Being country with second highest population in the world, India needs to determine priority issues for future research on ageing and redefine methodologies to undertake such studies. Earlier studies on ageing enable us to understand issues concerning the elderly, especially their problems. However, besides being exploratory, descriptive and localized, most of the studies focus on the urban elderly mostly male retirees/pensioners. The elderly are viewed as mere passive receivers of care. Now the profiles of the elderly population are undergoing a big change with a shift in issues concerns and aspirations. Today, a big proportion of the elderly intends to lead active life to earn sense of fulfilment for themselves, their family and the community. These changes affect quality of their life both directly and indirectly. Consequently, it is imperative to prioritize research efforts and evolve alternative methodologies to conduct meaningful issues related to ageing.

Researches consistently reflect that elderly in general and elderly workers in particular suffer from negative perceptions of their capabilities and desires for continued work. Recently, however, with changes occurring in context of employment markets and new researches suggest that the tide may be turning in favour of elderly workers. One key reason for examining the current situation for elderly workers is that many businesses start to worry about finding enough workers to fill the void of intend caused with elderly workers. They now consider employing elderly a positive step to safe guard the interest of the organizations. The AARP too begin to recognize and reward companies that prove them "elderly worker friendly."

The words like "work," "retirement," "volunteer," and also those related to the ageing (e.g., "seniors") tend to oversimplify the reality, which is more complex .They may serve as barriers to change. To combat negative image of the elderly as mere frail, dependent elderly underpinning a grim view of their future, society too willingly promote their positive image of the "active senior" usually indefatigable, healthy, usually wealthy, and eternally young in spirit. Both the images have limitations. New language, imagery, and stories need to be evolved to help elderly and the general public to re-envision the role and value of elders and also the meaning and purpose of later years in a person's life. Today's elderly live longer and remain healthy for longer periods of time the previous generations did. Currently cohorts of elderly workers are facing new pressures to continue work beyond the conventional age of retirement. Some continue to work because they enjoy it and expect new meaning, structure and purpose that work can provide to life .They want to continue work in order to receive costly health benefits. They want to work also to supplement inadequate pension that they are receiving. Some, of course, work because they can ill afford retirement. And, finally, new researches that view across generations of workers reveal that at least in some instances, employers prefer elderly workers to younger workers in view of their contribution about their utility and contribution to their business.The Government of India is committed to ensure conducive environment to the elderly to secure the goals of economic and emotional security. It recognizes that all institutions of civil society, individuals and community should act as equal and necessary partners to achieve this goal.

In this backdrop, when we review of the Indian legal system it reveals that our legal system enacts different legislations to deal with provisions in favour of the elderly. The Constitution of India specifies laws for the territory of India is concerned. The Article 21 of the Constitution announces for the elderly the fundamental right, called "Right to Life and Personal Liberty". Further Perusal of the Article 41 of the

Constitution, announces one of the directive principles, by which it enunciates the responsibility of the state, to make effective provisions within the limits of its economic development and capacity to secure the right to work, to education and to public assistance in cases like unemployment, old age sickness etc.

The aged who are employed in the organized sector in government service are given economic protection on retirement through the Pension Act, The Employees' Provident Fund and Miscellaneous Provisions Act, 1952.This is another mode to provide social and economic security for elderly workers who have given the best part of their life to industry. The payment of Gratuity Act, 1972, provides some more retirement benefits in addition to the PF and the Family Pensions benefits to employees in the organized sector. This certainly helps the aged to survive in their later life.

Recently the parliament enacted the Maintenance and Welfare of Parents and Senior Citizens Act, 2007.The name of the Act is descriptive and it conveys that parents and senior citizens should receive care and attention from their children. The Perusal of the Act further reveals that it is a short legislation with only 32 sections. It ensures that maintenance of old persons by their families will be a matter of right for the parents. It makes clear that it is a duty of children to take care of their parents.

In order to provide economic and social security in the real sprit, the Government of India goes a step further to launch the National Old-Age Pension Scheme. Its objective is to provide monetary relief and benefits to the destitute aged people so that they can survive happily and with relaxed mind in later years.

The careful analysis of the above referred legislations, policies and other schemes launched by the government reveals that they appear to be working well in theory to safeguard elderly. But the factual positions of their implementation pose a picture. In spite of all ideal provisions, we come across deplorable conditions of the aged people in almost all the states in India.

Several times, violation of the most precious constitutional right, right to life, has been reported. Each time it is rectified by intervention of the judiciary. The judiciary should intervene and ensure justice to elderly. Injustice may occur to elderly only when the government fails to implement the provisions in correct way. The National Policy of Older Persons was announced a way back in 1999 and it had very noble objective. But even after time beyond a decade, the same is not implemented by the government.

The first point that draws our attention is pension given to elderly .The amount paid to the retired elderly by way of their pension is not adequate. It is too meagre an amount for the elderly to hardly meet their expenses. There is enormous hike in the prices of all commodities including medicines. In such a situation the pension amount would not be sufficient to survive. Such may be a case for the elderly workers in the organized sector. The situation would be worse for the aged in the unorganized sector. They do not get even meagre amount as pension. They have to meet all these expenses on their own. The gratuity and the provident fund make sumptuous amount disbursed after retirement. While observing the mechanism, one will experience acute problem to get their own money from the respective government department. As the elderly aged has to wander office to office for days for the amount and in some cases they are seen even begging for the said amount. The rebate in payment of tax is availed by a very few elderly, as every elderly does not have that much income to avail the rebate.

As consequences of such conditions today we find many elderly persons working in their retirement age. They either wish to continue with their existing job or search for new jobs. Searching for a new job would not be easy task at this age, since we do not have re-employment policy in the organized sectors. As a part of nongovernmental effort website for elderly www.jobsforelderly.in launched in 2007 by Mehta, revealed that there were number of elderly who uploaded their bio-data on the website to get the job. In a period of three months there were hundreds of bio-data uploaded to get a job. The elderly who wanted jobs after retirement were educated and they were retried from organized sectors. The data revealed that most of the elderly had retired from decent jobs also, wanted to work after retirement.

Hence, it is imperative that the present study focuses on silver workers who are working in their retirement age. Such a study will help us to understand their importance at workplaces. Their vast experience of work would fetch respect for them, or they would be exploited by employers. The elderly have the right to work, and the civil society has to respect his/her and dignity in return. By undertaking such a research, the government and civil society will be able to provide a better work environment to its silver workers.

The rapid growth of the elderly population, and the wide diversity of their profiles with inter-related environmental influences of varied nature demand need significant consideration of researchers, policy planners and service providers. A research agenda on the ageing in the 21st century is evolved by the United Nations Programme on ageing .The International Association of Gerontology contributes to clarify it and implement public policies on the ageing, and influence also to the direction indicated and priorities for scientific gerontology. Thus, it is necessary to study issues related to the labour force participation (LFP) of older persons in view of its impact on the welfare of the elderly, households, society and the economy of the nation. Most of the researches are devoted to the elderly in developed countries, because the ratio of the old-age dependency is reported ratios are higher in them relatively to that in of developing countries. However, in countries like India, the ratio will rise is presumed to rise in coming decades. Moreover, developing countries do not have a well-developed and comprehensive pension system to offer. In addition, the joint family system is falling under strain. In light of these factors, a study of labour market behaviour of the elderly gains is important. Hence, there is a pressing need to re-examine the existing both formal and informal systems available to deal the challenges arising out of the 'Age Quake'. The World Health Organization pose an argument that countries can afford to get old provided if governments, international organizations and civil society enact "active ageing" policies and programmes to enhance the health status, participation and security of elderly. So it the time to plan and to act, Policies and programmes need to be framed addressing to which is based on the rights, needs, preferences and capacities of elderly. They also need to review embrace perspectives on course of life significance of earlier life experiences on the way individual's age. Therefore the main aim of the study is to help the elderly to create a social legacy claiming profound importance in the present context. Added years of their life would give them this chance and at large. There is a need for them to come to terms with the world at large in a way that would create their integrity with world and to their life give them psychological incentive.

1.13.2 JUSTIFICATION OF THE SAMPLE OF THE STUDY

Since the last century, human civilization has witnessed silent revolution, unseen and unheard by many. Although its impact is subtle, it is of utmost significant to everyone. The biggest achievement of the last century was longevity that results in increasing of ageing population worldwide. A man ages continuously through an irreversible biological process. It also occurs socially as perceived by the members of the society. Economically it occurs when a person retires from the workforce and chronologically it happens with passage of time. The survival of an increasing people beyond their traditional adult roles leads to population ageing.

The incredible increase in life expectancy may be termed as one of the greatest triumphs of human civilization. But it poses one of the tough challenges to be met by modern society. The term "old" is always related to physical incapacity, biological deterioration and also economical unproductively, disabilities and psychological failures. A healthy lifestyle is required during old age also. But in the Indian context, there exist three different trends that are seriously threatening the chances of meeting such needs. These are rapidly growing elderly population on one hand and gradual erosion of the traditional joint family system on the other .In addition there is inability of the government to sustain the incremental burden of pension expenses for its own employees. Hence, the possibility of government support for any other section of the elderly population in the society may be ruled out (Vaidyanathan 2003).

However, an aged person has right to decide about personal needs and aspirations, depending upon his capacity. Only sound social security system can protect such rights by assuring regular income during the post-retirement years. But developing such a system in the Indian context would prove a herculean task, as majority of the elderly do not enjoy currently any type of old-age income security. Neither the government nor the public sector alone can formulate the system. The private sector too cannot develop it in isolation. Joint approaches and strategies will be required to design and build up a robust old-age income security system (WHO 2002). The prerequisites for building such a system are effective economic environment, availability of financial instruments and a satisfactory regulatory model. These factors will help to win confidence of investors which is must required for smooth transition to long-term instrument.

Population ageing is a worldwide phenomenon. In India, the trend results in various challenges on account of gradual erosion of the traditional joint family system and the inability of government to support any section of the elderly population beyond retired government employees on pension. In recent years, India has undergone enormous changes on account of increased urbanization, industrialization and globalization. Across the world, several countries are experiencing population ageing. The growth rate of the elderly population is reported more rapid in developing countries like India than that in developed countries. Apart from demographic transitions, socio-economic and political changes together with increased individualism alter living conditions for the elderly.

Around one-eighth of the world's elderly population live in India. Most of them do not avail coverage of pension system. So they have to rely mostly on family arrangements or their own savings. In the past the elderly were highly respected members in a family in traditional Indian society. Taking care of them was considered among basic responsibilities of a family. Majority of the elderly who lived with their children preferred living with them and it was their desirable choice. .However, growth of 'individualism' in modern life led them to alienation and isolation in their families and society. Migration from rural areas too resulted in growth of more nuclear families in towns and cities.

As a result things become more difficult for the elderly. Policy planners never felt a need seriously to focus on this important area. Lack of attention on their part would not allow them support development of policies that would encourage and facilitate fullest participation of elderly in family, neighborhood and society. The traditional methods of old age income security would not cope with the realities of increased life span and spiraling medical expenses. Hence, there is a pressing need to reexamine existing formal and informal systems available to deal the challenges that arise out of the 'Age Quake'. Coupled with high growth rate of the elderly population, rapid changes are noticed not only in their profiles, but also in their personal, familial, neighborhood and societal environment. It intensifies a need further to evolve alternative approaches and methodological refinements to study issues related to ageing in a more sensitive manner. There is great deal of literature available on the subject of ageing but most of them inflict of it does a disservice to elderly. They neglect or addresses only in passing, the changing ways that elderly affect in society. Minimum attention is granted to the wealth of knowledge, expertise, skills and wisdom that elderly possess and that is made to educate younger generations.

Today, elderly are relatively more active and independent .It is owing to health consciousness, medical interventions, and their easy accessibility to medical facilities. However most of them are dependent on the younger generation for physical care and financial security. Hence they are forced and are forced to adjust in a society in which that stereotype prevails for the ageing referring to their as deteriorated physical and mental health. The existing studies mostly reveal negative aspects of ageing like the elderly are passive receivers of care, and they do not possess skills and talents to offer to the family and society. It is time that research needs to be geared to look at the positive aspects of the ageing that would ensure them happier in later years. In India, as elsewhere, elderly need to remain integrated in society, and they should be able to live with dignity and security. Further they should be able to pursue opportunities for self-development and participate actively in the formation of policies that concern them.

Two major effects of the globalization is realized in the form of breaking up of traditional joint family system and increasing economic burden on the elderly. It leads to increased marginalization of the elderly. It is important that government and society understand the rights and needs of the elderly and frame suitable policies and legislations to implement them effectively. The ageing needs to be viewed as positive experience for the elderly. A review of age-related issues presented in literature, media and researches would reveal that the majority only can attempt to bracket the elderly as dependent on family and society. Such unfavourable stereotypes of the ageing can serve to further marginalize the elderly in modern Indian society dominated mostly by the young-adult society. In order to create age-integrated society, negative views about the elderly need to reviewed and revised. The elderly need to be regarded as an integral part of society and their contribution should be given due recognition. It is equally important that the elderly prevent their obsolescence on their own by overcoming their negativity as far as possible to convert into positive outlook to others. 'As you think, so you are' is an aphorism that indicates the influence of mind over body. Considering steady increase in longevity, they must learn to accept the fact that professional retirement does not signify an end of active life. The studies on high longevity and heterogeneity among the elderly in fact reveal that there is increasing section of elderly who are still healthy and active. Well even into their 80s and 90s, they continue to lead productive life and they are eager about it. These people can serve a 'resource group' to make valuable contributions to society provided appropriate policies and programmes are developed to integrate them in developmental process.

Old age should be viewed from perspective of elderly participation and continuity of roles and functions and not of their disengagement and withdrawal. Unbiased perceptions about them will foster positive view of the ageing and reorient the existing stereotype that elderly invariably as mere liabilities. Efforts are urgently required to provide to them favourable environment and would facilitate them to enhance productivity and self-development. Importance of improving self-esteem and self-image, a primary requirement for successful ageing, cannot be overlooked. We need to inculcate a positive attitude. Considering the multi-dimensional aspects that constitute successful ageing and multiple determinants that influence it, some important questions may surface such as: How do we define successful ageing? What factors influence it? Are there variations in successful ageing among individuals with respect to class, gender or other strata of the elderly? What measures need to be taken to promote successful ageing?

Today, the elderly demand that society should not only ensure for their independence and participation, but also provide them care, fulfilment and dignity. Limited understanding of factors influencing their quality of life is largely responsible for the fact that the elderly are denied dignified existence. After all, last stage of life holds as much potential for growth and development as the earlier stages would do. Diversity among the elderly and varied interrelated influencing aspects of their environment should receive significant consideration of researchers and policy planners. The World Assembly on Ageing held in 1982 gave significant impetus to gerontological research; and it has recently gained importance. Further, the announcements of policies like National Health Policy, National Population Policy and National Policy on Older Persons too lead to far more awareness and consciousness among researchers, policy makers and others, resulting in an increased focus on age-related issues. In this light, the United Nations (2002) carry feeling that "There is a need to assess the 'state of the art' of existing knowledge, as it varies across countries and regions, and to identify priority gaps in information necessary for policy development." As the second most populous country in the world, it is important for us to assess the status of research on ageing in our country and identify existing gaps. It calls for attention of researchers as well as policy makers and others associated with issues of ageing. Such exercises would help us to prioritize issues for future research and refine methodologies to undertake such studies in better manner. An opportunity has to be created for the elderly to create a social legacy of profound importance. Added years of their life give them a chance. Their experiences in life give them capability. They need to come to terms with the world in a way that allows them integrity to life and gives them the psychological incentive.

In conclusion, it appears that population ageing is one of the most important and challenging issues in this millennium. It may infer that in this country, the ageing process has been largely influenced by socio-economic development of society. However, the problems call for serious thinking on a part that the government and civil society can play. In this context, the present research would like to find the reasons of silvers workers for working after retirement

1.13.3 SIGNIFICANCE OF THE STUDY IN THE DEPARTMENT OF EXTENSION AND COMMUNICATION

Department of Extension and Communication at the Faculty of Family and Community Sciences, The Maharaja Sayajirao University of Baroda, seeks to train its student to work on the various issues related to human development. In past number of studies were undertaken for the benefit of women and children on development issues like health education and income generation, women empowerment, human rights etcetera.

The students of department also work with the vulnerable sections of the society in the field courses. The elderly constitute vulnerable section of society and students of the department conduct field work with this group as a part of adult education course. So it makes it interconnecting that elderly was selected as the sample of this study. Conducting this study is more pertinent in department of extension and communication as it will help in designing the course curriculum of the courses like adult and non formal education of the department in order to make the field work more effective and need based.

Department undertakes various projects through its curriculum to cater to vulnerable section of the society. Elderly population is an emerging group in society that needs special care and attention. This group faces number of problems which can be tackled meaningfully through researches and action projects in the department.

1.13.4 JUSTIFICATION OF THE VARIABLES

1. Age

Age is a major variable that is used to indicate individuals' age differences. Increasing age signifies seniority and physical deterioration. This means age has an oppositional relationship with health levels of the elderly. When the elderly get older, their ability to work decreases according to increasing age. The study of Soontranuet et al., (1991) reveals that the proportion of the elderly's responsibility to their family decreases according to increasing age. It is in accord with the studies of Nirom (1987), Ruttanavijit (1995), and Keukulnurak (1997) which found that most elderly people who work are in the age group of 60-64 years old and they will reduce their work when getting older. Pittayanon (1992) indicates that age is an indicator of labour participation. There is a low rate of very old age people working because of their weak health.

Although in this study age is used as an indicator for working ability; that is people who work in the governmental sector and the state enterprise sector retire when they are 60 years old, it does not mean that people aged 60 or over are not able to work. The scientific research that studies the aging process or aging revealed that the elderly are able to retain their activeness for their lifetime, especially those aged between 60 and 75. They are healthy enough to do activities on their own (Khotrakul, 1993). It accords with the study of Hemathorn and Silapasuwan (1983 cited in Nirom, 1987) that found that early old aged people or those aged between 60 and 69 have active bodies and were able to do more efficient work than those who were aged 70 and over. The elderly aged from 80 years old were in the group that has the least ability to do activities. It can be said that the age of the elderly is relational to their ability to work. Keukulnurak (1997) found that both male and female elderly aged between 60 and 69 worked in the agricultural sector more than other age groups. The elderly aged over 80 did other work more than agricultural work because agricultural work required a lot of strenuous labour. Khotrakul (1993) revealed that those who did not work in the governmental sector tended to work until the time they thought it was enough for them. And those whose work requires physical energy, such as farmers or labourers, often retire before they are 60 years old.

The age at which any individual retires will reflect their circumstances, choices, and constraints. Hansson et al. (1997) argued retirement is rarely based on one influence alone, but that several variables affect the decision. According to Patrickson and Ranzijn (2004), individuals have 'bounded choices' about retirement, each needing to take into account the constraints of their financial position, health situation, and motivation to work. Employers contribute to these bounded choices by their offering, or not, suitable employment, and governments also contribute with policies and incentives concerning taxation, superannuation, and age pension benefits. In contrast, Parnes and Sommers (1994) described some elderly who were 'shunning retirement', based on their good health, continued psychological commitment to work, and dislike of retirement.

2. Education Qualification

Education is an indicator of an individual's ability to work, including opportunity to work, payment, and characteristics of the jobs. In addition, education has a positive relationship to economic systems. Those who receive high education have a better opportunity to get a good job; they will be well paid; and they are able to earn enough for their living costs (Chumjit, 1987). The studies of Amornsirisomboon (1992) and Keukulnurak (1997) found that education was related to both male and female elderly working. The rate of the elderly who finished grade 4 was higher than those finishing other grades. It accords with the study of The National Statistical Office (1998) in which the highest proportion of working elderly was from the group of those who had primary education. The second highest was those who had lower education than early primary school and lowest was those who did not receive any education. While Ruttanavijit (1995) found that education was not related to the elderly working, Boonnak (1994) in her study of the education of the elderly in Bangkok found that the more the elderly had higher education the more they wanted to work.

The rate of those who had higher education or over was 36.3 percent; those who finished junior high school was 30.9 percent; and those who finished primary school was 24.5 percent, respectively. Pittayanon (1992) revealed that education has an influence on labour participation. Those who have high education participate in the labour force more than those who have low education because the former consider that they should use the knowledge gained from their education for their own benefit. Education affects different occupations of the elderly. While most elderly who have high education work in the non-agricultural sector, those who have low education work more in the agricultural sector (Nirom, 1987). The study of Boonyanupong and Boonyanupong (1990) found that both the elderly who lived in the urban and rural areas began their work after they finished primary school. This was because in the past there was no indicator that specified that age and knowledge were requirements for work. As a result of the fact that there was a transferral of occupational knowledge from individual to individual, such as parents, familial members or owners of the business, the elderly in the past did not have high education (Boonyanupong and Boonyanupong, 1990).

3. Health Status

Health is a major factor that affects behaviours and roles of individuals of every gender and age. Changes in physical conditions and deteriorating bodily functions make old age people have more health problems than other age groups (Chariyaratpaisarn, 2000). Ruttanavijit's study of elderly people in the Central region and Northeastern region of Thailand (1995) revealed that elderly people's physical abilities are related to their work. The rate of those who have good physical abilities is higher than those who do not have good bodily functions. It accords with Chayovan's study of the community's response to elderly people's health problems (1995). Chayovan found that the number of the elderly who worked in the past year were those who had less health problems and was higher than those who did not work because the work status of the elderly was a selection. That is, the elderly who were able to work were those who had good health or did not have health problems. However, the study of Ruttanavijit (1995) found that sickness was not related to the work of the elderly.

A lot of research studies revealed that 70 – 80 percent of the causes that make the elderly stop working are health problems (Chayovan and Wongsit, 1987). The study of Nirom (1987) found that health conditions of the elderly were the major factor that allowed the elderly to work in the agricultural sector. Some people who were old but healthy were able to work. It was also found that health conditions were indicators that specified elderly people's abilities to work. Most of those who had good health worked in agricultural and non-agricultural sectors. The second highest were those who had medium health problems and the last were those who had bad health problems.

Another important health factor is the health of the worker's partner (Talaga and Beehr 1995). Talaga and Beehr (1995) and Wolcott (1998) found if their partner is in poor health, men will continue to work to provide greater financial resources, while women will tend to leave the workforce, in order to directly care for their sick partner.

4. Type of Family

When considering family structure, which is able to indicate working conditions, it is found that male elderly and female elderly living in nuclear family households work more than those living in extended family households and unrelated individuals households. The fact is that nuclear family households consists of husband and/or wife, and unmarried child, so children make the elderly take more responsibility for the couple and the children than the elderly living in an extended family household and unrelated individuals household (National Statistical Office, 2001). The studies of Amornsirisomboon (1992) and Keukulnurak (1997) found that most of the working old age people were married. This echoes the study of Boonnak (1994) that 58.2 percent of people who want to work were married people; 33.6 percent were those were widowers or divorcees; and 7 percent were single people. It accords with the study of The National Statisticial Office. Marital status is related to the working of the elderly. Old age people who are single and those who are married are of the highest numbers. Pittayanon (1992) reveals that the most important variable of married women's participation in the labour force is the husband's income. Women from well-to-do families spend most of their time raising their children and doing house work. In contrast, the study of Rakwanich (1993 cited in Ruttanavijit, 1995) indicates that the highest numbers of the working elderly are those who are single. The second highest are those who are married and those who are widowers, divorced, or separated.

5. Economic Status

One of the important factors concerning the retirement decision is that of the individual's Economic status. An individual's economic status includes issues of savings, both personal and superannuation, housing ownership, other investments, dependence of others (children, elderly parents, sick relatives), expected income stream from combined pension and superannuation, and adequacy of health insurance (Karoly and Rogowski 1994; Wise 1996; Patrickson and Ranzijn 2004). If finances are very healthy, then the decision to retire may be possible at any age or stage. On the contrary, if finances are very unhealthy, the option to retire may not be realistic at a particular point in time. One effect of longer life expectancy is that people commonly having children later in life, and hence, they may still be financially responsible for children at the traditional retirement age of 65 years. In addition, these same people may have parents that are still alive and if they are, their health care costs are likely to be greater and to go on for longer. In other words, the 'older Baby Boomers are already becoming financially sandwiched in their need to provide for two other generations' (O'Neill 1998, p. 178). Both these financial imperatives, plus the strong likelihood that they will live longer than their parents did due to healthier lifestyles and improvements in medicine, may push workers to continue working or attempt to return to the workforce. Moreover, the likelihood that government-funded social service payments will dwindle and individuals will need far more to financially fend for themselves, suggests that some elderly will be forced to continue working because they will be unable to live on their accumulated savings, superannuation and pension (Schwartz 1999). Evidence from the USA supports this possibility, as that country's economic crisis recently resulted in some elderly not being able to retire, and some retirees returning to work, because of their reduced retirement savings and investments (Kadlec 2002; Clement 2004). In contrast, other research suggests that financial considerations were not the most important motivator in the decision to retire. For example, Leonard (1999, p. 28) reported a study finding a growing number of employers were asking elderly to remain on the job, and many of these elderly were staying on, not because of financial needs, but because their work colleagues had become like family to them, and 'their pride and self-esteem are also linked to the notion that they are making a contribution to society'. Likewise, Gardyn (2000) argued money was not the main motivator for elderly continuing to work, instead, the main motivators were found to be the desire to keep active and to maintain social interaction with others and to feel productive.

1.14 Objectives of the Study

(A) Objectives related to Silver Workers

1. To study the profiles of silver workers working in Vadodara city.

2. To study the reasons of silver workers to work after retirement with respect to
   a. Personal reasons
   b. Familial reasons
   c. Financial reasons
   d. Work related reasons

3. To study the differences in the reasons of silver workers to work after retirement in relation to the selected variables:
   a. Age
   b. Educational qualification
   c. Last Designation
   d. Present salary
   e. Health status
   f. Type of family

4. To study the influence of work on silver workers

5. To study the differences in influence of work on silver workers in relation to the selected variables:
   a. Age
   b. Type of work (Present)
   c. Present designation
   d. Health status

6. To study the problems faced by silver workers at their workplace

7. To study the difference in the problems faced by silver workers at their workplace in relation to the selected variables:
   a. Age
   b. Educational qualification

    c. Present salary
    d. Health status
    e. Present designation
    f. Perceptions about old age

8. To study the satisfaction of silver workers in relation to their work status

9. To study the differences in satisfaction amongst silver workers in relation to the selected variables:
    a. Type of work (present)
    b. Present salary
    c. Present designation

(B) Objectives Related to Employers

10. To study the profiles of organizations employing silver workers

11. To study the reasons of employers for recruiting silver workers in their organizations/companies/institutions/firms/business houses/corporate.

12. To study benefits of employing silver workers in their organizations/companies/institutions/firms/business houses/corporate.

13. To study the problems faced by employers by employing silver workers in their organizations/companies/institutions/firms/business houses/corporate.

1.15 Null Hypotheses of the Study

1. There will be no significant differences in the reason of silver workers to work after retirement in relation to the selected variables:
    a. Age
    b. Educational qualification
    c. Last designation
    d. Present salary
    e. Health status
    f. Type of Family

2. There will be no significant differences in influence of work on silver workers in relation to the selected variables:

   a. Age
   b. Type of work (Present)
   c. Present designation
   d. Health status

3. There will be no significant difference in the problems faced by silver workers at their workplace in relation to the selected variables:

   a. Age
   b. Educational qualification
   c. Present Salary
   d. Health status
   e. Present designation
   f. Perceptions about old age

4. There will be no significant differences in satisfaction amongst silver workers in relation to the selected variables:

   a. Type of work (Present)
   b. Present salary
   c. Present designation

1.16 Delimitations of the Study

1. The study is delimited to retired silver workers (58 and above) residing in Vadodara City
2. The study is delimited to silver workers reasons, influence, perception, problems and satisfaction of silver workers working after retirement

1.17 Assumptions of the Study

1. Most of the silver workers were working after retirement
2. There are various reasons of silver workers to work after retirement

1.18 Operational Definition of the Study

1. **Silver Workers:** In the present study, they are those people who work after retirement. These people fall in the age group of 58 years and above residing in Vadodara City.

2. **Employers:** In the present study, they are those people who recruit the silver workers in the organization, corporate, business houses and firms post their retirement

CHAPTER - 2

REVIEW OF LITERATURE

This chapter will provide a background to and a context for the investigation of the topic of silver workers working post retirement, which is of key importance in the present-day industrialized world that is facing a rapidly aging population and concomitant labour force shortages, through a review of relevant literature. The review conducted aimed to identify research that examined the reasons of working beyond retirement. In this study retirement age is defined as the accepted retirement age in the country where the study took place. This is generally the age at which individuals become eligible for the state pension. This chapter is having exclusive studies which compared retired people and people employed over traditional retirement ages to focus specifically on the effect of working beyond the normative retirement age.

The present study therefore aims at studying the reasons why elder work after retirement. The study limits its scope to elderly people in India, several studies are conducted on various issues concerning society, culture, economies, politics, and health etc. In society the area of social life, good attention is paid to issues concerning women and children. But it's regretting fact that elderly have received scant attention from researchers and as a result, not many researches are conducted focussing on their issues. One may call it lack of sensitivity of the Indian society to their elders or neglect paid to elders in a society once they cease to be productive member in a society. The reason may be whatever, it is hardly noticed that elders in our society suffer neglect and helpless and their expectations are not duly attended. Government and public agencies like non government organizations etcetera do not appear to carry out social responsibilities about them. The result is that a few studies are available on elderly people. Against if, there are many other countries who display sensitivity to elders.

It is witnessed universally that for ages the sense of politics that is implied in popular expressions "Right is Right" and survival remains the reality for all living beings. In the context of the human history, politics prevails in a form of tug of war between two sections the powerful and weak. These two groups are constantly at strike for advantage over each other and the weak are always losing to suffer derivation this occurs at different grounds like social, cultural and political. At social level, the weak who suffer include the old, women and children popularly known as the weaker sections. These humans are easily exploited to their helplessness described as beautiful losers: old or elderly people form a sizeable part of beautiful losers in human society.

In India several studies are conducted related to health status, recreation, but very few studies have been carried related to reasons of elderly working after retirement; consequently significant numbers of studies are carried out in foreign countries which have relevance to the elderly, specifically to the present study. The literature related to the available research studies is reviewed for the purpose of preparing a ground for the present study. The review is presented under following heads

2.1 Studies Related to Reasons of Silver Workers to Work after Retirement

2.2 Studies Related to Employment Status of Silver Workers

2.3 Studies related Factors Influencing Silver Workers to Work beyond Retirement Age

2.4 Studies Related to Employers Perspectives Towards Recruting Silver Workers

2.5 Studies Related to Perceptions of Silver Workes Related to Retirement

2.6 Studies related to Problems of Silver Workers Working Beyond Retirement Age

Total Studies:

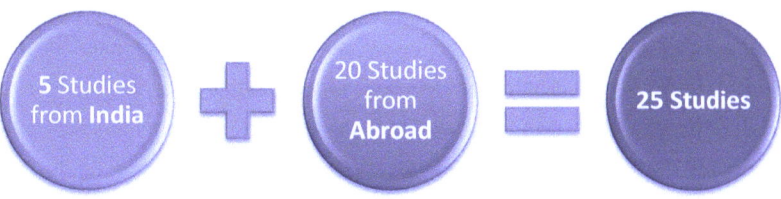

Years: 2002 to 2010

The purpose of this kind of presentation of the available literature is to prepare useful ground for the present study with due classification on the related aspects and issues. It may help correct understanding of the issues that are dealt in the present study. Further some of the heads above mention one phrase "silver workers. It refers to elderly people who work after retirement some of the research studies conducted abroad focus chiefly on some of the compel elders to work after retirement. They arose of the factors such as demographic factors, lack of information, and attitude and interest level on part of elders. The studies summarized below will explain he reasons in the light of these factors.

2.1 Studies related to Reasons of Silver Workers to Work after Retirement

Brown et al., (2010) conducted a research study on "Working in Retirement: A 21st Century Phenomenon". The main aim was to define what it means to be working in retirement and how employers might best meet the needs of elderly, to the advantage of workers and of the employers themselves. The sample of the study involved 1,382 participants aged 50 and older. The data collected by the FWI'S nationally representative study of the U.S was used for the study.

The major findings of the study revealed that 75 percent of workers who aged 50 years above expected to get post retirement jobs in future. Further it was observed that people worked after retirement for variety of reasons, which included one to avail opportunity to earn more money with which they could have more comfortable life in retirement and because they would be bored if they were not working. Those working in retirement were highly satisfied .They could keep them engaged in their work. They even rated their workplace more positively than those who were not yet retired.

A significant number of such employees showed preference for transition to self employment as retirement jobs. While those worked in retirement worked for a fewer hours, on an average than those who were not yet retired. Majority of elders working in retirement have reported working full time and they wanted to work for the same or even more hours.

Finally the study suggested that these working retirees represented a new paradigm for thinking about work throughout an individual's lifespan in terms of flexible careers. Flexible careers is supposed to recognize that people's values, needs and aspirations with respect to work change as individuals move through different life stages .It may allow multiple exit and re-entry points.

(http://familiesandwork.org/site/research/reports/workinginretirement.pdf)

Dittrich, Busch and Micheel (2008) conducted a study on "Working beyond retirement age in Germany: The employee's perspective". The aim of the study was to focus on old person's willingness to continue working after reaching legal retirement age. The sample survey was conducted by the Infratest in Germany with 1,500 employees (blue collar workers, white collar workers and civil servants) they were of the age between 55 and 64 years. The variables of the study included gender, job status, job demand, job reward, job position, working time, family Income, size of a company, health, expected work ability, and specifically motivation worth willing for a prolonged working life.

The findings of the study revealed that factors related to desire to continue working indicated to a family income. Lower income would arouse higher desire to continue working. Further smaller would be the firms size the higher would be desire to continue working; work classification would also count as important factor. There was also non-linear interaction effect for work hours. The positive effect of work motivation on work ability was strongest for those respondents who were working part time. (http://economicscience.net/files/Working%20beyond-retirement-age-in_Germany_20-10-10.pdf)

Ling and Fernandez (2006) conducted a study on "Labour Force Participation of Elderly Persons in Penang". The main objective of the study was to examine demographic and socio-economic profile of the elderly and the factors that influenced the labour force participation of senior citizens i.e. the choice to be "in" or "out" of the labour force. The sample of the study comprised of 328 respondents of the age falling between 55 and 89 years. The sample selected for this study consisted of 142 respondents who participated in the labour force, whereas the remaining 186 respondents did not form a part of labour force. The sample consisted of individuals of different races in the state of Penag. So the questionnaire was prepared in two languages i.e. English as well as in mandarin, a language spoken pre-dominantly by the Chinese population in Penag .Two types of sampling namely purposive and opportunity sampling were used to identify possible participants who were over an age of 55. The variables to study included the factors like (i) demographic factors like age, gender, marital status, number of children and race, (ii) human capital variables like education level and health status, (iii) work-related variables such as sector of employment, individual's former employment status and spouse's labour force participation status and (iv) financial considerations which would include spouse's monthly income, financial security that was derived from non-labour income and also monthly expenses.

The findings in this study indicated that gender, high monthly expenses, previous employment status of an individual and the spouse's labour force participation status had significant positive relationship with the labour force participation. The human capital variables like education and health were positively related to the labour force participation but were statistically insignificant. The factors which had a significant negative relationship with the labour force participation of the elderly were age, spouse's income, financial security and low monthly expenses.

http://www.globalresearch.com.my/proceeding/icber2010_proceeding/PAPER_138_LaborForce

Abraham and Houseman (2004) conducted a study on Work and Retirement Plans among Older Americans. The aim of the study was to examine factors that influenced work and retirement plans of older Americans' and also to know whether or not these plans were realized. The analysis was based on the data received from the HRS; .The study was conducted as a panel study that included representative samples of Americans who were born between 1931 and 1941. The panel members were interviewed biennially since 1992. The analysis was restricted to those individuals who were working for at least 20 hours per week and at least for 1,000 hours in a year at the time of the survey, and these claimed significant labour force attachment.

The findings of the study revealed that good number of people expressed interest in working at older ages. Among elderly interviewed for the survey quarter planned to stop work altogether and 18 percent planned to reduce hours of work. A need to change jobs was felt a major obstacle by older Americans who sought to reduce their work hours and remain employed. While nearly as many older working Americans said that they had plans to reduce their work hours and even to retire fully.

The study also reported that elderly might have faced substantial barriers in changing jobs. They are mainly age discrimination in employment and lack of information about job opportunities and also options for skills training. In this scenario, policies framed to eradicate age discrimination may provide information on employment and training opportunities. It may also increase possibility of job transitions .It thus, exert positive effects about employment among seniors.

2.2 Studies related to Employment Status of Silver Workers

Yesudian and Singh (2009) conducted a study on Working Elders in India: A Gender Specific Situation Analysis. The objective of this study were, to study the trend of elderly population's work participation in India, to study the pattern of work participation among the elders in India and its various regions, and to explore the demographic and socio-economic characteristics of these working elders.

The first objective various sources of information such as Census 2001 and 61st National Sample Survey were used. The 61st round of NSSO survey focused on employment and unemployment situation in India. It was conducted from July 2004 to June 2005 covering 1,24,680 households comprising of 79306 from rural and 45376 from urban areas. Some socio-economic characteristics of the aged were also used from NSSO 60th round data. The NSSO survey covered all the regions of India, with the exception of some interior areas of Nagaland and Andaman and Nicobar Islands, and Leh (Ladakh) and Kargil districts of Jammu and Kashmir.

Individuals aged 60 and above were considered as elderly in this study. In India the retirement age for formal or organized jobs for central and state governments varies from 55 to 60.Work participation according to Indian Census is defined as 'participation in any economically productive activity with or without compensation, wages or profit.

Findings of the study revealed that more than half (51.8 percent) of the elderly population in India depends on someone economically. Among them majority (77.9 percent) depends on their own children. Economical dependency is high (73 percent) among elderly women, both in rural as well as in urban areas. Schedule tribe (ST) elderly men and women are much more involved in labour force than the other ethnic groups. At the national level the work participation rate is declining. However, female work participation is increasing for elderly women. Age-specific work participation rate highlights, the higher proportion of economically active male workers in the 60-65 years age group. Hence this study has explored the elderly person's work participation over the decades and also explored the background characteristics of these elderly workers. It also found some determinants which contribute to gender-specific work participation in old age

Giang and Pfau (2006) conducted a study on a gender perspective on elderly work in Vietnam. The main objective of this study was to examine the current status and determinants of employment for the Vietnamese elderly.

The sample of the study consisted of 39,071 people in 12,020 household, in which the number of elderly people and the household were 3,865 and 2.883 respectively. Summary was carried out to collect the data. The survey is organized by household, but it also included some characteristics for individuals in the household, such as age, gender, relationship to the household head, marital status, working status, wage or salary, health, and educational attainment. Variables of the study included working status, age, marital status, and educational level, and the household characteristics include residential areas, residential regions, household living arrangements, household composition, household income quintile, as well as receipt of social security benefits and remittances.

It was evident from the findings of the study that 44 percent of the elderly were working in 2006 .The prosperity of males to have higher employment rates was found across all the category groups. Majority of the elderly were living with their children on the other hand 22 percent of the elderly were living in the household with only elderly (including elderly living alone). The findings further showed that elderly living in the household receiving social security or remittances generally had lower rates of employment than did non-recipients for both genders. There was higher tendency to work at a statically significant level among younger elderly, married elderly, elderly in centre regions and rural areas, elderly in houses holds with less working aged people, elderly in low income households and elderly in households not receiving social security.

Characteristics which do not play a significant role for both genders include educational level and remittance receipt. The study was concluded pointing that elderly were left behind with more responsibilities under limited social and financial sources, which in turn may force them to work in order to earn a living. (http://mpra.ub.uni-muenchen.de/24946/4/MPRA_paper_24946.pdf)

Delong (2006) conducted a study on "The Paradox of the 'Working Retired' – Identifying Barriers to Increased Labour Force Participation for Elderly in the U.S.". The main aim of the study was to assess any real changes in the labour force participation rate over time and state of the aging workforce today. The sample of the study consisted of 2,719 respondents in the age group of 55 and 70. The study was conducted during the first quarter of the year 2006. It consisted of an interactive online survey fielded by the zoby international.

The findings of the study revealed that, overall 38 percent of the respondents were retired and were not working for money, or they had not worked outside the home earlier for almost 15 years. This group included about 15 percent of the respondents in the age of 55-70 years. These persons were availing retirement benefits, and also either returned to the workforce or were actively searching work.

It was revealed from the study that the respondents having an age between 55- 59 years complained about "age bias" for about 39 percent of the time, whereas those in the age of 60-65 years –olds and 66-70 years olds identified age bias as mere a barrier for about 42 percent and 60 percent of the time respectively.

Those who were currently in the workplace who were about 72 percent and in the age group of 55 to 59 called work as need for raising "income to live on" as primary reason for working. This group was followed by those who expressed it as the desire to "maintain lifestyle (43 percent) and "build additional retirement savings" (41 percent). Among those of 60 to 65 years, a need for "income to live on" (60 percent) was still the most frequently mentioned reason for working.

What followed this reasons was a shift in priorities which appeared as the desire to "stay active and engaged" (54 percent) and "do meaningful work" (43 percent), these reasons were in second and third places. Elderly who were 66 to 70 year old, this shift in priorities was merely dramatic, with 72 percent of them who said like "want to stay active and engaged" as the most frequently mentioned reason for working. The second choice for them was "want the opportunity to do meaningful work" (47 percent) and third choice was like "enjoy social interaction with colleagues" (42 percent). A choice like "Need income to live on" trailed a fourth place and it was given by 37 percent of those 66 to70 years' olds.

The findings further revealed that majority of all three groups made it clear tht they were interested in part-time work only. Almost all the respondents of the study expressed they expected to live up to a median age of "81 to 85 years ." About 44 percent of old workers in age group of 55 to 59 years were not confident that they will have enough money to live comfortably past age 85. Those ageing 60 to 65 and 66 to 70 were considerably more confident (69 percent) on an issue of retirement security, although their confidence might be unfounded.

Therefore from this research it can be concluded that the motivations for work would not change for every person in similar way. For some, the motivational drive was economic gain never all the time and for many others economic motives would be preference next to a need to accomplish something meaningful in life their early sixties.(http://group.aomonline.org/cms/Meetings/Atlanta/Workshop06/Streams/Aging/CMS%20AgingWorkforcePaper-DeLong-FINAL6-21-06.pdf)

Kaldi (2005) conducted a study on "Employment status of the elderly referring to the social security organization of Tehran city". The main aim of the study was to examine the employment status of the elderly workers over an age of 60. The respondents selected for study were employed elderly in Tehran. They were all retired men on pension who were also receiving benefits from the social security organization from 1996 to 2003. They were selected as the statistical population of the study .The reason for keeping the years between 1996 and 2003 was to get information on the latest group of workers who retired according to the current regulations. The sample respondents consisted of 15 persons selected from each office. It made a group of total of 450 persons coming to 30 social security offices in Tehran. The survey was carried out on the employment status of these elderly in reference to the social security organization in Tehran. A questionnaire followed with interview was the method adopted for collecting information from the pre-determined sample respondents.

The major findings of the study revealed that the elderly person's interviewers in 60 to 65 years age group (20 percent) in 66 to 70 years age group (28 percent) and in 71-75 years age group (12 percent) who were interviewed on the issue declared that their income was not sufficient in terms of their life expenses. Only 1 percent of the interviewees who were above 75 years old have preferred this option. Totally, 71 percent of the interviewees declared that their income was not enough to meet their life expenses.

Among the elderly workers interviewed those in 60 to 65 years old group(18 percent) ,in the 66 to 70 years age group (19 percent) ,71 to 75 years age group (11 percent) had a full time job, whereas only 0.9 percent in above 75 years old group were in part time jobs.

About the recruitment condition interviewees, in total 77 percent of them informed that they had a contract based job and some 20 percent had temporary jobs, only 2 percent of them had permanent jobs. Totally, 58 percent of the interviewees declared that most essential problem for them was lack of earning opportunities in life, 19 percent of them said that it was lack of attention from family and society, and 7 percent reported that it was physical or mental inabilities that affected their chances for jobs adversely.

The question was "why they continue working in the elderly period". In response to it more than half (60 percent) of them replied, that it was because they could not earn enough money during their earlier life. Net to that more than half (57 percent) declared that since the pension was their only income they had no enough money to meet the life expenses and so they had to work to earn enough livelihood. Therefore, 58 percent of the interviewees believed that main problem was not earning their livelihood and more than one fourth of them considered that the main worry was to arrange for survival in future as they had no sufficient income.

The study concludes with a remark that different needs of the elderly should be studied properly with an objective to improve their living status by providing them enough facilities. This subject can be incorporated under the social policy framework by compiling comprehensive plans for the elderly welfare through providing proper services that are adapted to their needs (www.me-jaa.com/mejaa4/sso.pdf)

Kangsasitiam (2004) conducted a study on "Household structure and elderly working status" This research aimed to analyze household factors affecting employment status of the elderly in Kanchanaburi province (Thailand). The sample group used in this study was male and female elderly aged over 60 living in Kanchanaburi province in 2001. The total number was 3,985 elderly. multinominal logistic regression was used for analyzing statistical data. Variables of the study included age, gender, marital status, education, health, house head status, household structure, household financial status, migration, and living area.

Findings of the study revealed that age group of most old age people was between 60 and 69 years old, the second highest people aged between 70 and 79, and the least people aged over 80. In the matter of marital status, it was found that majority of elderly (62 percent) were married One third of the elderly were widowed, divorced, and separate. The proportion of divorced and separated (35 percent) was higher than the other age group. In the matter of educational level, most of elderly had primary education (59 percent). The proportion of elderly having secondary school education and higher was the least (15 percent). Other elderly who did not receive education were (36 percent).

Further findings of the study revealed that working status of the elderly categorized according to gender, the ratio of female elderly (61 percent) who did not work was a lot higher than the male elderly (37 percent). In the matter of the elderly who were working, most of them work in the agricultural sector. The ratio of male elderly (52 percent) working in the agricultural sector was about two times higher than that of the female elderly (27 percent).

In the matter of working status categorized according to age group, the elderly in the younger age group worked more than the elderly in the older age group. The elderly in the older age group work less. The elderly aged between 60 and 69 were in the least group that does not work.

The working status of the elderly categorized according to household structure, more than half of the elderly living alone (53 percent) and extended family household (55 percent) do not work. The ratio of the elderly living in nuclear family household who does not work represented the lowest ratio of the elderly, which was 38 percent. As for the elderly who work, most of the elderly work in the agricultural sector. The percentages of the elderly living in nuclear family household, the elderly living in extended family household, and the elderly living alone were as follows: 48 percent, 35 percent, and 32 percent respectively.

The finding of the study indicated that household factors were related to the working and non-working status of the elderly. Therefore, the elderly should be encouraged to participate in the work that is suitable to their ability. (http://ipsr.healthrepository.org/bitstream/123456789/307/3/THCT2004_Yukolnee%20Kangs asitiam_eng.pdf)

Brown (2003) conducted a study on staying ahead of the curve in Washington DC. The study aimed to explore elderly vision of retirement and to better understand the types of jobs that workers want to do who plan to work in retirement.

The sample of the study consisted of 2,001 respondents between in the age group of 50 to 70 years. They who were employed either on full time or part time basis. The interviews were conducted with them on phone by the roper ASW from April to June 2003 using the random digit dialling method.

The findings of the study revealed that the most important considerations of job for working retired persons were "keeps you mentally fit" (74 percent) makes you feel useful (70 percent) is fun or enjoyable (86 percent) and lets you feel interact with other people (61 percent).These considerations also served as the most important reasons to elders to work after retirement. When asked to mention one factor defining their decision to work after retirement, the respondents said that, it was money needed. Among those who were actually working in their retirement has the same reasons and rated them as decisive, with a slight change of ranking .The reason of productive or useful was rated first it was followed by the reasons to stay mentally active, physically active and need of money.

This research study clearly identifies financial need as the primary reason that respondents chose to work even after retirement. The study also showed that the reason was non-financial too. The study also showed that the non-financial benefits of work would certainly influence their decision to remain in labour force. (http://assets.aarp.org/rgcenter/econ/multiwork_2003_1.pdf)

Dhillon and Ladusingh (2001) who focused their study on "Economic Activity in Post Retirement Life in India" .The study analyzes work participation in post retirement life of 60 plus old persons in by primary, secondary and territorial sectors . The study also examines trends in working-life-expectancies to evaluate association between longevity and post retirement economic activities in India. It is found that the average length of working life of the 60 plus in India is 9.8 years for males and 3.9 years for females. Though the life expectancy at the 60 plus age for males has enhanced by 2.9 years over a period of thirty years 1971 to 2001, ,the working life expectancy has increased only marginally by just 0.1 years during the same reference period. On the other hand for the females, against improvement of 4.2 years in longevity at the 60 plus age, there have been a gain of 2.4 years has been noticed in their working life. Work participation of working old persons has shifted from the primary sectors to the formal sectors. It indicated an increase in their productive activities. The economic tables obtained from the Census of the years 1971, 1981, 1991, and 2001 were analyzed to compute a rate of the trend in age-specific work participation by sex and by sectors of employment.

In addition to it the sample registration systems based on the abridged life-tables for the years 1970 to 1975, 1980 to 1985, 1989 to 1993 and 1999 to 2003 were obtained from the registrar general of India and used to construct the working life tables. The census data provide information on the rates of work participation by age group. Based on it age specific work participation by sex were computed for the primary, secondary and territory sectors each separately. The primary sector in

India includes cultivators, agricultural labourers, livestock, forestry, fishing, hunting and plantations, orchards and allied activities, mining and quarrying. The secondary sector included manufacturing, processing, servicing and repairs at consumer Industry and other than consumer Industry, and constructions. The territory sector included trade and commerce, transport storage and communications and others services.

Based on this study, the findings suggested that in terms of the relationship between life and working life expectancies. The longevity does not promote post retirement work participation of the males. However, for females it is the other way round, because as their participation in economic activities increased in terms of working life expectancy over specified time. However, the overall, improvement in the longevity does not necessarily extend the working life of the person in the 60 plus age in India. When the ratio of WLE was compared to LE it was found that for males 73.9 per cent of their remaining life in 1971 was spent working. This percentage declined to 60.1 percent by the 2001. What contributed to this decrease on major part was a decline in older men's work participation in the primary sector. The work participation of elderly male persons shifted from the primary sector to the formal sector. It was a sign of higher productivity on their part in the post retirement period than it was earlier. Still, elderly male persons work participation was predominant in the primary sector as there were not many jobs in the formal sector or they lacked of skills required for those jobs. When it comes to work participation of women over 60 years they spent, 10.5 percent of the remaining life gainfully through work participation in 1971.In 2001, it increased to 21.1 percent. Although the female working life expectancy marked an increased in all sectors, it was still far behind of the males working life expectancy. A possible reason would be under reporting of work participation of most women as they were involved in unpaid household work

2.3 Studies related Factors Influencing Silver Workers to Work beyond Retirement Age

Agewell Research and Advocacy Centre (2008) conducted a research study on "Assessment of the Impact of Economic Slowdown on Older persons of India". The broad objective of the study was to assess an impact of economic slowdown on older persons in the recent time.

The sample of the study included 500 respondents who were of the age of 55+years. They were selected from five regions' of India North, South, East, West and Central India. Direct and in depth interviews were conducted with these respondents by administering semi structured schedules.

The results of the study revealed that majority of the elderly believed that the economy was in fact suffering set back and many of them were finding it very hard to address their needs. Even their daily life too was affected severely due to decrease in their day to day income. Further it was revealed that good number of elderly persons started making radical changes in their financial condition such as getting gainful occupational engagement and by reducing their expenses on recreational facilities and luxuries.

It was noticed that almost half of government as well as private employees in the age group of 55 to 60 postponed their plans to opt for voluntary retirement scheme (vrs) .However the respondents of age between 65 and 70 were less likely to be affected than those of the ages 55 to 60. The respondents said that they had taken adequate steps to cope with a slowing economy or increasing prices.

The results indicated that economic problems forced some decisions on the elderly. It appeared that older persons had fewer decisions left to make, because their expenditure and economic activities had already been restricted to necessities given their fixed incomes.

Cameron and Waldegrave (2008) conducted a study on work, retirement and well being among the older New Zealanders. Main objective was to study the lifetime work experiences of New Zealanders of the age of 65 to 84 years, and also to present analyses of their associations with —satisfaction of work and with overall wellbeing.

The data used as indicators for work in the EWAS Survey were derived from questions related to three phases of the working life of the respondents: (i) first main jobs; (ii) principal jobs during their midlife; and (iii) their most recent principal job. The data were also collected about their significant absences from the workforce (of more than six months duration), their retirement, and their recent work engagement.

The findings of the study revealed that work and wellbeing of New Zealanders ageing from 65 to 84 has confirmed many with lifetime experiences of older people in case of, both in and out of the workforce. It was surveyed about older New Zealanders that the first principal job for nearly all was full-time paid work. It began at a median age of 16.2 years. Women in Newzealand were significantly more likely to be homemakers or they were engaged in part-time paid work during midlife, they were less likely to be engaged in full-time paid work.

In terms of their most recent job, significantly many of the respondents reported that men were in full-time paid work, with similar proportions of each gender in part-time paid work. The range of occupations from respondents 'first job through to their midlife occupation and on to their current or most recent occupation showed considerable stability. Younger age cohorts and women were more likely to have experienced two or more extended periods outside the workforce. The most cited reasons for these periods outside the workforce were family responsibilities (mostly by women), poor health, and injury or disablement.

The median retirement age was significantly higher for those in older age cohorts, and significantly lower for women than for men. But in contrast with international literature, there were no significant differences in retirement age by education. However, education was significantly associated with work after retirement. It suggested that while education would not affect the age of retirement, it does affect the continued participation of older people in worker related activities after retirement. Women were found to be significantly more likely to be involved in voluntary work. Bit would be both as their last principal job and their job after retirement.

A matter of self-reported satisfaction of old people with work was found to have no relation with lifetime work experiences and absences from the workforce measured in this survey. However, self-reported satisfaction with work was found to be significantly associated with overall wellbeing. This suggests that a way to encourage further wellbeing for them would be to generate satisfaction with work amongst those who have already retired. Finally, two important associations with overall wellbeing were identified. Firstly a period beyond of more than one year spent outside the workforce was negatively associated with overall wellbeing and it was the case only for men.

Spending time outside the workforce was not related with satisfaction with work. But it may have an effect through lower economic standard of living in later life. It or may be related even to poor health .Therefore, it has an effect through health dimension of overall wellbeing. The dynamics of this effect should be investigated further as to particular why it is significant only for men.

Secondly, retirement by choice was associated with higher level of overall wellbeing. It confirms some findings in the international literature that indicate that higher levels of well-being are noticed among those who prefer to be in their current work role. Again, retirement by choice was not significantly associated with satisfaction with work, so further investigation is required to determine mechanism by which work roles and the control over them would affect overall wellbeing.
(https://www.waikato.ac.nz/wfass/populationstudiescentre/docs/ewas/ewas-chp6.pdf)

Uppal and Sarma (2007) conducted a study on "Aging Health and Labour Market Activities the case of India". The study explores intricate relationship between the health status of the elderly and their labour market participation in rural and urban parts of India. The sample for the study was drawn from a nationally representative survey." The 1995/96 National Sample Survey" using probit regression and propensity score matching techniques.

The major findings of the study indicated that decision to participate in labour market on the parts of the age 60 and above in India in particular, are affected with disabilities and chronic illnesses on the probability of working. Results further showed that disabilities and chronic illnesses exerted negative effects on probability of their working. The effect is more visible in rural areas. The data revealed that approximately 21 percent of the elderly in urban and rural areas and 39 percent in rural areas were working. It was most likely because they did not have sufficient means to survive. The result obtained from the models showed that adverse health shocks disabilities and chronic illnesses had negative impact on the elder's employment. Since they did not have adequate means of support or a job to raise earning and bad health would lead them further to much lower levels of well-being .In the absence of a broad based pension system, only 10 percent of them covered for this situation might be mitigated by providing assistive technology or accommodation of those with disabilities by prospective employers. This is being likely to increase employment for such elderly persons.

Calvo (2006) conducted a study on does working longer make people healthier and happier. The main aim was to study the impact of late life paid work on physical and psychological well being of workers.

For the study the longitudinal data was drawn from the Health and Retirement Study (HRS) and the RAND-HRS data base. The sample analyzed was composed of individual aged between 59 and 69 years who were working either or not working and were alive in the year 2002.

The findings of the study showed that longer working life exerted had beneficial effects on individuals' physical and psychological well being .The findings revealed that if one had an undesirable job does not change the favorable effects of aid work on self rated health. However, it had an impact on follow up mood indicators and mortality .It could be said that higher job satisfaction was associated with improved mood.

The study suggests that on the whole longer working life will help most people to keep up maintain their well-being. While working longer appears beneficial to most people, for some it will likely to have negative consequences. The type of a job seems to be a critical factor. It may be feared that with undesirable jobs potential favorable effects of work cab be washed out. Another critical factor would be an opportunity to continue working which too would minimize negative consequences.

Friedli (2003) conducted study on Transition to Retirement and Ageing Change and Persistence of Personal Identities in Thun Switzerland. The main aim of the study was to assess (1) The content of identity: The question if and how retired working people had a different ways to define or characterize themselves than other employed people. (2) The age identity (subjective age): The question of how old people feel, and what predictors and implications can be found for younger or older age identity. The sample of the study comprised of 792 respondents of the age 58 to70. A standardize questionnaire was developed keeping in view to collect the data that would be required for the study.

The major findings of the study revealed that for the respondent's profession remained important consideration for self-description after retirement, and it could not be replaced with their new identity as being retired. Retired persons estimated more domains of self-description. It means that identity diversity was perceived higher for the retired than for those who were not yet retired. Further, the findings of the study revealed that higher identity, correlated with a high satisfaction across different life domains. This finding gives significant implications of psychological theories related to development of older people it strongly disproves strongly a view that a state of disengagement would be inherent to successful or even normal aging.

There is a tendency to feel younger than one's real age. It implies a motivational component and therefore, probably be seen as special case of self-enhancement. The finding provides a possible theoretical framework for further research. To explore relationships between various predictors and subjective age, a predictive structural model of subjective age was developed; it included aspects of personality, behaviour and body. (http://ethesis.unifr.ch/theses/downloads.php?file=TeuscherU.pdf)

Bansal and Sharma (2003) conducted a study on Retirement: An Emerging Challenge for the Planners. The aim of the study was to analyze and identify; various social and psychological factors that influence the level of happiness among retired people .For empirical analysis of measurement of well being a primary survey was done among elderly males in the Haryana state of India. The purpose was to collect relevant data with help of a questionnaire. The questionnaire was designed in such way so that maximum information on various characteristics of the respondents may be obtained. The information obtained social, psychological and physiological conditions of elderly males were useful and relevant for the present study. It indicated that retired/aged males who engaged themselves in some kind of social, economic, political or religious activities felt happier than those who did not do anything. The results of the analysis clearly indicated that work has its own reward. The results led further policy implication that more efforts should be made. It was observed that to engage the retirees/aged people in some activity or the other. "Individuals who kept themselves physically and mentally active were likely to feel more satisfied than others who led passive life. Therefore, it is useful to help old people develop a programme involving activities like social work and extending various types of help in the household. It was further argued that those who survived longer were individuals who had kept themselves physically and mentally active."

The finding of the study revealed that retired people could lead happier life provided they: (i) engaged themselves in various social, economic, religious activities: (ii) mentally prepared themselves for life after retirement well in advance and made necessary plans in that direction; (iii) who made efforts to reduce their needs and resultant expenditures' (iv) took proper care of their health, and (v) tried to remain less dependent on others.

2.4 Studies related to Employers Perspective towards Recruiting Silver Workers

Mermin, Johnson and Toder (2008) conducted a study on "Will Employers Want Ageing Boomers?"The main aim of the study was to examine employer demand for elderly currently and explores how this demand would be changing over time. The study focuses on the issues like personal and social benefits of increased work put on by older adults and the reasons why boomers were likely to work longer than younger generations, and also whether employers prefer to have elderly.

The finding of the study revealed that 30 occupations in which most persons over 65 years and above were employed age 65 were employed for nearly half (48 percent) of all employed older adults. The three occupations that employed the largest numbers of older adults were retail salespersons, farmers and ranchers (agricultural management positions) and the immediate supervisors and managers of retail sales workers. The top 30 occupations included nursing and home health aides, registered nurses, physicians and surgeons, and personal and home care aides. These occupations altogether employed more than 4 percent of workers who aged 65 and above. Adults of an age 65 or older made up about 31 percent of funeral service workers, and thus the occupation claimed with the highest share of elderly. Further, more than one in five workers employed as crossing guards, farmers and ranchers, models, demonstrators, and product promoters were of an age of 65 or more. Other occupations in which older adults made up beyond 9 percent of the workforce were tax preparers, clergy, property managers, real estate brokers, and bus drivers.

About 36 percent of workers aged 65 or above were employed as managers or professionals, 17 percent of them worked in service occupations. Some 15 percent of old workers work in sales and 14 percent worked in office and administrative support occupations. Another 17 percent of old workers worked in blue collar occupations that included construction, factory, and transportation jobs.

Most employers' surveys indicated that firms generally value elderly' knowledge and experience and reliability, and work ethics. About 47 percent of the employers said it was very true that late-career employees possessed "high level of skills related to what is needed for their jobs," as compared with 38 percent of mid-career employees and 21 percent of early-career employees. Because late-career employees held at their back many years' of experience in their respective positions. It is however, not clear from these survey how employers viewed elderly possessing limited experience. (http://www.urban.org/uploadedPDF/411705_aging_boomers.pdf)

Swanberg, Sharon and Mckechine (2007) conducted a cross-generational study on generational differences in perception of elderly' capabilities .The objective of the study was to examine perception of elderly across four generations, and also to study the effects of these perceptions on elderly. The sample of the study comprised of respondents who were employees in 388 stores and in 37 districts of a national retail chain.

The findings of the study revealed that elderly belonging to both the traditionalist generation and the baby boom generation were very positive about them and their company. They believed that they were as more reliable than younger workers, and were more productive and loyal to their companies. Indeed they earned the highest scores for employee's engagement.

Further it was observed that the older generations were more positive in their responses regarding older employee's ability to work better with younger supervisors. Finally, in terms of perceptions that elderly were "just as likely be promoted as younger workers the responses given by two older generations did not differ significantly.

The findings in terms of psychological well being of employees the two older generations perceived equal opportunities for elderly. They were significantly higher kind well being than those who perceived unfair advantage for younger workers.

In general, elderly belonging to both the traditionalist's generation and the baby boom generation were very positive about them and also for the company they worked for. They perceived themselves as more reliable than younger workers. They also believed that they were more productive, and great loyal to their companies. Indeed they claimed the highest scores of employees' engagement. Such findings suggested that the lens of "generation" was proved useful for understanding that some level of conflicts might occur between workers of the older and the younger generation. These were but a few of the within-generation differences in matter of thinking about people's values, attitudes, and work styles at workplaces in present time.

Brown (2006) conducted a study on "Business Executives' Attitudes Towards the Ageing Workforce: Aware but not Prepared? The purpose of this study was to understand business executive's views towards 50 + workers and corporate America's preparedness for the ageing of workforce. Chief executive officers and other "c"-level executives, senior vice presidents, vice presidents, and general manager's respondents for the online survey the conducted between July 10 and July 23, 2006. The sample for study was derived from the Business Week Market

Advisory Board. It is an online panel of approximately 17,800 readers of the Business Week and McGraw-Hill publication and also online registrants. The registration for the survey was floated through email to randomly selected respondents of panel members. All respondents hailed from companies that have a staff of at least 100 employees worldwide. Among these companies more than half (56 percent) were bigger organizations with at least 1,000 employees. In order to ensure that the study would collect the opinions of those who influence workforce-related decisions, the survey access kept restricted focus to those who reported that they were holding responsibility of managing employees and that they could influence decisions related to recruitment as well as matters of compensation or other financial matters.

The results of the study focus to those revealed that more 83 percent of the respondents reported that workers who were reaching conventionally determined age of approaching retirement would play a greater role in the U.S. workforce over the next decade than they did in previous decades.

Nearly 74 percent of the respondents strongly or somewhat agreed positively that the U.S. economy might experience shortage of skilled workers over the next decade. Whereas some 79 percent of them agreed that knowledge and experience that older employees carried away when they retire from jobs or leave the organization on any grounds would cause damage.

Some companies would prefer to retain old workers in view of their knowledge and skills that they have cultivated with long experience of working for the company in this matter only 16 percent of them reported that their company adopted formal policies or programs to encourage employees who were approaching retirement to continue working.

There were only 14 percent of the respondents who believed that their companies were much committed to retaining experienced employees who were approaching the retirement age. They rated each of their characteristics as quite important for the company .Majority of executives evaluated qualities of old workers such "experience" (91 percent), "knowledge" (78 percent), ability to "mentor other workers" (71 percent), and "valuable insights into customer or business needs" (63 percent) and rated them as valuable for the company's progress and success.

Undoubtedly, each of these traits contributes specifically to customer service and retention. Therefore, these traits were identified priority by 40 percent of respondents as the top priority of their organizations.

There was also a group of executives (52 percent) who held a belief that old age workers formed group that felt bit "uncomfortable with the technology",49 percent of them indicated that elderly were bit "inflexible," and 44 percent of them felt that they had "difficulty at reporting to younger supervisors. These executives called their attitude as the disadvantage of employing workers 50 plus

The findings of the study further revealed that most business executives were generally aware that the U.S. workforce is aging and that many firms would face risk of talent shortages and significant loss of knowledge as increasing number of old workers reach conventional age of retirement. However a few of these corporate leaders reported that their organization had taken adequate steps to counteract such demographic shift in the workforce (http://assets.aarp.org/rgcenter/econ/aging_workforce.pdf)

Center for Aging and Community of the University of Indianapolis, U.S.A (2006) conducted a study on "Gray matters: Opportunities and Challenges for Indian's Ageing Workforce". The main aim of the study was to gain a better understanding of how Indiana employers were preparing for the anticipated shortage of skilled labour due to the impending retirement of the baby boomers. The study also investigated an extent to which organizations perceived the pending loss of these employees as important factor to affect their business operations. The sample of the study consisted of Indiana employers who were surveyed online .It made a group of more than 50 employees. The survey was conducted by the CAC for the period from March-May 2006. Over 400 employers responded to the survey,

The findings of the study revealed that 55 percent of the respondents indicated that their organizations would be very likely to adopt a strategy to rehire retired persons to cope the loss. Over 41 percent and 43 percent of the respondents indicated that their organizations would likely have retiring workers to mentor their replacements or to write operating procedures describing their jobs before they retire. Further about 20 percent of them considered steps such as hiring replacements and about 18 percent of them considered to train their replacements.

Only 21 percent of the respondents indicated that their organization would be very likely to use this strategy. Only 11 percent of the respondents indicated that they were very likely to rehire the retired workers as either a full-time or part-time employee .Some 10 percent of the employers approved two other retention strategies. An offer to rehire the retired workers under a contract was rated by 9 percent of the respondents and reducing responsibility as an adopted strategy was endorsed by 9 percent of the employees offering benefits like promotion, or offering financial incentives, or sabbatical leave were considered as very likely to be used by less than 5 percent of respondents of the survey.

Comparing perceptions of older respondents to younger ones as reflected from their questions of the survey when younger responsible were asked about their willingness to participate in training. Nearly 10 percent (9 percent) of them reported that elderly had very poor to poor willingness to participate in training. On the other hand, only (2 percent) of the older respondents felt that elderly had very little willingness to participate. Likewise about 66 percent of the older respondents, expressed about good willingness on elderly part and some 50 percent of the younger respondents on the other part felt that elderly had very good willingness to participate in training.

As today elderly usually delay formal retirement, employers get more and more opportunities to take advantage of their experience and maturity. However, the levels of sophistication and effort as HR practices vary considerably among employers. In general, larger firms appear to be more focused on finding solutions than smaller one do. A selected number of employers, often considered as "employers of choice," were found to be engaged in variety of initiatives to accommodate and embrace an aging workforce. (http://cac.uindy.edu/media/GrayMattersI.pdf)

2.5 Studies related to Perceptions of Silver Workers towards Working and Workplace after Retirement

Wyatt (2009) conducted a study on "Effect of the Economic Crisis on Employee Attitudes towards Retirement". The study aimed to focus on employees' retirement timing .Sample of the study consisted of 2,232 active employees and 904 retirees of non-government organizations with 1,000 or more employees to gauge the effect of the economic crisis on Americans.

Findings revealed that more than two-thirds of workers aged 50 and over (69 percent) believed that they will need to save significantly more for retirement as a result of the economic crisis. One-third of workers (34 percent) had increased their planned retirement age in the last 12 months. Elderly were most likely to increase the length of their working career, with 44 percent of workers aged 50 and over planning to work longer compared with 38 percent of those in their 40s and only 25 percent of workers under 40.

Fifty-four percent of workers aged 50 to 64 who planned to postpone retirement said they will work at least three years longer than expected. Three-quarters of workers aged 50 to 64 (76 percent) cited the decline in the value of their 401(k) plans as a key reason they would retire later.

The average planned retirement age for all employees was 65 years old. Elderly, however, plan to work longer. Half of those aged 50 and over expected to work past age 65. One-quarter of workers (26 percent) expected to retire before age 65 compared with 41 percent.

It was concluded that all Americans had been affected by the economic crisis, but sharp declines in stock prices will had more immediate impact on elderly. With reduced account balances, a shorter window to recover their losses and less confidence in their ability to afford a comfortable retirement, many were likely to work longer than planned.

Reynolds, Ridley and Horn (2005) conducted a study on "A Work-Filled Retirement: Workers' Changing Views on Employment and Leisure". The main aim was to study current perceptions of the treatment of elderly in the workplace.

A total of 1,232 adults were interviewed for this survey .Respondents who worked full or part time, or who were unemployed and looking for work were interview. The sample for this survey was stratified to ensure all regions, as defined by the U.S.

Interviews were conducted at Center for Survey Research and Analysis (CSRA's) interviewing facility in Storrs, Connecticut, using a Computer-assisted telephone interviewing system Professional survey interviewers who were trained in standard protocols for administering survey instruments conducted all CSRA surveys.

Findings of the study revealed that those born between 1946 and 1964, boomers were almost twice as likely as non-boomers to believe they will be working part time for extra money. A majority of workers look forward to a productive retirement focused on working out of interest or for enjoyment, supplementing their incomes, or starting new businesses that contribute to the economy. Others expected to remain active through volunteer activities. However, workers were not as certain as they were five years ago that they will be able to retire when they want. Personal savings were the most commonly cited source of primary retirement income after employers sponsored pension plans more than half think they were doing a good job of saving for retirement.

Findings of this study indicated that growing presence of older workers in the labour force is likely to force changes in employers' policies and workplace practices. Policymakers should look for solutions that facilitate a work-filled retirement for employees that choose it, meet the needs of employers for a steady supply of qualified workers, and address the need of all workers for retirement security. (http://www.retirementplanblog.com/WT16-Retirement.pdf)

2.6 Studies related to Problems faced by Silver Workers

Punia and Punia (2002) conducted a study on Socio-emotional and Psychological Problems of Retired Elderly in Haryana: A Comprehensive View. Main objective of the study was to find out the types and extent of problems faced by old people. The participants were retired old men and women (above 58 years) from Hisar,

Bhiwani and Sirsa districts of Haryana state, covering whole of Bagar pocket. A sample of 80 people from each district city participated in the study, finally 240 elderly constituted the sample. A personal interview schedule was administered to the sample of retired personnel to obtain socio-demographic information. Higher proportions of the respondents were of 58 to 67 yrs of age group and had education upto post graduation level. A majority of families possessed medium and low socioeconomic status. More than fifty percent of the selected respondent had large family size and had a monthly income range of Rs. 3000 to 6000. Personal interview schedule and a standardized old age adjustment problem inventory (Husain and Kaur, 1995) were used to gather information on family demography and different types of problems faced by old people. This inventory measures the following areas: (a) Health (b) Home (c) Social (d) Marital (e) Emotional (F) Financial. The respondents were asked to tick 'Yes' or 'No' for all 125 statements score, more the problems. The statistical analysis for measuring the type and extent of the problems of the elderly were frequency and percentage and for differences in the problems faced by old male and old female, the 'Z' value was calculated.

In conclusion, compared to retired males, retired females faced more problems in old age and this may be possible due to the fact that her medical needs are also given second priority. In the joint family system, she faces psychological pressure and hostile feelings from the daughter in-law as the control of family moves from her to the daughter-in-law. By nature the female is more submissive and after initial squirmishes adjust even though unwillingly in most cases. The male on the other hand, has been the main wage earner and has enjoyed the position of supreme dominance in the house and does not face these problems. Further it was found that after retirement there is feeling among the aged that every one's attitude toward them has changed. The old people felt lonely and perceived avoided in their life. Almost all had financial problems perceived a loss of status accompanied by a sense of alienation and hopelessness. There is a need for counselling of old as well as the second generation to make relations more cordial.

Conclusion

Studies conducted on elderly in India showed that majority of the researchers aimed at finding the current status of silver workers, problems that they face after retirement, effects on health post retirement. From the reviewed literature it was found that solely the reasons of silver workers working after retirement was not studied in Indian context. There is no data available on the reasons, perceptions, problems and satisfaction of silver workers to work after retirement. There was dearth of researches studies to find out which were the reasons that insisted them to work after retirement, also the influencing factors, what were the problems that they faced while working after retirement, what do employers think about the such elderly who work after retirement, do they recruit them.

Studies conducted in other countries than in India on elderly revealed that-

1. Majority of the studies were conducted to find out the status of retired elderly.
2. Current perceptions of elderly towards workplace
3. Impact of late life paid work on physical and psychological well being of elderly workers and types and extents of problems faced by elderly
4. Explore the elderly vision of retirement and to better understand the types of jobs they want to do in retirement.
5. Employers demands and views for elderly and explores how this demand would be changing over time.
6. Future of work and workplace transformation with an emphasis on the provision of flexible working arrangements
7. Sample of the studies were mainly elderly aged 60 years and older and employers were chief executives and senior vice presidents
8. Tools used for data collection were Questionnaire, Interview Schedule, Rating Scales, Online Survey, Telephonic Interviews
9. Almost every study reported that elderly do work after their retirement. Knowledge and
10. Age, Gender, Educational Level, Sector of Employment, Financial Security ,Spouse Employment Participation, Family Income , Health Status were the variables studies by the majority of the researchers experience that older

employees is carried away when they retire from jobs or leave the organization on any grounds would cause damage

However it was also observed that no studies were found which solely focuses on the reasons, problems, perceptions and factors that influence elderly to work after retirement. Therefore it can be concluded from the review of related literature that there is need to undertake research study which can throw light on reason of silver workers to work after retirement, problems that they face while working, factors that influence them to work, their perceptions about retirement and also about the view points of employers in terms of recruiting them

CHAPTER – 3
METHODOLOGY

Given the study is exploratory research to first investigating the target group, for analysis, both quantitative and qualitative methods have been applied. This study aims at quantifying the qualitative data gained from open ended questions. This is not a pure qualitative analysis. Therefore in a first approximation, all given answers were listed and frequencies were counted. Then categories were created, numbers assigned and percentages were obtained. On the one hand, there are quantitative analyses of subjective ratings using percentage scale or numerically anchored scales. On other hand, there are open ended questions which demand free non supported statements from the respondents. These statements were coded and quantified in a subsequent step. This study considers appropriate analyses for these different approaches and quantitative data were imported into SPSS and Excel as shown in chapter 4.

As the qualitative part of this study generated a large amount of textual material certain systematic methodological conducive to tits condensation were referred to interpretation of open ended questions. The following analysis explores the association between job search duration and types of factors such as reasons, problems, perceptions, satisfaction, their suggestions and factors that influence silver workers to work after retirement. It also included the employers who recruit retired silver workers for jobs/work.

Figure 4 gives an overview of the general procedure of this study. Research question was what are silver workers like? What do they do, how they think and what they have to say?

Figure 4: Overview of the Study

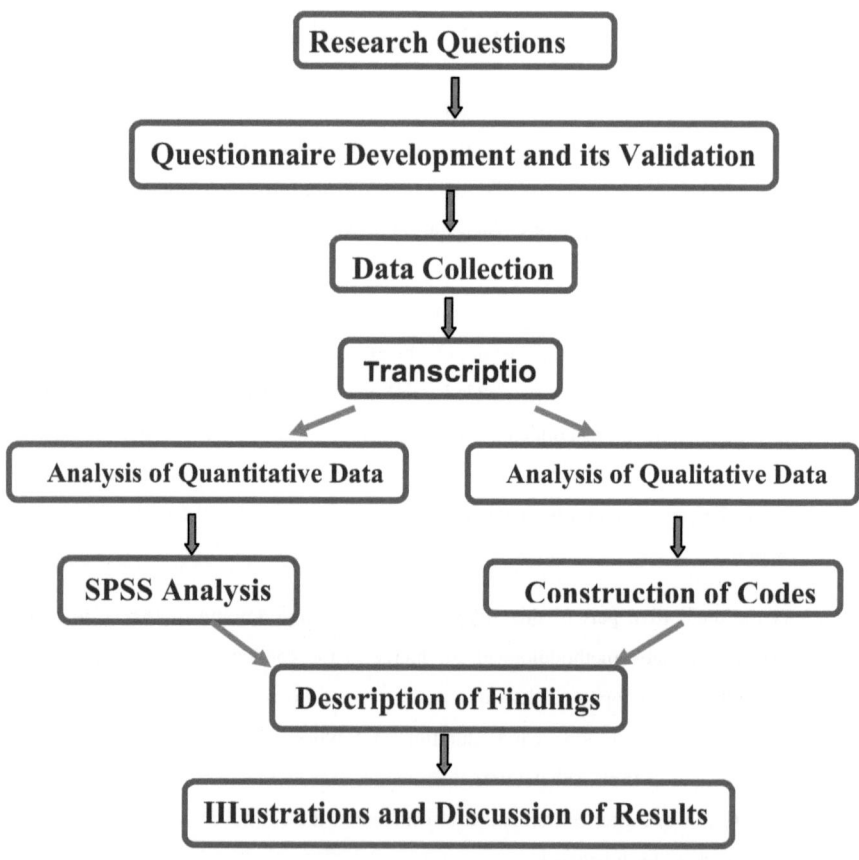

The present chapter describes the steps in methodology. This chapter is divided into the two sections:

(A) Methodology for Quantitative Data, and
(B) Methodology for Qualitative Data

(A) METHODOLOGY FOR QUANTITATIVE DATA

    3.1   Pilot Study

    3.2   Population of the Study

    3.3   Sampling Unit

3.4 Sampling Frame

3.5 Sample Size and Selection Procedure of the sample (Silver workers and Employers)

3.6 Construction of the Research Tools

3.7 Validity of the Research Tools

3.8 Reliability of the Research Tools

3.9 Pre-testing of the Research Tools

3.10 Procedure of Data Collection

3.11 Scoring and Categorization of the Data of Silver Workers

3.12 Scoring and Categorization of the Data of Employers

3.13 Plan of Statistical Analysis of the Data

(B) METHODOLOGY FOR QUALITATIVE DATA

3.14 Sampling Unit

3.15 Sample Frame

3.16 Sample Size

3.17 Process of Conducting Interviews

3.18 Analysis of the Interviewed Data

3.1 Pilot Study

The present pilot study was undertaken with objective of identifying the silver workers working after retirement and their reasons for working after retirement. The reason for conducting the pilot study was to study the feasibility of conducting a study on working silver workers.

The sample comprised of 30 silver workers (58 years of age and above) residing in Vadodara city. Purposive sampling method was used to select the sample. The questionnaire was constructed to collect the data from the silver workers to find out their reasons and problems, factors that influence them to work after retirement. Their work satisfaction, suggestions of working after retirement

3.1.1 FINDINGS OF THE PILOT STUDY

The information was collected in terms of educational qualification, gender, and age, family income, type of job, reasons for working after retirement, problems and benefits of working after retirement, expected maximum age of silver workers to work after retirement.

- Major findings of the pilot study revealed that high majority of silver workers were male and only 2 percent were female .Regarding the level of education, silver workers with graduation degree were 52 percent whereas 44 percent had masters degree, technicians or similar and those with graduation were 4 percent.

- Further the findings of the study revealed that 64 percent silver workers were in 60-65 years old age group, 32 percent were in 66-70 years old group and 71-75 years old group were 4 percent.

- Majority of the silver workers (60%) lived with their families whereas 35 percent were living with their spouses and 5 percent lived alone.

- Majority (70%) of silver workers reported that they were working part time, and 30 percent were working full time.

- Majority (65%) of silver workers were self employed. While 25 percent of them reported that they were working in private sector, businesses and 10 percent in other organizations.

- High majority (80%) of the silver workers had monthly family income between Rs.20,000 to Rs.50,000 whereas 20 percent had between Rs.50,000 and 70,000 per annum.

- To the question of what were the reasons of your working after retirement" majority (60%) of the silver workers reported that for staying active and engaged after retirement, whereas 30 percent revealed that they had not earned enough money during their earlier life, and now had to earn to pay their life expenses. Very few (10%) of them declared that their pensions was their income which was not enough to pay the life expense and hence now they worked.

- The distance from their residence to work place for a majority (65%) was between 5 and 10 kilometres, whereas 5 percent of them reported the distance as between 10 to 15 kilometres.

- When asked about the problems they faced while working after retirement a majority (60%) reported being mistreated because of age by younger colleagues, whereas 35 percent believed that they were paid less salary/income and very few (5%) felt neglected when their salary was determined or promotions were decided.

- Silver workers reported financial security, remaining active and updated, financial independence, social interactions and remaining healthy were the benefits of working after retirement.

- Majority (70%) of the silver workers reported that they will continue to work till the age 75 years, whereas 20 percent of silver workers reported that they work till they are physically capable enough to work, while a few (10%) reported that they were willing to work till 80 years of age.

3.1.2 CONCLUSION OF THE PILOT STUDY

It can be concluded that the motivations for work do not change for everyone in the same way. For some, the drive for economic gain never goes away, but for many others economic motives fall behind the need to accomplish something meaningful in their early sixties. One of the best ways to accommodate these changes is to look for more creative ways to structured work. Many factors today seem to be encouraging elderly workers to stay in the workforce, but, in practice, individuals still face major barriers to working longer than previous generations. It is not to develop effective theories about the employment of elderly until the dynamics that are currently driving elderly workers into retirement sooner than they had planned are truly understood.

The study was concluded with a remark that different needs of the silver workers should be studied to improve their living status by providing them with facilities. This subject can be implemented under social policy framework by compiling comprehensive plans for silver workers welfare through providing proper services that are adapted to their needs.

Based on these findings, policies can be formulated for the silver workers, in which will emphasize the importance of policies to implement a comprehensive social security scheme to cope with an expected aging population, as well as to create jobs for working-age people in the still relatively young country.

Hence, it is imperative to study about elderly working after their retirement such a study will help us understand their importance at workplace. The vast experience of theirs fetches respect for them or are they exploited by the employers. The seniors have the right to work, and the civil society and dignity in return. By undertaking such a research, the government and civil society will be able to provide a better work environment to a large work force of elderly.

Therefore, it can be concluded from the results of the pilot study that a research on **"A Study on Silver Workers Residing in Vadodara City"** can be undertaken

3.2 Population of the Study

The population of the present study comprised of silver workers those who are officially retired (58 and above) working for productive purpose/still working and earning after their retirement. The other group of sample consisted of employers from Vadodara city who have recruited those silver workers in their offices/institution/firms and business houses residing in Vadodara city of Gujarat State.

3.3 Sampling Unit

Sampling unit refers to the geographical area from where the samples are drawn. In the present study, samples of silver workers who were working after their retirement and the employers who recruit these retired silver workers were drawn from the Vadodara city of Gujarat state.

3.4 Sampling Frame

The elderly working post retirement, who is termed as silver workers in the present study and that comprised the sampling frame for the present study. The selected samples were working in the various organizations companies, private banks, firms, and corporate of Vadodara city of Gujarat State.

At the same time, the sampling frame also included the employers who recruit these retired silver workers on jobs post retirement in the different organizations of Vadodara city of Gujarat State. With regards to the acquisition of sample, large organizations were systematically contacted who supposedly maintained contact with their retirees. Some silver workers were identified with the help of these organizations. However most silver workers were acquired using personal contacts known to the researcher or from interviewees in a snow ball process. While the employers were identified with the help of silver workers or through the personal contacts of the researcher.

3.5 Sample Size and Selection Procedure of the Sample (Silver Workers and Employers)

The sample of the present study comprised of two types of respondents one were the silver workers and other were the employers who employed silver workers. (See Figure)

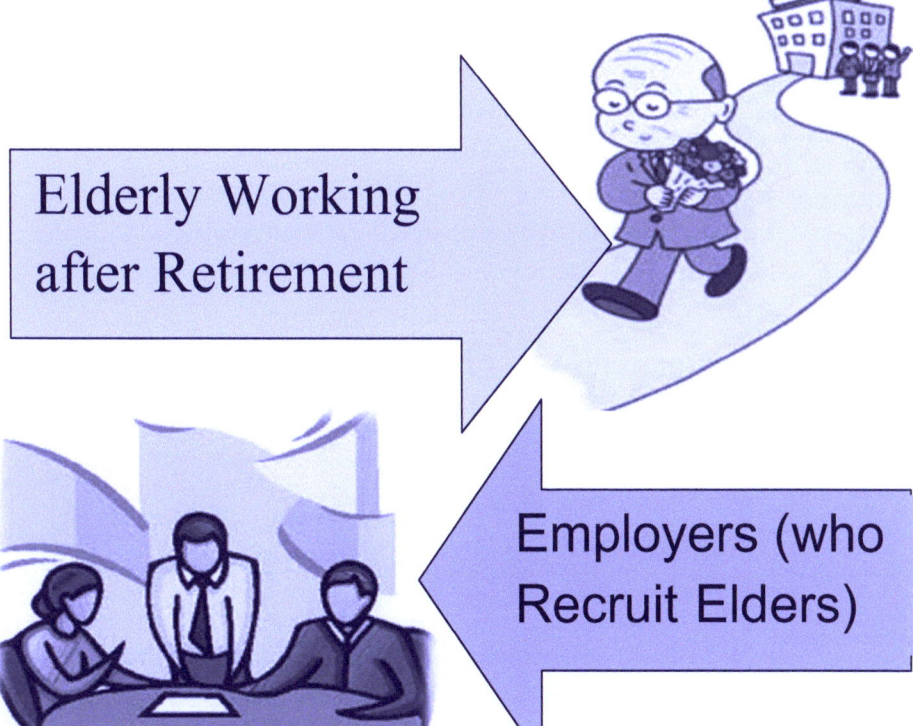

In total there were three hundred and fifty respondents from which three hundred were silver workers who were working post retirement and fifty were the employers who recruit those retired silver workers in their organizations, corporate, banks, companies, firms and colleges from Vadodara city of Gujarat State.

In order to indentify an employer which is the second sample of the study, the researcher approached the same organization where the silver workers were found working during their retirement. The size of the organisation (i.e number of employees) was one important factor in shaping the experience, ethos and practice of employers.

A purposive sampling method was used to draw the sample. Researcher identified banks/corporate/organizations/companies/firms functioning actively and recruiting silver workers and the organization recruiting those silver workers after retirement in Vadodara city. Researcher visited those banks/corporate/organizations/companies/firms and asked about silver workers who were recruited there after retirement. Almost fifty silver workers were identified initially those who were working after their retirement.

Those silver workers provided the names and addresses of the other silver workers whom they knew. The names and addresses of silver workers were also collected from colleagues, friends, relatives, neighbours, who knew silver workers those who were working after retirement. Same organizations were approached by the researcher in order to identify the employers .The snowball sampling technique was used to identify the sample.

3.5.1 SAMPLE SIZE FOR QUALITATIVE DATA

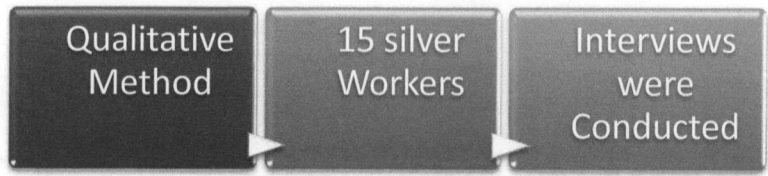

It was decided to use in-depth interviewing as the main method to collect data for the study since an interpretative approach (qualitative in nature) was adopted for the investigation. The central concern of the interpretative research understands human experiences at a holistic level. Because of the nature of this type of research, investigations are often connected with methods such as interviewing, participant observation and the collection of relevant documents. Maykut and Morehouse 1994 state that the data of qualitative inquiry is most often people's words and actions, and thus requires methods that allow the researcher to capture language and behaviour. The most useful ways of gathering these forms of data are participant observation, in interviews and the collection of relevant documents. Observation and interview data is collected by the researcher in the form of field notes which are later transcribed for use in data analysis. Same procedure and method was adopted to gather the sample for qualitative data. The sample for qualitative analysis total fifteen interviews were individually conducted with the silver workers.

3.6 Construction of Research Tools

The present study was an exploratory research. Therefore, survey method was preferred for studying the reasons of silver workers and for the employers who recruit them. The questionnaire, perception scale and rating scales were the tools used for data collection. In addition to obtain a picture of ideal working situation during retirement open ended question were incorporated. The main aim to incorporate open ended questions was to attract unfiltered impressions of the silver workers descriptions of their circumstances and experiences. The tools were constructed keeping in mind various purposes after reviewing related literature desired from books, journals and other literatures. As a first step, main topics for survey were defined such as former professional career, motivation for working during retirement, changing profession when entering retirement, and type of work in retirement. The pilot study helped the researcher to frame the questionnaire. The tools were prepared in English and then translated into Gujarati for better comprehension of the silver workers and to ensure ease in communication.

3.6.1 DESCRIPTION OF RESEARCH TOOL USED FOR SILVER WORKERS

A questionnaire consisting of six sections was prepared to study the reasons, perceptions, problems, their work related satisfaction and factors that influence silver workers, to work after retirement. The sections, content and response system used in the research tool of silver workers are detailed in the table below:

Table1: Description of Research Tools of the Silver Workers

(Refer Appendix-1)

Sections		Content	Response System
Section-1	Part-A	Background Information of the Silver Workers	Check list cum Questionnaire
	Part-B	Details About the Family	Check list cum Questionnaire
	Part –C	Present Occupational Status	Check list cum Questionnaire
	Part-D	Work History	Check list cum Questionnaire
	Part –E	Health Status	Checklist
Section-2	Part-A	Reasons of Working after Retirement	4-Point Rating Scale
	Part-B	Perceptions about Retirement	3-Point Rating Scale
Section -3		Influence of Work on Silver Workers	3-Point Rating Scale
Section -4		Problems Faced by Silver Workers at Workplace	4-Point Rating Scale
Section -5		Satisfaction at Workplace	3-Point Rating Scale
Section -6		Suggestions	Open Ended Questions and checklist

The research tools used for data collection of silver workers are as follows:

3.6.1.1. Section-1: Profile of the Silver Workers

In this research tools used for silver workers has been spilt in five parts namely, Part –A, Part-B, Part –C, Part-D and Part-E.

Part -A of Section-1 Background Information: It consisted of questions related to the background information of the silver workers such as:

- Age
- Sex
- Educational qualification
- Marital status
- Type of house
- Leisure time activities

Part -B of Section-1 Details about Family: This section comprised items related to the details related to the families of silver workers like:

- Type of family
- Number of family members

Details about family members like:
- Silver workers relationship with them
- Their occupational status
- Income
- Marital status
- Physical or mental disabilities
- Sources of families income

Part -C of Section-1 Present Occupational Status: This section included questions related to the:

- Organizations/firm/company/corporate/bank/college/institute in which silver workers were presently working,
- Their employment status
- Designation
- Type of work

- Income/salary
- Type of duties
- Working hours
- Distance of workplace
- Problems they faced while searching present job
- Reasons of doing present job/work etcetera

Part -D of Section-1 Work History: This section consisted the question related to first job of the silver workers that is the job they were doing before retirement such as:

- Designation
- Type of organization they were working in before retirement
- Employment status
- Designation
- Income
- Type of work

Part -E of Section-1 Health Status: To find out the health status of silver workers, a checklist consisting nine items was prepared including the possible health problems which could occur in the old age. Silver workers had to tick mark against the health problems they were facing. The tool developed by Kikani (1993), Department of Foods and Nutrition, The M.S University, Vadodara was adopted by the researcher. The nutritionist and experts from Geriatrics were also consulted for preparation of the proforma.

3.6.1.2. Section-2 Reasons of Working after Retirement and Perception about Retirement

Part -A of Section-2 Reasons of Working after Retirement: This section included the items which can be possible reason for silver workers to work after retirement:

- Financial reasons
- Familial reasons
- Work related reasons

- Personal reasons

The statements were prepared after reading and reviewing of books and previous researches conducted in the same area and also research articles, on the subject etcetera. Some of the statements are modified from another similar study for preparing this tool for present study. It is four point rating scale .Silver workers were required to mark against the statements, wherein they had to indicate the extent of reasons for working after retirement as perceived by them. The content and number of statements under each aspect are as follows:

Table 2: Content and Number of Statements under each Aspect.

Aspects	No. of Statements
Financial	10
Familial	11
Work	7
Personal	8
Total	**36**

Part -B of Section-2 Perceptions about Retirement: This section consisted of 46 statements representing positive and negative perceptions about retirement namely:

- Decreasing physical and mental strength
- Retirement and reduced income
- Retirement and society
- Worries of being retired
- Adapting social role in flexible way
- Fear of growing age and isolation

The statements were prepared after reading and reviewing of books and previous researches conducted in the same area and also research articles, on the subject etcetera. Some of the statements are modified from other similar studies. It is three point rating scale .Silver workers were required to mark against the statements, wherein they had to indicate the extent of perceptions about retirement as perceived by them.

Table 3: Content and Number of Statements under each Aspect.

Aspects	No. of Statements
Favourable	17
Unfavourable	29
Total	**46**

3.6.1.3. Section -3 Influence of Work on Silver Workers

This section included the items on influence of work on silver workers .The main aim to design this section was to know the influence positive or negative influence of "Work" on silver workers due to their working life after retirement. Twenty four statements were prepared after reading and reviewing of books and previous researches conducted in the same or related areas and also research articles on the subject etcetera. It is a three- point rating scale. The content covered under this section included statement related to the influence of work on silver worker's like:

- Physical and mental well being
- Family
- Income
- Leisure time
- Silver workers job related goals
- Silver workers equation with family and society

The silver workers were asked to tick mark against the statements which indicated the influence of work on them.

3.6.1.4. Section -4 Problems Faced by Silver Workers at Workplace

A list of possible problems which could be faced by silver workers while working after retirement and problems they face due to workplace were listed in the tool. The problems were related to physical, social, financial or familial problems, problems related to:

- Work given to them
- Designation

- Equation with authorities
- Working with younger generation
- Working/Adapting new technologies
- Reduced income
- Infrastructure of workplace
- Distance of workplace
- Working hours

Above mentioned could be the problems that can be faced by silver workers due to work or because of workplace. A four point rating scale was designed to study the extent of problems faced by silver workers. It included twenty five statements. The silver workers were asked to tick mark against the statements which indicated certain problems which might affect their working life

3.6.1.5. Section -5 Satisfaction at Workplace

This section consisted of 12 statements related to satisfaction of silver workers related to:

- Opportunity to work
- Welfare facilities in the organization they work
- Advancement of their work skills
- Work value system
- Nature of their work and salary/income
- Readdressal of grievances

A three point rating scale was designed to study the extent of satisfaction by silver workers related to their work and workplace. The silver workers were asked to tick mark against the statements which indicated their extent of satisfaction.

3.6.1.6. Section -6 Suggestions

This section included checklist and open ended questionnaire to seek suggestion of silver workers about:

- Specific personnel policies that can be framed for silver workers
- Their suggestion about preparation for retirement

- Services which they think important for silver workers
- Services that employers can provide to silver workers that can make their working in later life attractive

3.6.2 DESCRIPTION OF RESEARCH TOOLS USED FOR EMPLOYERS

A questionnaire consisting two sections was prepared to study reasons, advantages and disadvantages, qualities, factors that influence the employers towards recruiting silver workers. The sections, contents and response system used in the research tools of employers are detailed below:

Table 4: Description of Research Tools of the Employers

(Refer Appendix-2)

Sections	Content	Response System
Section -1	Background Information of the Organization/companies/institution/firms/corporate/business house	Check list cum questionnaire
Section-2	Information related to silver workers working in their Organization/companies/institution/firms/corporate/business house	3 point rating scale and intensity Indices

3.6.2.1 Research tool used for data collection of Employers

Section 1 consisted of questions related to the background information of the Employers to include:

- Age
- Sex
- Designation
- Experience
- Organization's details like type of organization
- Objectives/mission
- Financial resources of the organization
- Number of silver workers working in their organization

Section 2 Consisted of questions related to the employees such as:

- Qualities of silver workers
- Advantages of recruiting silver workers
- Disadvantages of recruiting silver workers
- Factors that influence employees to work after their retirement
- Formal policies to retain retired employees into work sector

3.7 Validity of the Research Tools

To check the validity of the research tools, the questionnaires were sent for review by experts from the following institutions:

- Dean, Faculty of Family and Community Sciences, The Maharaja Sayajirao University of Baroda, Vadodara
- Head, Faculty of Family and Community Sciences, The Maharaja Sayajirao University of Baroda, Vadodara
- Associate Professor, Department of Extension and Communication, Faculty of Faculty of Family and Community Sciences, The Maharaja Sayajirao University of Baroda, Vadodara
- Associate Professor, Department of Psychology, Faculty of Education and Psychology, The Maharaja Sayajirao University of Baroda, Vadodara
- Associate Professor, Department of English, Faculty of Arts, The Maharaja Sayajirao University of Baroda, Vadodara
- Associate Professor, Department of Statistics, Faculty of Science, The Maharaja Sayajirao University of Baroda, Vadodara
- Associate Professor, Faculty of Social Work, The Maharaja Sayajirao University of Baroda, Vadodara

The experts were requested to check the questionnaire for:
- Content validity
- Nature of the statements
- Clarity of language and ideas
- Appropriateness of the response system

The suggestions given by experts were incorporated in the tool

3.8 Reliability of the Research Tools

The test- retest method was used for measuring the reliability of the questionnaire. The tool was administered on five silver workers and five employers in Vadodara city. To measure the reliability of the tool, it was administered again on the same persons after a gap of fifteens days. The coefficient of correlation between the two sets of scores was calculated to find out the reliability of the tool by using the following formula:

$$r = \frac{\sum xy}{\sqrt{\sum x^2 \sum y^2}}$$

Where, r = Coefficient of correlation
X = Score of First test
Y = Score of Second test
The tool reliability was found 0.92

3.9 Pre-testing of the Research Tools

The prepared questionnaires were pre-tested on ten silver workers and ten employers in the Vadodara city. The researcher simplified some terms that respondents could not follow. Silver workers and employers selected for pre-testing of the tool took about thirty to thirty five minutes to fill the questionnaire.

3.10 Procedure of Data Collection

The data were collected from 300 silver workers and 50 employers who recruit those retired silver workers in their organizations, firms, corporate, business houses, from different areas of Vadodara city during December 2012 to May 2013. With regards to acquisition of respondents, large organisations were systematically contacted who supposedly maintained contacts with their retirees. Some respondents were acquired using personal contacts known to the researcher or from respondents in a snow ball process. Thus making the study's sample a cumulative sample. A large number of silver workers were identified through companies/organizations/corporate/institutes/firms/colleges who were recruiting retired silver workers. A permission to collect data from silver workers as well as employers was sought from the various authorities of the concerned organizations. The silver workers and employers were contacted and the data was collected by meeting them according to their convenience of time and place. The questionnaires were distributed to silver workers. They were collected back after a week or fifteen days.

Many a times, silver workers took more than 30 to 35 minutes to fill the questionnaire as it required them to do some thinking on the items and relating it to their working practise and experiences. Interview method was used to collect data from those silver workers, who faced difficulty in reading or were not used to filling questionnaire. Six to seven hundred questionnaires were distributed amongst the silver workers as well as employers out of which 378 in total were returned.

- Various reasons were found for not returning the questionnaire such as:
- Losing the questionnaire
- Unwilling or uninterested in the study/in filling questionnaire
- Not filling the questionnaire after many reminders
- Few silver workers found the questionnaire too lengthy and some question about which they were hesitant to answer

Interview schedule was prepared as tool for the employers and interview method was used to collect the data. Tools were prepared in English language. Employers took around fifteen to twenty minutes to answer the questions.

No major difficulties were faced during the data collection and it was completed peacefully. Majority of the silver workers and employers were interested in the study as it was related to them.

3.11 Scoring and Categorization of the Data of Silver Workers

Different types of scoring procedures were used for giving weightage to various items of all the parts of the tools used to collect information regarding the variables of the study. The scoring pattern and categorization of the silver workers and employer are discussed separately in the following lines:

3.11.1 CATEGORIZATION OF VARIABLES

The tool contains questions regarding profile of the silver workers. The categorization of the Independent and Dependent variables for a silver worker was done as follows

Table 5: Categorization of Independent Variables for Silver Workers

Variables	Basis	Categories
1. Age	58-66 years	Young-Old
	67-74 years	Old
2. Educational Qualification	Graduate to Doctorate	Higher Level of Education
	Higher Secondary to Diploma	Moderate Level of Education
	Primary to Secondary	Low Level of Education
3. Designation	Class I	
	Class II	Higher order Designation
	Class III	Middle order Designation
	Class IV	Low order Designation
4. Present Salary	Less than 17,000 Rupees	Low Income Group
	17,000 Rupees	Middle Income Group
	More than 17,000 Rupees	High Income Group
5. Health Status	0-1 Health Problems	Healthy
	2-4 Health Problems	Somewhat Healthy
	More than 4 Health Problems	Less Healthy
6. Type of Family	Living Alone	Living Alone
	Living with Partner	Living with Spouse
	Living with Children	Living with Family
7. Type of Work	8 hours	Full Time
	Less than 8 hours	Part Time
8. Perceptions about Retirement	Above Mean	Most Favourable
	Mean and Below Mean	Favourable and Less favourable

Table 6: Categorization of Dependent Variables for Silver Workers

Variables	Basis	Categories
1. **Reasons of Working**	Above Mean	More Number of Reasons
	Mean	Moderate Number of Reasons
	Below Mean	Less Number of Reasons
2. **Influence of Work**	Above Mean	High Level of Influence
	Mean	Moderate Level of Influence
	Below Mean	Low Level of Influence
3. **Problems at Workplace**	Above Mean	More number of problems
	Mean	Moderate number of Problems
	Below Mean	Less number of Problems
4. **Satisfaction at Workplace**	Above Mean	High satisfaction
	Mean	Moderate Satisfaction
	Below Mean	Less Satisfaction

3.11.2 REASONS TO WORK AFTER RETIREMENT

To measure the reasons of silver workers to work after retirement, the scores were given to the silver workers as shown in the (Appendix 1, Section 2-A). The minimum and maximum possible ranged from 1 to 36. However, the scores achieved by the respondents ranged from 1 to 36 and they were categorized as follows:

Aspect Wise total Obtainable Scores:

Aspects	Number of Statements	Maximum Obtainable Scores	Minimum Obtainable Scores
Financial	10	30	10
Familial	11	33	11
Work	7	21	7
Personal	8	24	8
Total	36	108	36

The range of intensity indices were calculated overall and aspect wise to measure the extent of reasons of the silver workers to work after retirement. To describe the extents of reasons, the range of intensity indices were decided as follows:

The range of intensity indices were decided as follows:

Extent of Reasons	Scores	Range of Intensity Indices
Great Extent	3	2.51-3.00
Some Extent	2	1.51-2.50
Less Extent	1	1.00-1.50

Range of the scores for describing the reasons of silver workers to work after retirement was decided as follows:

Type of Reasons	Score
Less Number of Reasons	36-60
Moderate Number of Reasons	61-85
More Number of Reasons	86-108

Range of mean scores for describing the reasons of silver workers to work after retirement were decided as follows:

Range of Mean Scores	Categories
Less Number of Reasons	Below Mean
Moderate Number of Reasons	Mean
More Number of Reasons	Above Mean

3.11.3 PERCEPTIONS ABOUT RETIREMENT

The perception scale was developed to measure the intensity of the perceptions of silver workers about retirement. It was a 3 point scale. The scoring of the responses on a scale was done as follows:

Scoring pattern according to the nature of statements in the perception scale regarding silver worker's perception about retirement

Nature of Statement	Agree to Great Extent	Agree to Some Extent	Agree to Less Extent
Positive	3	2	1
Negative	1	2	3

The total numbers of statements were 46. The minimum and maximum obtainable scores ranged from 46-138. Range of scores describing the perceptions of silver workers regarding retirement was decided as follows:

Type of Perceptions	Score
Less Favourable	46-76
Favourable	77-107
Most Favourable	108-138

Aspect Wise Obtainable Scores were as follows

Perceptions about Retirement	Number of Statements	Maximum Obtainable Scores	Minimum Obtainable Scores
Favourable	17	51	17
Less favourable	29	87	29

The range of intensity indices were calculated overall and aspect wise to measure the extent of perceptions about retirement of the silver workers. To describe the extents of perceptions, the range of intensity indices were decided as follows:

Range of Intensity Indices:

Extent of Perceptions	Scores	Range of Intensity Indices
Great Extent	3	2.51-3.50
Some Extent	2	1.51-2.50
Less Extent	1	1.00-1.50

Categories for describing the perceptions of silver workers regarding retirement was decided as follows:

Range of Mean Scores	Categories
Favourable and Less Favourable	Mean and Below Mean
Most Favourable	Above Mean

3.11.4 INFLUENCE OF WORK ON SILVER WORKERS

To measure the influence of work on silver workers, a three point scale was developed. The overall intensity indices were calculated to measure the extent of influence of work on silver workers. The total number of statements in the scale was 24 and the possible obtainable score ranged from 24-72.

Obtainable Scores were as follows

Content	Number of Statements	Maximum Obtainable Scores	Minimum Obtainable Scores
Influence of work	24	72	24

To describe the extent of work, the obtainable scores and range of intensity indices were decided as follows:

Range of Intensity Indices:

Extent of Influence	Scores	Range of Intensity Indices
Great Extent	3	2.51-3.00
Some Extent	2	1.51-2.50
Less Extent	1	1.00-1.50

Range of the scores for describing the intensity of influence of work was decided as follows:

Extent of Influence	Score
Low Level of Influence	24-40
Moderate Level of Influence	41-57
High Level of Influence	58-72

To find out overall and item wise influence of work intensity indices were calculated. Range of mean scores for describing the intensity of influence of work was decided as follows:

Categories	Basis
Low Level of Influence	Below Mean
Moderate Level of Influence	Mean
High Level of Influence	Above Mean

3.11.5 PROBLEMS FACED BY SILVER WORKERS AT WORKPLACE

To measure the extent of problems faced by silver workers at workplace a four point rating scale was prepared which included twenty five statements. The maximum obtainable score was hundred and minimum obtainable score was twenty five. The scoring of the statements in the scale was done as follows:

Obtainable Scores were as follows:

Content	Number of Statements	Maximum Obtainable Scores	Minimum Obtainable Scores
Problems faced by silver workers at their workplace	25	75	25

The intensity indices were found out overall and item wise to measure the extent of problems faced by silver workers at workplace. The categorization of intensity indices was as follows:

The range of intensity indices were decided as follows:

Extent of Problems	Score	Range of Intensity Indices
Great Extent	3	2.51-3.00
Some Extent	2	1.51-2.50
Less Extent	1	1.00-1.50

Range of the scores for describing the intensity of problems at workplace was decided as follows:

Type of Problems	Score
Less Problems	25- 41
Moderate Problems	42-58
More Problems	59-75

Categories for describing the intensity of problems at workplace were decided as follows:

Categories	Basis
Less Problems	Below Mean
Moderate Problems	Mean
More Problems	Above Mean

3.11.6 SATISFACTION AT WORKPLACE

To measure the extent of satisfaction of silver workers at workplace a three point rating scale was prepared which included twelve statements. The maximum obtainable score was thirty six and minimum obtainable score was twelve. The scoring of the statements in the scale was done as follows:

Obtainable Scores were as follows:

Content	Number of Statements	Maximum Obtainable Scores	Minimum Obtainable Scores
Satisfaction of Work	12	36	12

The intensity indices were found out overall and item wise to measure the extent of satisfaction of silver workers at workplace. The range of intensity indices was as follows:

The range of intensity indices were decided as follows:

Extent of Influence	Scores	Range of Intensity Indices
Great Extent	3	2.51-3.00
Some Extent	2	1.51-2.50
Less Extent	1	1.00-1.50

Range of the scores for describing the intensity of satisfaction of silver workers at workplace was decided as follows:

Type of Satisfaction	Score
Less Satisfaction	12-20
Moderate Satisfaction	21-29
High Satisfaction	30-36

To find out overall and item wise satisfaction of silver workers at workplace intensity indices were calculated. Range of the mean scores for describing the intensity of satisfaction of silver workers at workplace was decided as follows:

Categories	Basis
Less Satisfaction	Below Mean
Moderate Satisfaction	Mean
High Satisfaction	Above Mean

3.12 Scoring and Categorization of Data of Employers

3.12.1 QUALITIES OF RECRUITING SILVER WORKERS

To measure qualities that employers considered while recruiting silver worker, a three point scale was developed. The overall intensity indices were calculated to measure the extent. To describe the qualities, the obtainable scores and range of intensity indices were decided as follows:

Obtainable Scores were as follows

Content	Number of Statements	Maximum Obtainable Scores	Minimum Obtainable Scores
Qualities of the Employees	22	66	22

The intensity indices were found out overall and item wise to measure the extent of qualities of an employee. The categorization of intensity indices was as follows:

Range of Intensity Indices:

Extent	Scores	Range of Intensity Indices
Great Extent	3	2.51-3.00
Some Extent	2	1.51-2.50
Less Extent	1	1.00-1.50

Range of scores for describing the qualities of the employees was decided as follows:

Extent	Scores
Great Extent	22-36
Some Extent	37-51
Less Extent	52-66

3.12.2 ADVANTAGES OF RECRUITING SILVER WORKERS

To measure advantages that employers takes into consideration while recruiting silver workers, a three point scale was developed. The overall intensity indices were calculated to measure the extent. To describe the advantages, the obtainable scores and range of intensity indices were decided as follows:

Obtainable Scores were as follows

Content	Number of Statements	Maximum Obtainable Scores	Minimum Obtainable Scores
Advantages	18	54	18

Range of Intensity Indices:

Extent	Scores	Range of Intensity Indices
Great Extent	3	2.51-3.00
Some Extent	2	1.51-2.50
Less Extent	1	1.00-1.50

Range of scores for describing the advantages of employing silver workers was decided as follows:

Extent	Scores
Great Extent	18-30
Some Extent	31-43
Less Extent	44-56

3.12.3 DISADVANTAGES OF RECRUITING SILVER WORKERS

To measure disadvantages that employers takes into consideration while recruiting silver workers, a three point scale was developed. The overall intensity indices were calculated to measure the extent. To describe the disadvantages, the obtainable scores and range of intensity indices were decided as follows:

Obtainable Scores were as follows

Content	Number of Statements	Maximum Obtainable Scores	Minimum Obtainable Scores
Disadvantages	17	51	17

Range of Intensity Indices:

Extent	Scores	Range of Intensity Indices
Great Extent	3	2.51-3.00
Some Extent	2	1.51-2.50
Less Extent	1	1.00-1.50

Range of scores for describing the disadvantages of employing silver workers was decided as follows:

Extent	Scores
Great Extent	17-28
Some Extent	29-40
Less Extent	41-52

3.12.4 INFLUENTIAL FACTORS IN RECRUITING SILVER WORKERS

To measure the factors that influence the employers takes while recruiting silver worker, a three point scale was developed. The overall intensity indices were calculated to measure the extent. To describe the influential factors, the obtainable scores and range of intensity indices were decided as follows:

Obtainable Scores were as follows

Content	Number of Statements	Maximum Obtainable Scores	Minimum Obtainable Scores
Influential Factors	10	30	10

Range of Intensity Indices:

Extent	Scores	Range of Intensity Indices
Great Extent	3	2.51-3.00
Some Extent	2	1.51-2.50
Less Extent	1	1.00-1.50

Range of scores for describing the influential factors in employing silver workers was decided as follows:

Extent	Scores
Great Extent	10-16
Some Extent	17-23
Less Extent	24-30

3.13 Statistical Analysis of the Data

A statistical package for social sciences (SPSS) was used to analyze the data. Different statistical measures for various purposes used were as follows:

Table 7: Plan for Statistical Analysis of the Data of Silver Workers

No.	Purpose	Statistical Measure
1	Background Information of the Silver Workers	Frequencies, Percentage and Intensity Indices
2	Reasons and Perceptions of Silver Workers to work After Retirement	T-Test, ANOVA (F-test) Intensity Indices
3	Influence of work on Silver Workers	T-Test, ANOVA (F-test) Intensity Indices
4	Problems faced by Silver workers at work place	T-Test, ANOVA (F-test) Intensity Indices
5	Satisfaction at Workplace	T-Test, ANOVA (F-test) Intensity Indices
6	Suggestions	Intensity Indices

Formula used for t-test:

$$t = \frac{(\overline{x_1} - \overline{x_2})}{\sqrt{\frac{S_p^2}{n_1} + \frac{S_p^2}{n_2}}}$$

$$S_p = \sqrt{\frac{(n_1-1)S_1^2 + (n_2-1)S_2^2}{n_1 + n_2 - 2}}$$

Where,

$\overline{x_1}$ = mean of Group 1

$\overline{x_2}$ = mean of group 2

n_1 = number of group 1

n_2 = number of group 2

df = $n_1 + n_2 - 2$

S1 = SD Group 1

S2 = SD Group 2

Sp = Pooled Variance

Formula used for ANOVA (F-test)

F = $\dfrac{\text{Large Variance}}{\text{Small Variance}}$

Or = $\dfrac{\text{Between Group Variance}}{\text{Within Group Variance}}$

Between group variance = Variance in the mean of each group from the total mean of all variance groups

Within group variance = Average variance of scores within groups

Formula used for Calculating Item Wise Intensity Indices:

Item Wise Intensity Indies = $\dfrac{\text{Total Score for an Item}}{\text{Total Number of Respondents}}$

Table 8: Plan for Statistical Analysis of the Data of Employers

No.	Purpose	Statistical Measure
1	Background Information related to silver workers working in their organization/companies/institution/firms/corporate/business house	Frequencies and Percentages
2	Information related to silver workers working in their organization/companies/institution/firms/corporate/business house	3 point rating Scale and intensity Indices

(B) METHODOLOGY FOR QUALITATIVE DATA

An in-depth interview method was used to collect qualitative data only from selected silver workers of Vadodara city:

The purpose of conducting in-depth interview was:

- To study the reasons of the silver workers to work after retirement.
- To study their perceptions about old age and retirement
- To obtain suggestions for the policies they wish should be framed for silver workers as well the kinds of jobs/work opportunities that should be created for them

3.14 Sampling Unit

The silver workers working in different organizations, firms, institutions, private banks, corporate based in Vadodara city were contacted for conducting in-depth interviews.

3.15 Sampling Frame

The selection of the samples was done using purposive sampling method. While distributing and collecting the questionnaires the silver workers were identified and selected on the basis of their willingness to share their experiences and perspectives. However, the prior permission from the respondents were oriented about the nature and objectives of the study. Then, according to the pre-decided time the researcher approached the silver workers to conduct the interview.

3.16 Sample Size

The fifteen silver workers selected from different organizations, firms, private banks, institutions, were interviewed for all relevant details through personal visits. The prior appointments were sought from these silver workers for the interviews.

3.17 Process of Conducting In-depth Interview

In the beginning, the interviewees were given a handout describing the nature of the study. They were assured of all confidentiality. The interviews were mainly conducted in English or Gujarati as per the preference and comfort of the participants. They were held at the respective organizations or at the residence keeping in mind the convenience of the silver workers. The interviewer introduced the topic to the silver workers and then they were asked to express and share their own experiences related to the topic of discussion. They were asked to share their views and perceptions without any hesitations. All the 15 in-depth interviews were conducted personally by the investigator. Each in-depth interview conducted focused on selected key issues of the study. The selected silver workers were able to discuss at length key issues of the study. It took almost 1 to 1 ½ hour during which almost all the key points were discussed by the silver workers and the interview was conducted with a note of gratitude. The notes were taken about discussed to record the response of the participants.

3.18 Analysis of the Interviewed Data

The notes maintained at the time of the interviews were transcribed and the data was finally recorded. The respondents were classified and coded under a particular questions or issues. Then under each question, the coded data obtained from the 15 interviews were clubbed on a comparative analysis table. It helped the researcher to categorize the qualitative findings under major sections. These sections are discussed in the following chapter.

CHAPTER – 4
FINDINGS AND DISCUSSION

The current demographic trend of an aging population and workforce will present researchers and policymakers with many challenges in the near future. Initiatives have been put forward to address this issue of great importance. Many of these initiatives are aimed at increasing the labour force participation of older individuals. In order for these policies and programs to succeed, the factors that are associated with prolonged workforce activity must be understood. This includes the phenomenon of return to work after retirement. The present study aims to fill a number of gaps in the literature through a comprehensive examination of this topic. Numerous variables and various interactions among these variables are investigated as potential correlates of the probability that one has engaged in post-retirement work.

Beyond a study of factors that are correlated with the likelihood of having been involved in work after retirement, this study is concerned with how return to paid work after retirement is associated with the health and well-being of silver workers. Elderly individuals whose health and happiness are compromised by their post-retirement work activity will be unlikely to sustain this activity for a lengthy period of time. On the other hand, elderly workers whose health and quality of life are benefiting from their work efforts after retirement will likely proceed with these efforts with much commitment and enthusiasm. Furthermore, it would be socially unjust to encourage productive work among retired individuals for the benefit of the larger society if this benefit is to be realized at the expense of their health and life satisfaction and other factors. For all of these reasons, there is a need to understand how post-retirement work is associated with the health and happiness of silver workers.

When people of 60 years and above decide to work after retirement they make a unique category of workers. They attract ever ones attention. Their existence in human society gives rise to variety of responses, reactions and apprehensions, because it connotes on greater part, to some kind of compulsion or willingness that prompt elderly to decide to work after retirement. Work due to social attention and assurance for security both economical and social. In this age, elderly aspire for psychological security with due attention. But the fact remains that despite age related limitations good number of persons in their age of sixty and beyond were hunting for work that would support them and get them some kind of support and in it turns helps them to remain physically and mentally active. Does it mean that they feel insecure in the present set-up of the economical, social and psychological condition of human society or it was their willingness to continue working after retirement?

In view of this reality, the present research seeks to conduct an enquiry into economical, social and psychological undercurrents in the reality today that prompt elderly decide to work even after they retire from their first employment. Does it turn out to be a kind of compulsion or because of familial responsibilities on their part or they wanted to do it out of their willingness or passion for work, or some other kind of considerations? The present research focuses on these issues to review the decisions of elderly to work after retirement. Popularly these workers are termed as "Silver Workers". The focus is laid on silver workers in the city of Vadodara to conduct a sample study on the related issues at large. Emerges from the responses and reflections of the silver workers against the questions asked to them. As a result we can obtain dial perspective on the silver workers decision to work after retirement

This chapter interprets specific results of silver workers experiences regarding transition to retirement and their post retirement activities. This included findings of retiree's reasons and conditions for post retirement work, as well as their ideas and perceptions about retirement and their organizational needs. The silver workers study provides an insight into circumstances of continued work during retirement. For instance, silver workers in this study have high level of educational level. Their former jobs often have been characterised by high complexity. In addition, silver workers subjectively had achieved their occupational goals to a very high degree. Therefore, they left a highly productive level of activation when they retired.

Secondly, the study consisted of the employers who were recruiting the silver workers. Although few organizations have taken steps to prepare for the potential loss of critical talent and knowledge as elderly retire, executives overwhelmingly report that their organizations value silver worker for their experience, knowledge, and insights. However, stereotypical notions of elderly worker inflexibility and difficulty with technology persist. Companies are testing innovative recruitment, retention, workforce planning, and flexible work solutions in an effort to attract the talent needed to maintain corporate productivity.

The present study was undertaken with a major objective of study the reasons that prompt silver workers to work after retirement .This chapter seeks to present an overview of the data collection and information collected from the respondents in order to frame findings for the purpose of the present study. The applied and explorative study of silver workers incorporates a wide variety of interests. So, the present study evolves multiple methodological approaches that would sound appropriate to its broad approach. The first approach is a theory based quantitative part. The second approach looks at the qualitative part to represent unbiased reflections of the respondents. These reflections were further coded and quantified subsequently for the purpose of review and analysis. It further looks into the perspectives of employers who employ silver workers at their organization, companies. Thus a kind of triangular perspective may be evolved on the ground of the data, information and responses and reflections obtained from a huge size of the sample comprising of three hundred silver workers and fifty employers as the respondents selected from city of Vadodara. It may be noted that only those silver workers were selected as the sample of the study that were recruited in any of the corporate, private banks, firm, agencies, organizations, private schools. The quantitative and qualitative findings are presented in the following order:

Part-1 Silver Workers

(A) Findings of the Quantitative Data

4.1 Profile of the selected Silver Workers

    4.1.1 Details about Family

    4.1.2 Silver Wokrers and their Present Occupation

    4.1.3 Work History

    4.1.4 Health Status

4.2 Overall and Aspects Wise Reasons of Silver Workers to Work after Retirement

4.3		Differences in the Reasons of Silver Workers to Work after Retirement in Relation to the Selected Variables
4.4		Item Wise Findings regarding Reasons Prompting Silver Workers to Work after Retirement
4.5		Perceptions of Silver Workers about Retirement
4.6		Item wise Findings Regarding Perceptions of Silver Workers about Retirement
4.7		Preparation for Retirement
4.8		Influence of Work on Silver Workers
4.9		Differences in the Influence of Work on Silver Workers in relation to the Selected Variables
4.10		Item Wise Findings Regarding Influence of Work on Silver Workers
4.11		Problems Confronted by Silver Workers due to work and Workplace
4.12		Differences in the Problems Confronted by the Silver Workers due to work and Workplace in relation to the Selected Variables
4.13		Item Wise Findings Related to Problems Confronted by the Silver Workers at their Workplace
4.14		Satisfaction of the Silver Workers related to Work and Workplace
4.15		Differences in the Satisfaction of Silver Workers related to Work and Workplace in relation to the Selected Variables
4.16		Item wise Findings of the Satisfaction of Silver Workers related to Work and Workplace
4.17		Suggestion by the Silver Workers

(B) Findings of the Qualitative Data

4.18		Profile of the Selected Silver Workers
4.19		Interviews Conducted with Selected Silver Workers

Part -2 Employers

Findings of the Quantitative Data

4.20 Profile of the Employers

4.21 Details about the Employees

4.22 Item wise Findings Regarding Influential Factors in Deciding the Time to Retire

4.23 Item Wise Findings Regarding Qualities Considered by the Employers While Employing Silver Workers

4.24 Item Wise Findings Regarding Advantages of the Employers while recruting Silver Workers

4.25 Item Wise Findings Regarding the Disadvantages of the Employers in Recruiting Silver Workers.

The quantitative data provides an objective perspective on silver workers. The qualitative data projects a subjective perspective on them through review of their reflections on related issues. Thus, the part I focuses on two basic dimension related to the subject of the research. The part II, on the other hand, projects yet one more objective dimensions of the employers who from the counterpart of the silver workers. It helps to avail neutral perspective on the subject of the research. The present study was conducted with the specific dimension of studying the reasons, problems, influencing factors, their satisfaction with the work they were presently doing. Silver workers themselves form most sensitive and sentimental segment of the society and their decision to work after retirement might be influenced by economical, social and psychological compulsions. In this light their profile would form interesting and significant part of the data required for the present study. They lead us to determine variable on the ground of which the reviews and analysis for the study may be valuable for the purpose.

Part-1 Silver Workers

(A) **Findings of the Quantitative Data**

4.1 Profile of the Selected Silver Workers

Table 9: Percentage Distribution of the Silver Workers According to their Background Information

(N=300)

Background Information	Category	F	%
Age	Young-Old	116	38.67
	Old	184	61.33
Sex	Male	294	98.00
	Female	6	2.00
Marital Status	Married	288	96.00
	Widow/Widower	7	2.33
	Single	4	1.33
	Divorcee	1	0.33
Educational Qualification	High Level	254	84.67
	Moderate Level	31	10.33
	Low Level	15	5.00
Religion	Hindu	286	95.33
	Jain	7	2.33
	Parsi	4	1.33
	Muslim	3	1.00
Caste	General	250	83.33
	SC/ST	37	12.33
	OBC	13	4.33

Table 9 shows that the majority of the selected, silver workers (61.33%) belonged to older age group, whereas little less than forty percent of them (38.67%) belonged to young-old age group. It means that higher percentages of silver workers belonged to older age group were working than those belonging to young old age group.

The findings of the data focus first on the profile of the silver workers selected for the present research. As the data reflects the silver workers were distributed in the groups of 'young-old' and 'old' in the ration of 60-40 percentage(As shown in Figure 5). It means that majority of them were belonging to old age group and remaining were in young-old age group. Kangsasitiam (2004) conducted a study on "Household structure and elderly working status". It indicates that the intensity of the subject on discussion would be relatively higher.

Further table 1 and Figure 6 revelas that sex indicates wide gap in distribution between males and females like a very high majority of the silver workers (98%) were male and just 2 percent of them were females. It clearly explains that a very few women silver workers prefer to work after retirement or it might be the case that they were getting less opportunities to work post retirement in comparison to male silver workers. Secondly high very majority of the silver workers were male and only six of them were female. It means that the issue on the discussion would be mostly male oriented according to the study conducetd by Preeti Dhillonv and Laishram Ladusingh (2001) who focused their study on Economic Activity in Post Retirement Life in India.

Table 1 and figure 7 revelas that marital status reveals that very high majority of the silver workers (96%) were married, whereas very low percentage (2.33%) of them were widow. About 1.33 percentages of the silver workers were single and only one of the silver worker was a divorcee.

In view of the marital status of the silver workers the data represents that very high majority of them were married and having their spouses' alive. The rest meagre minority of them were distributed among the other groups like widow/widower single and divorcee, which means that they were living alone and not with their spouses. Such status reflected that most of the silver workers had to carry out responsibility of a spouse and a family. There have been considerable changes in the levels of education among silver workers over the past several decades. Thanks to the expansion of the education system, there are now high majority of the silver workers who claimed that they were educated holding graduate/post graduate degrees. Some of them were moderately educated upto college level and a small number of them had studied upto matriculation

Further a focus was laid on level of education among the silver workers (As shown in Figure 8). It was revealed that very high majority (84.67%) of the silver workers had obtained high level of education; nearly 11 percentages (10.33%) of the silver workers had moderate level of education. Very low percentage (5%) of them had low level of education. It indicates that the silver workers with higher level of education were more inclined to work after retirement than the other two groups with moderate or low levels of education.

The level of education among the selected silver workers point at a fact that the minds were cultivated with good education they had gained and they possessed high sensitivity about the prevailing conditions of life they were facing. The level of knowledge enriched their minds with good capacity to know, understand and react to what was happening around. Further, knowledge and education enabled them to express them well and respond effectively to the queries put towards them. With good level of education, it may be expected that the silver workers would be able to voice their concerns more effectively and put across their ideas and views with relatively better quality. Education would prove significant in determining the sharpness of the qualitative data that were obtained from the silver workers through their responses in the form expressions and reflections to the issues discussed. Findings of Hung's (2003) study also shows that people who are academically educated are more willing to participate in the labor market than those who are not.

Religion as specified in the table 1 and Figure 9, it can be revealed that very high majority (95.33%) of the silver workers belonged to the Hindu faith. Little less than 3 percentages (2.33%) of them were Jain and very low percentages (1.33%) of them were Parsi and (1%). Muslims .Further table 1 indicates that silver workers from all religions were involved in post retirement work and the major part of the workforce was formed with Hindu persons.

Further, very high majority of the silver workers followed the Hinduism and the remaining small number of them was other faiths like the Jainism, the Parsi, and the Islam. Since religion contributes significantly to shape the psychology and the tendency of an individual's beliefs, responses and reactions too would be coloured with the system of the relevant philosophy. The data reflects that most of the silver workers possessed patterns of thinking and believing the Hinduism .Consequently, their responses and reactions would naturally be influenced with Hindu conventions and traditions.

Further it can be seen form table 1 and Figure 10 that as specified categories of the government of India very high majority (83.33%) of silver workers belonged to general caste, little more than 10 percentages (12.33%) of them belonged to SC/ST and nearly 5 percentages (4.33%) of silver worker belonged to OBC. The table reflects that silver workers from various caste groups formed the labour force.

Categories of caste are a recent classification of population that were specified by the government of India in view of equal distribution of opportunities of growth and quality of living among all segments of the population. These categories are applied through formal government acts and regulations to make available equal opportunities in education and jobs to the deprived classes. Under the noble notion of the 'Right to education' and 'Right to work' in the interest to ensuring social justice among all the classes of the population .The data displayed in the table represents that a good majority of the silver workers belonged to the 'General' category whereas relatively very small number of them belonged to the reserved categories of the 'SC/ST" and 'OBC" .This classification indicates that a good majority of them enjoyed good opportunities of education and jobs and for small number of them had their rights reserved in the matter of education and jobs. It further hints at the psychology that they lived with. The good majority of them were bit satisfied with the opportunities of education and jobs they had enjoyed. As small number of them may be carrying feeling of being deprived and neglected suffering injustice in the prevalent social and economical set-ups. In this manner, the data concerning the personal profile appear to clear the picture about socio economical and psychological dimension of the silver workers and it would prepare a suitable ground for specific kinds and quality of responses and reactions from them during interactions on their present conditions in view of their decision to work after retirement.

Table 10: Percentage Distribution of the Silver Workers According to their Native State

(N=300)

Native State	F	%
Gujarat	251	83.67
Maharashtra	16	5.33
Rajasthan	14	4.67
Madhya Pradesh	5	1.67
Chennai	9	3.00
Kerala	3	1.00
Uttar Pradesh	1	0.33
Assam	1	0.33

The table 10 and Figure 11 shows that a high majority (83.67%) of silver workers native place was Gujarat nearly 6 percent (5.33%) belonged to Maharashtra .Little less than 5 percent (4.67%) were from Rajasthan, there were less than 2 percentages of them who belonged to Madhya Pradesh and 3 percentages of them were from Chennai, followed by 1 percent from Kerala and just 1 silver work belonged to Uttar Pradesh and just one to Assam. The table reflects that though the silver workers had native places in other states they did not move back home but continued to work in Gujarat even after their retirement.

Another point that the data reflect on is the comfort level the silver workers experience at social level. First it represents that good majority of them belonged to the Gujarat state and some belonged to the states of Maharashtra, Rajasthan, Madhya Pradesh, Chennai, Kerala, Uttar Pradesh and Assam. For most of them, the nativity of Gujarat allowed them relatively more comfort level and relaxation while staying in Gujarat in terms of language dressing, style of living, food habits, conventions and tradition of the home state. Others might feel less comfortable in a state other than the home. However, there is high mobility and migration of people to other states for business and migration of people to other states for business and jobs. Since migration becomes inevitable for them on economic prospects they have to do some kind of compromise in the matters of language, food habits, dressing style, style of living etc. It also reveals that instead of doing such compromises and adjustments silver workers decided to stay back in Gujarat after their retirement. This shows that they might be getting good work opportunities in Gujarat than their native state

Table 11: Percentage Distribution of the Silver Workers According to the Type of House they Possess

(N=300)

Type of House	F	%
Bungalow/Tenement	206	68.67
Flat	65	21.67
Row House	29	9.67

In order to assess the comfort level of living, a survey was made about what property silver workers possessed. It can be seen from the table 11 that all (100%) the silver workers owning their own houses. Further, the table 3 and figure 12 shows that little less than seventy percent (68.67%) of the silver workers owned a bungalow or a tenement and little more than one fifth (21.67%) of the silver workers owned flats and nearly ten percent (9.67%) of them owned a row house. This shows that though the type of house may differ but the fact remained that each and every silver worker owned house. They had shelter to spend in their post retirement life comfortably.

It was revealed that good majority of them were the owners of bungalows or tenements and some of them owned flats. A small number of them had row houses. Thus, it is understood that majority of them possessed decent and comfortable dwellings, if not luxurious ones. It seems that they had managed a decent house from their income before retirement so they feel ease in this matter. It also indicated that silver workers were not working after retirement with the burden of purchasing a property as they were already having their own houses which shows a sign of financial stability

Table 12: Percentage Distribution of the Silver Workers According to the Type of Vehicle they Own and Drive.

(N=300)

Type of Vehicle they Own						Type of Vehicle they Drive					
Only Two Wheeler		Only Four Wheeler		Both		Only Two Wheeler		Only Four Wheeler		Both	
F	%	F	%	F	%	F	%	F	%	F	%
187	62.33	54	18.00	59	19.67	219	73.00	38	12.67	43	14.33

Almost high majority (99.33%) of the silver workers reported that they owned vehicles whereas only two of them admitted that did not own a vehicle. The table further shows that majority (62.33%) of silver workers owned two wheelers whereas 18 percent of them owned four wheelers. There were about twenty percent of them who owned both two and four wheelers. Table 12 also indicated that high majority (73%) of the silver workers were driving only two wheelers and almost thirteen percent (12.67%) of them were driving only four wheelers(As shown in Fugure 13, 14 and 15) . Little less than fifteen percent of them were driving both the kind of vehicles, two and four wheelers. The table reveals that almost all the silver workers owned vehicles and they were even driving their own vehicles.

Since the present time life is so speedy and busy that one had to manage a day's time well to be able to manage as many as jobs possible. At times, he/she has to run to distant places. So he/she needs a vehicle to facilitate his/her quick movements. In the present age a vehicle becomes an inevitable need for a person, particularly one wants to work more to raise some more income. Having a vehicle makes a lot of difference to improve work and improves prospects or more income. It also reveals that silver workers were physically fit enough to drive on their own and they did not depend to others for going out.

Table 13: Percentage Distribution of the Silver Workers According to their Purpose of Driving

(N=298)

Purpose	F	%
Work/Job	298	99.33
Social Purposes	251	83.67
Household Task	206	68.67
Doctor's Visit	137	45.67

Table 13 and Figure 16 shows that almost all the (99.33%) of silver workers used to drive for work/job except two of them, little more than eighty percentages (83.67%) used to drive for social purposes, nearly seventy percentages of them (68.67%) used to drive for household task, and 45.67 percentages of them used to drive for doctor's visit. This table indicated that age or health was not the barrier for silver workers to drive as almost all of them were independently driving while going for job/work. Further the table also shows that silver workers were actively driving for other day to day activities.

In view of the purpose of driving, almost all of the silver workers informed that they used vehicles to reach places of work and for purpose of job or work. High majority viewed owing vehicles as a matter of social pride and they moved on vehicles for social purposes, like meeting relatives and attending social occasions. Majority of them said they needed to drive vehicles for household task like fetching grocery and to arrange for daily needs. About half of the silver workers drove vehicles on health ground like to visit doctors or approaching hospitals and like. Thus, it is understood that most silver workers used vehicles on valid reasons as a facility to help their routine task.

Table 14: Percentage Distribution of the Silver Workers According to their Participation in Number of Leisure time Activities

(N=300)

Activities	F	%
More (11 to 20 Activities)	180	60.00
Less (10 or Less than 10 Activities)	120	40.00

Table 14 and Figure 17 shows that 60 percent of the silver workers were participating in more number of leisure time activities. While 40 percent of them were participating in less number of leisure time activities. It clearly shows that majority of the silver workers were actively involved in leisure time activities along with their present job after retirement.

Leisure time activities are common with all persons. They start them as something to do when they are free from routine duties and task. They view it as pastime activities to give them a good change of mind from routine burdens and tensions. Slowly, these activities come to be habit or even addiction for most persons without which they would feel void and uncomfortable. In one way, leisure time activities indicate a human tendency to try out something new as interest and hobbies. It is noticed that one may involve in more than one activity as his/her time permits .The data indicates that good number of the silver workers admitted that they were participating in more activities of eleven to twelve different kinds, whereas considerably small numbers of them informed to be participating in less than ten different activities. This reveals that in spite of remaining busy the day long silver workers do find time for leisure time activities, which shows their enthusiasm and fitness and love towards their life. On whole it is good sign that majority of the silver workers preferred to keep themselves busy in some meaningful activities.

Table 15: Percentage Distribution of the Silver Workers According to their Participation in Specific Leisure time Activities

(N=300)

Activities		F	%
Read	Newspaper	282	94.00
	Magazine	123	41.00
	Books	117	39.00
Listen	Music	202	67.33
	Bhajans	138	46.00
	Religious Lectures	115	38.33
	Political Lectures	106	35.33
	Health Lectures	104	34.67
	Educational Lectures	61	20.33
	Social Lectures	44	14.67
Visit	Relatives	190	63.33
	Temple	189	63.00
	Garden	177	59.00
	Restaurants	101	33.67
	Theatre/Cinema	98	32.67
	Neighbours	75	25.00
	Club/Mahila Mandal	36	12.00
Play	Indoor	77	25.67
	Outdoor	15	5.00
Walk		254	84.67
Household Work		238	79.33
Sleep		168	56.00
Computer		164	54.67
Yoga/Meditation		113	37.67
Grandchildren		109	36.33
Creative Work		14	4.67

Table 15 specifies the kinds of leisure time activities that silver workers were found to be involved with. These activities range from reading ,listening, writing, playing, walking, household work, sleeping, working on computers, practising yoga/mediation, enjoying the company of grandchildren, some kind of creative work etc. the table indicates preferences to some kind of activity by the silver workers participation. Accordingly high majority (94%) of silver workers were participating in reading activities such as news paper reading. Followed by listening to music in which silver workers showed high interest (67.33%). Little more than sixty percentages (63.33%) of the silver workers were interested in visiting relatives and majority (84.67%) of them prefer walking. High majority (79.33%) of them said they were interested to do household work in their leisure time. More than fifty percentages of them liked to sleep, or work on computers, yoga or meditation, playing or spending time with grandchildren from other kinds of the leisure time activities that one third of them preferred. A very less percentages (4.67%) of them were involved in some kind of creative work.

Figure 5: Percentage Distribution of the Silver Workers according to their Age

(N=300)

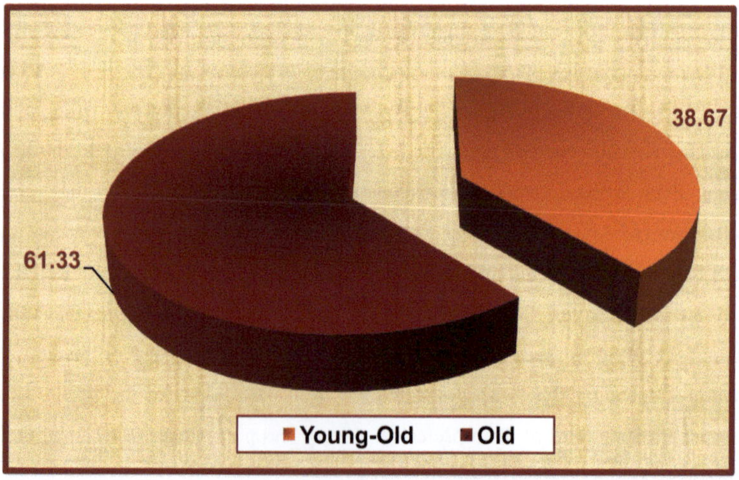

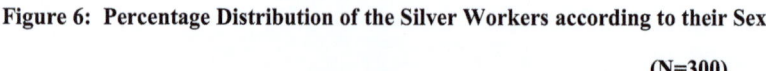

Figure 6: Percentage Distribution of the Silver Workers according to their Sex

(N=300)

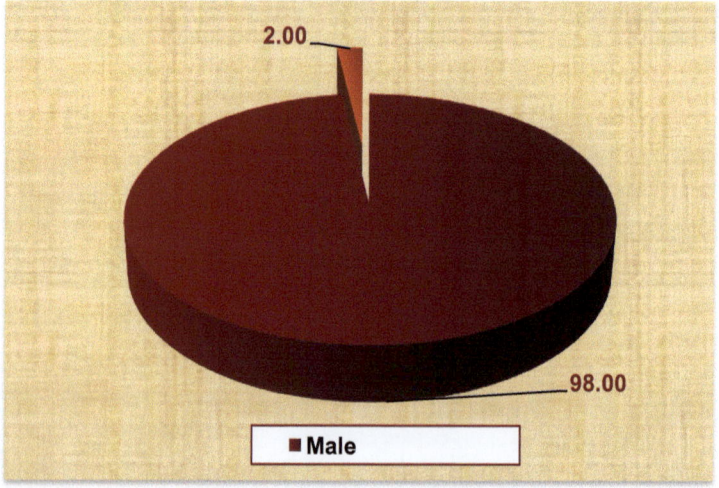

Figure 7: Percentage Distribution of the Silver Workers according to their Marital Status

(N=300)

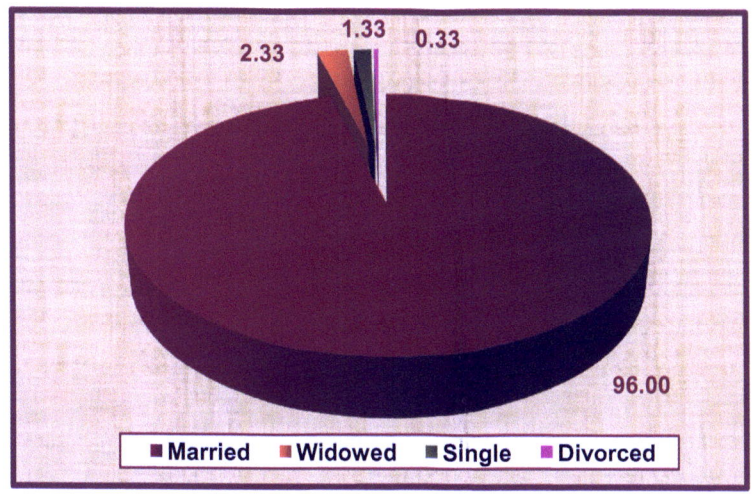

Figure 8: Percentage Distribution of the Silver Workers according to htier Educational Qualification

(N=300)

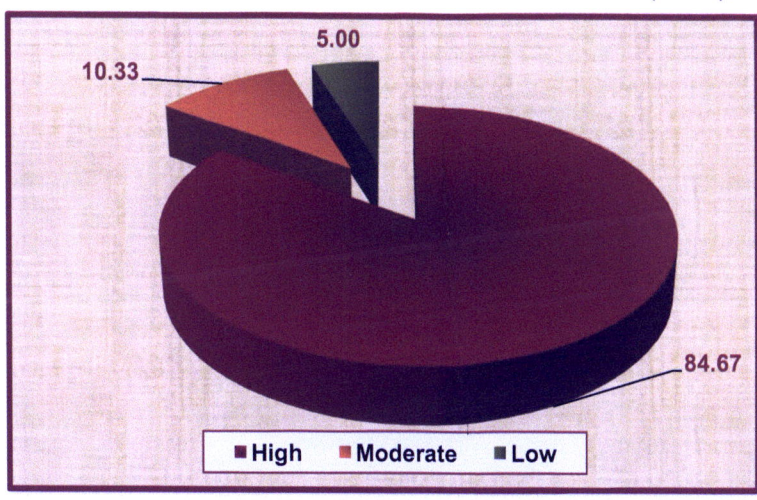

Figure 9: Percentage Distribution of the Silver Workers according to their Religion

(N=300)

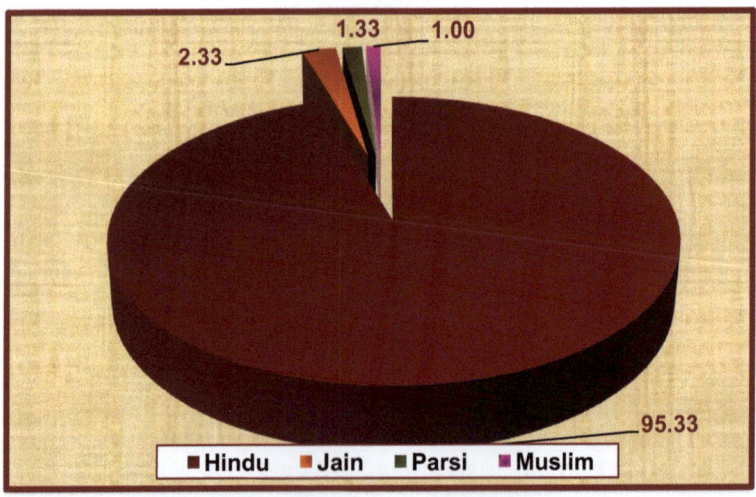

Figure 10: Percentage Distribution of the Silver Workers according to their Caste

(N=300)

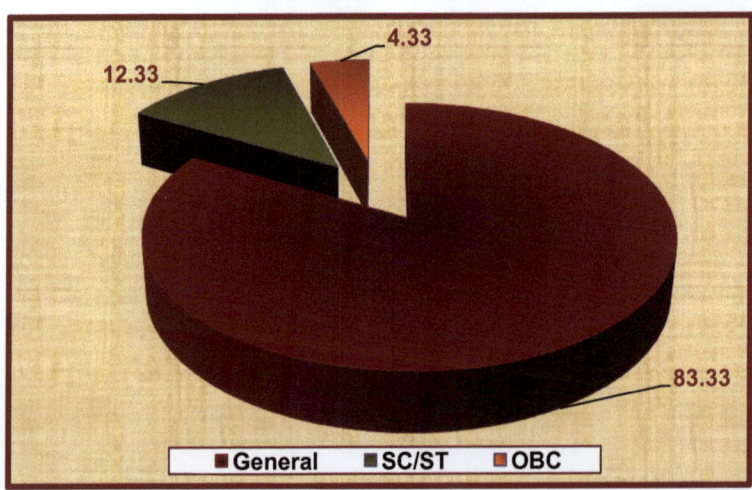

Figure 11: Percentage Distribution of the Silver Workers according to their Native Place

(N=300)

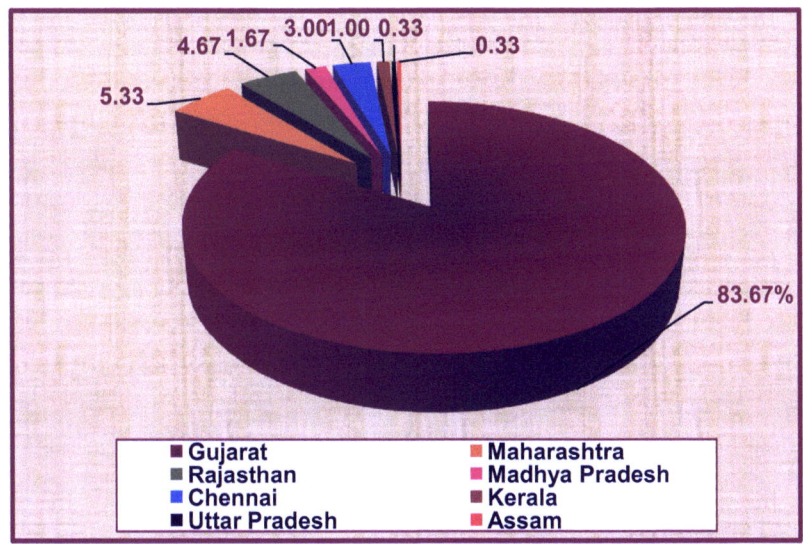

Figure 12: Percentage Distribution of the Silver Workers according to their Type of House

(N=300)

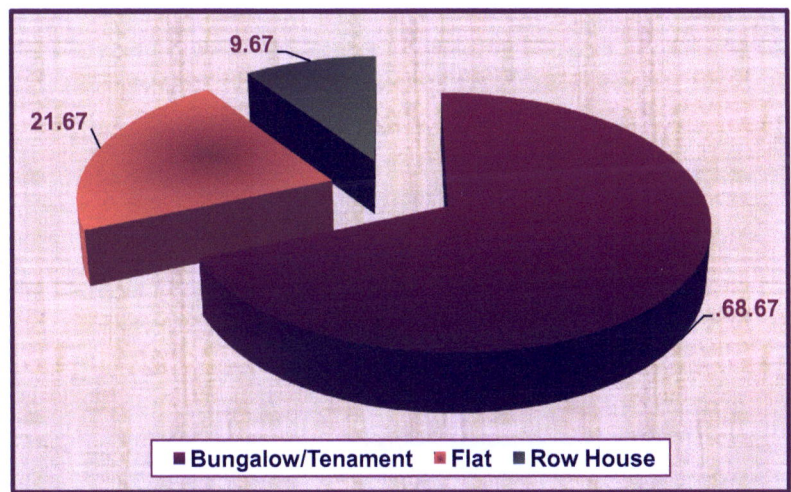

Figure 13: Percentage Distribution of the Silver Workers according to Vehicle they Own

(N=300)

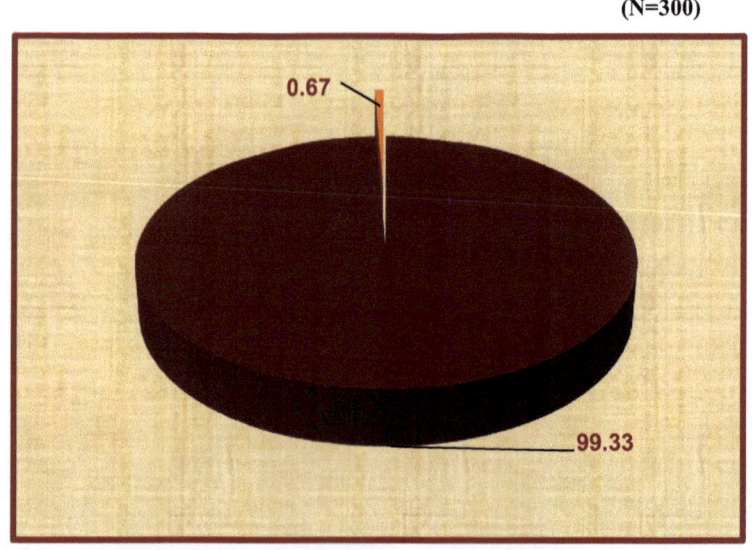

Figure 14: Percentage Distribution of Silver Workers according to the Type of Vehicle they Own

(N=300)

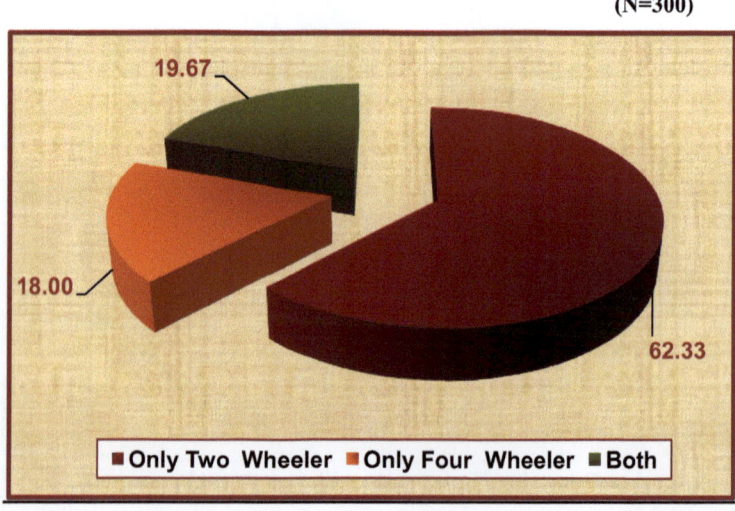

Figure 15: Percentage Distribution of Silver Workers according to the Type of Vehicle they Drive

(N=300)

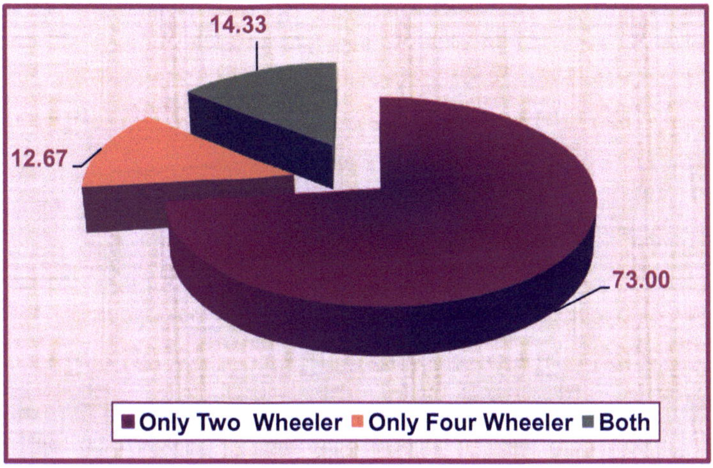

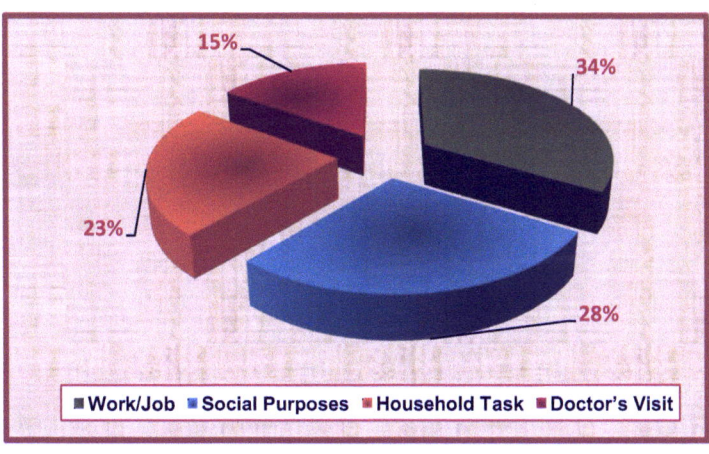

Figure 16: Percentage Distribution of Silver Workers according to their Purpose of Driving

(N=300)

Figure 17: Percentage Distribution of Silver Workers according to their Leisure Time Activities

(N=300)

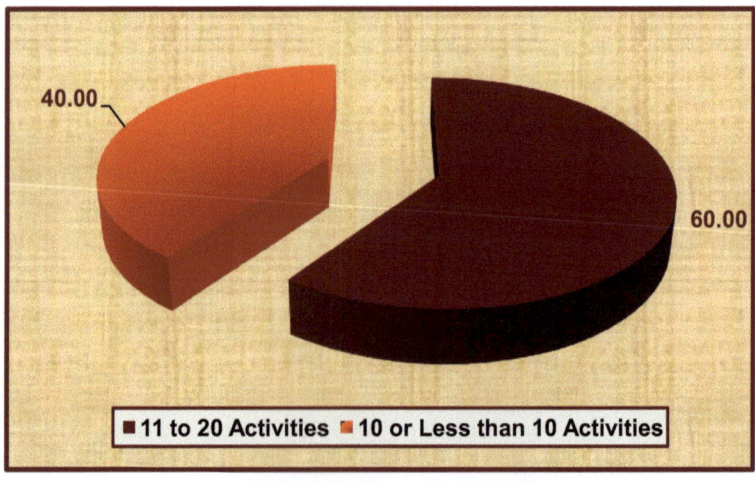

4.1.1 DETAILS ABOUT FAMILY

A family is a social unit to which a person is attached throughout his life. He deserves comfort and solace from his family. In an old age when a person retires from his job he feels lonely and in that condition a family is a valuable asset to him.

Table 16: Percentage Distribution of the Silver Workers According to their Type of Family

(N=300)

Type of Family	F	%
Living with Family	189	63.00
Living with Spouse	104	34.67
Living Alone	7	2.33

Table 16 and Figure 18 reveals that majority (63%) of silver workers were living with their families. Nearly thirty five percentages of them were living with their spouses and very fewer percentages of the silver workers (2.33%) were living alone. It was revealed the silver workers living with families preferred more to work than those living with the spouse or living alone.

Man being a social animal does need a family. It is in a family that he fells stable, secured and comfortable. It this sense, the data collected in view of the families of the silver workers reflects how stable and secured they feel with their families to add to his comfort level. The data reflects that a good majority of the silver workers were staying with their families and about one third of them were living with their spouses. A few of them were staying alone. This indicates that high majority of them enjoyed social stability and secured comfortable living with their families. Further, high majority of them were living either with families or with spouses and were married and few of them were divorced or widow or even unmarried. The marital status may imply the extent of responsibility and caring sense of their part.

Table 17: Percentage Distribution of the Silver Workers According to their Relation between Type of Family and Marital Status

(N=300)

Type of Family	Married		Single		Divorced		Widowed	
	F	%	F	%	F	%	F	%
Living with Family (N=189)	184	97.35	-	-	1	0.52	4	2.11
Living with Spouse (N=104)	104	100	-	-	-	-	-	-
Living Alone (N-7)	-	-	4	57.14	-	-	3	4.28

Table 17 and Figure 19 shows that high majority of the silver worker were living with family and they were married. A small percentage of them were living alone and they were widowed and divorcee

The marital status of being divorced or widow would get in the some kind of dissatisfaction, regret or complaining nature against them, those with single status would get some kind of carefree/ careless or even reckless attitude to others. The silver workers having marital status appeared to carry some kind of pressure that would ample them to search for job after retirement and they might be having responsibilities towards their spouse, children education and marriage. Since divorce or widowed or single among the silver workers were not much pressurized by their families to work after retirement their decision to work after retirement would be prompted by the consideration other than the familial or economical reasons. For such silver workers the reason to work after retirement can be to kill their time or might be as they did not want to depend on other for financial requirement. Thus a family can serve a source of support and solace to an elderly person, while on the other hand it can be a factor to cause anxiety to him/her.

Table 18: Percentage Distribution of the Silver Workers According to their Size of Family

(N=300)

Size	F	%
Large (4 to 6 members)	153	51.00
Small (1 to 3 members)	147	49.00

Table 18 and Figure 20 shows that almost half percentages of the silver workers belonged to large families and nearly fifty percent (49%) of them belonged to small families. It was revealed that the difference between the types of families of the silver workers was very small.

In this sense a size of a family matters. A bigger family can assure good support and solace to an elderly person and on the other hand, it can also cause anxiety and pressure to him/her. With a smaller family these contradictory experiences would reduce relatively. As the data represents the silver workers were found belonging to these two groups on almost equal grounds. Those having a bigger family of four to six members formed almost 51 percent of them and those having a small family of 1 to 3 members formed about 49 percent of them. This explains that the feeing and benefits of a family was almost equally divided among them and so it can be understood that their responses would bear reactions and reflections would be divided with mixed feelings. Such mixed reactions and reflections can be further applied to the factors that prompted them to work after retirement. In this sense, it can be inferred that decision to work after retirement would be compulsion for the half of them and for the remaining half it could be a choice or willing in the interest of activeness, fitness updating skills and knowledge and also sharing knowledge and experience to contribute to others growth

Table 19: Percentage Distribution of Silver Workers According to the Educational Qualification of their Spouse (Husband/Wife)

Educational Qualification	Husband (N=6)		Wife (N=282)	
	F	%	F	%
Under Graduate	1	16.67	86	30.49
Graduate	3	50.00	103	36.52
Post Graduate	2	33.33	93	32.97

Table 19 and Figure 21 reveals that in case of female silver workers, half of them had husbands holding graduate degrees. Little more than one third of them had husbands holding post graduate degrees. A very small percentage of the women silver workers had husbands who had studied up to undergraduate level. While in case of male silver workers, almost 37 percentage of the silver worker's spouse (wife) were educated up to graduate level and one third of them the spouse (wife) were under graduates. For about thirty three (32.97%) percentage of the silver workers spouse (wife) had studies with post graduate degree (as shown in Fiigure 22).

Another significant is related to a family is a level of education among spouse and other members would display approach and attitude towards those members of a family. Education is indicative of level of understanding, approach and attitude that members of a family would display in interactions and decision making on routine matters and on special occasions. If an elderly person in a family retires after a full tenure of working for 35 to 40 years and then at an advanced age he/she decides to work even after retirement, what would it reflect? Would members in his/her family resent to his/her working after retirement? Even if he/she has a strong desire to work after retirement on consideration other than socio economical compulsion members in his/her family would first resent to his/her decision and then they would agree to him/her on some assurance and conviction related to health and comfort. In this consideration, the data presented focus on the level of education among the spouses and other members in the silver workers families. Accordingly, the silver workers spouses either the husband or wife, were considerably educated with half of them possessing graduate degrees and the one third possessing even post graduate degrees' small number of the spouses had studied below the level of graduation. It was a good sign that none of the spouses was illiterate. This status of education reflects relatively positive attitude among them addressing correctly the pressures on them and liking they desire for.

Table 20: Percentage Distribution of Silver Workers According to the Occupational Status of their Spouse (Husband/wife)

Occupational Status	Husband (N=6)		Wife (N=282)	
	F	%	F	%
Working	4	66.66	204	72.34
Not Working	-	-	75	26.59
Retired	2	33.33	3	1.06

Table 20 and Figure 23 reflect on the occupational status of the spouses of the silver workers. Majority (66.66%) of the female silver worker's husbands were working and little more than thirty percent (33.33%) of them had husbands who were retired .The table and Fugure 24 further reveals that majority (72.34%) of the male silver worker spouses were house wife's, whereas for little more than twenty five percent (26.59%) of them the spouses were retired. For a very less percentage (1.06%) of them the spouses were working.

From above table it can be revealed that almost good majority of the spouses were working and a few were even retired. Only one fourth of them were not Woking. This further reflects that working spouses can better understand the decision that would afflict the counterpart and play supportive role to support him/her in their decision to work. This also reveals that silver workers having working spouse might develop a sense of inferiority complex, or they feel finically dependent, because of which they chose to continue working after retirement. It can also be the other way that silver workers were taking it in a positive way to have a working spouse as they get an encouragement from to keep themselves working post retirement.

Table 21: Percentage Distribution of Silver Workers According to the Sex of their Children and their Marital Status

Children			Marital Status			
			Married		Unmarried	
	F	%	F	%	F	%
Sons (N=314)	314	60.38	278	88.53	36	11.46
Daughters (N=206)	206	39.61	182	88.34	24	11.65

Table 21 shows that majority (60.38%) of the silver worker had sons and forty percent of them (39.61%) were having daughters. It can be further revealed for the above table and Figure 25shows that for high majority of silver worker (88.53%) sons were married. Whereas little more than one tenth percent of silver worker's (11.46%) sons were unmarried (As shown in Figure 26). Further it was revealed that high majority (88.34%) of the silver workers daughters were married, whereas nearly 12 percent of them (11.65%) the daughters were unmarried. It reveals that there were silver workers who still had responsibilities of getting their sons/daughters married.

Above table reflects in the children to include sons, daughters and daughters-in-law in the silver workers families. As silver workers had more of sons almost 60 percent and less of daughters and most of them were married. It reflects that majority of their sons and daughters were settled in life. Further, as shown in the table 19 in findings chapter, high majority of sons were working and employed with some organization and a small group would imply a kind of responsibility on the silver workers. Among daughters, almost sixty percent were not working or still students and only forty percent were employed.

Table 22: Percentage Distribution of Silver Workers According to the Occupational Status of their Sons, Daughters and Daughters-in-Law

Occupational Status	Sons (N= 314)		Daughters (N=206)		Daughters-in-Law (N= 278)	
	F	%	F	%	F	%
Working/Employed	291	92.67	82	39.80	113	40.64
Not working/Student	23	7.32	124	60.19	165	59.35

Table 22 and aFigures 27, 28 and 29 reveals the occupational status of the silver workers sons, daughters and daughters-in-law. High majority of the silver worker had son's working and very less (7.32%) of them were not working/students .Further, it was revealed that for nearly forty percentages (39.80%) of them, the daughters were working and almost 61 percentages of them the daughters were not working. While nearly 41 percentages of the silver workers the daughter-in-laws were working and little less than 60 percentages of them the daughters-in-law were not working

Daughters in law were either working or not working in the same proportion of about 60-40 percent. Such a status reflects a mixed kind of attitude and support that the silver workers would receive from their children in their decision to work after retirement as well as this data also leads to conclusion that as most of the silver workers children were working , they did not had much financial burden of their children. So the reason to work after retirement would not be mainly to help the children.

Table 23: Percentage Distribution of the Silver Workers According to their Sources of Family Income per Month

(N=300)

Sources of Income	F	%
Pension	165	55.00
Interest from Fixed Deposit	89	29.67
Interest from Investments	66	22.00
Rental Income	23	7.67

As the table 23 and Figure 30 shows ,more than half (55%) of the silver workers were found to be receiving pension and less than thirty percent (29.67%) had income in form of interest of fixed deposits. While 22 percentages of them had interest raised from their investments and a few of them (7.67%) were earning through their rental income. This shows that all of them had limited sources of income

There follows in a person's life next to the immediate concern of a family economic concern that turns out to be inevitable on the living conditions in the present time. Money is an urgent matter that no one can ignore. It affects ones life and quality of his living intensely. Money can improve or mar quality of living making a person happy or miserable. The pressure of money works so intensely that a man is much afflicted with tension of having no money, hunger ,deprivation and deteriorating health and he may be compelled to commit suicide. Lack of money causes conditions in a person's life that can be neither shared with anyone nor can be tolerated by him/her. He/she runs a condition of suffocation and tension that he is unable to share with his family or friends. But for those who have stable financial condition and well to do even after retirement face number of problems as they develop a sense of inferiority complex. They lose their confidence and feels isolated from the society and in some cases they also bears change in attitude and behaviour of family members due to their retirement. It is like a swamp into which he/she plunges himself out of carving for survival so ones psychological condition may turn fatal to his life. When we think of an elderly person who looks for work after retirement this would be the first doubt to arise in our mind. The silver workers conditions of living may be perceived as confronting problems of money inviting such depressing feelings.

It is known from the data that good majority of the silver workers were surviving on the pension they were receiving on the ground of the first job. Some of them had income from fixed deposits with banks. Some had invested money and they were getting dividend against them. A few of them owned houses and they raised some income to survive life in the time of soaring prices. It becomes clear that they could meet the two ends of income and expenditure. For those silver workers who were not having enough savings as well those who were not receiving pensions it might be difficult for them to have decent life, they need to earn more and so they do need a job even after retirement. With limited source of income, they were compelled to decide to work after retirement.

Such a picture reflects our economic constraints that prompted the silver workers to work after retirement. On the other there were also silver workers who seems to be finically stable as they were having savings and income from other sources as well pension they chose to work after retirement which clearly shows that financial need was not the only reasons for them to work after retirement.

Figure18: Percentage Distribution of the Silver Workers according to their Type of Family

(N=300)

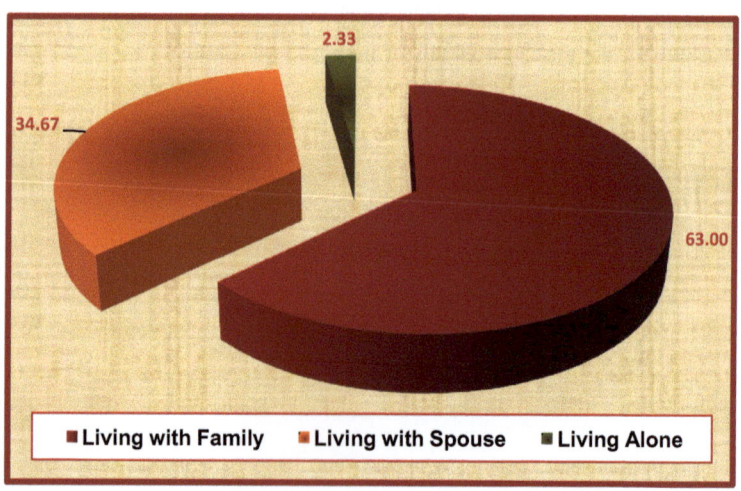

Figure 19: Percentage Distribution of the Silver Workers according to their Marital Status

(N=300)

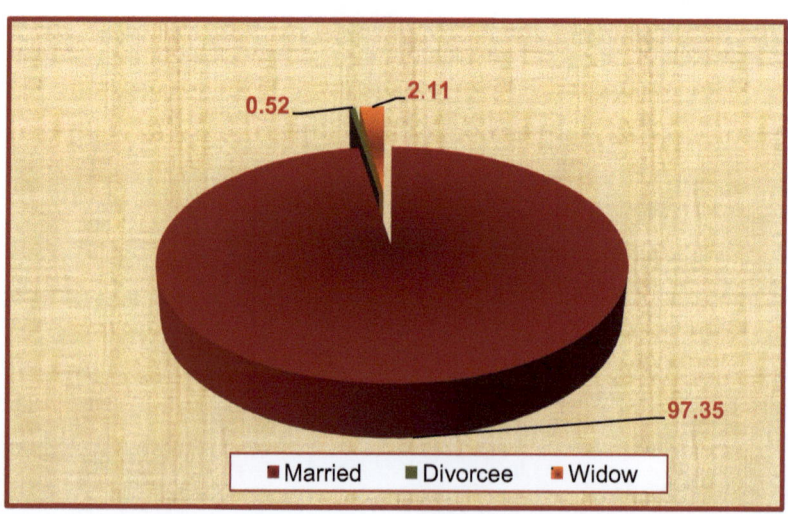

Figure 20: Percentage Distribution of the Silver Workers according to their Size of Family

(N=300)

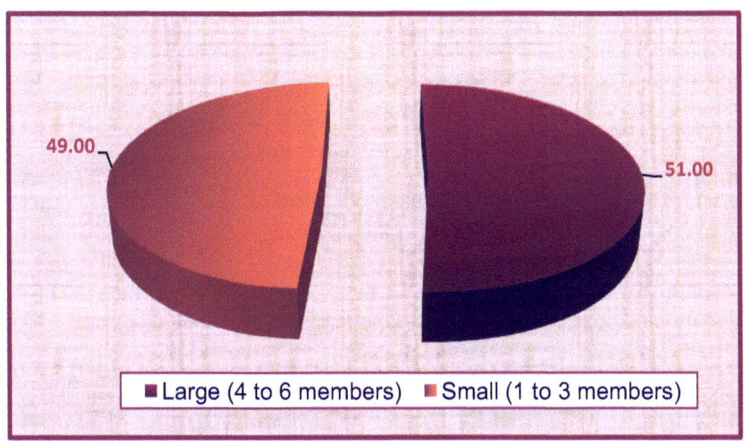

Figure 21: Percentage Distribution of the silver workers according to the Educational Qualification of Spouse (Husband)

(N=6)

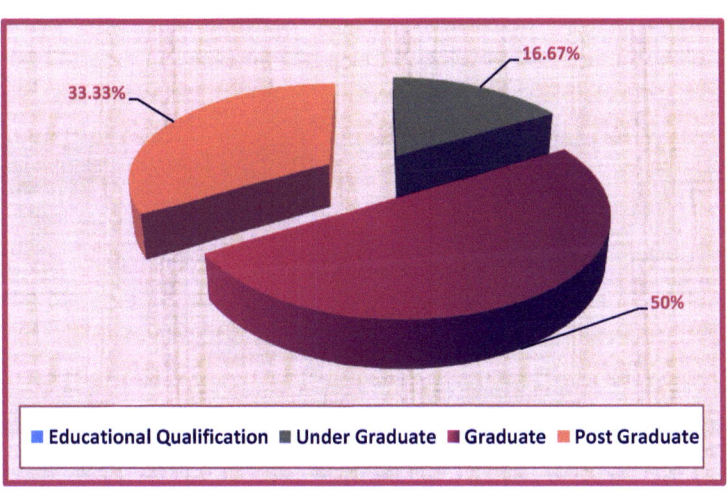

Figure 22: Percentage Distribution of the Silver Workers according to the Educational Qualification of Spouse (Wife)

(N=282)

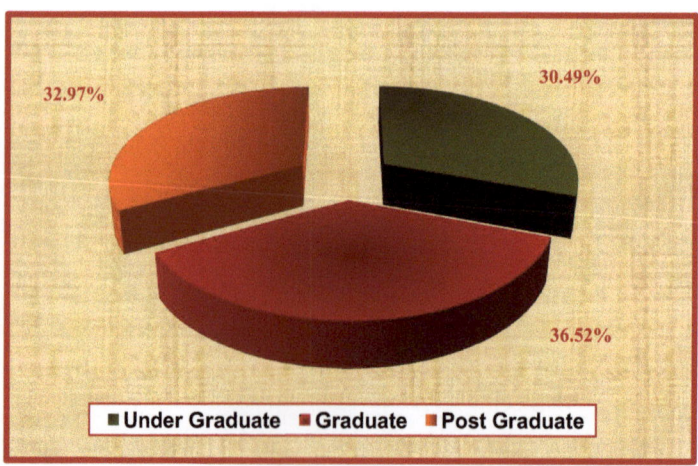

Figure 23: Percentage Distribution of the Silver Workers according to the Occupational Status of Spouse (Husband)

(N=6)

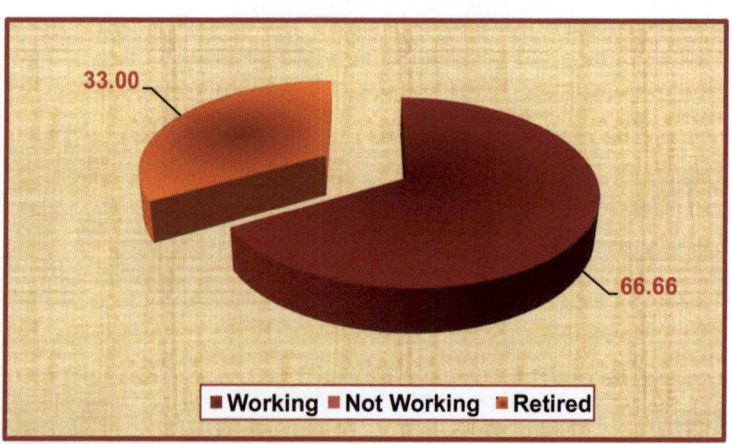

Figure 24: Percentage Distribution of the Silver Workers according to the Occupational Status of Spouse (Wife)

(N=282)

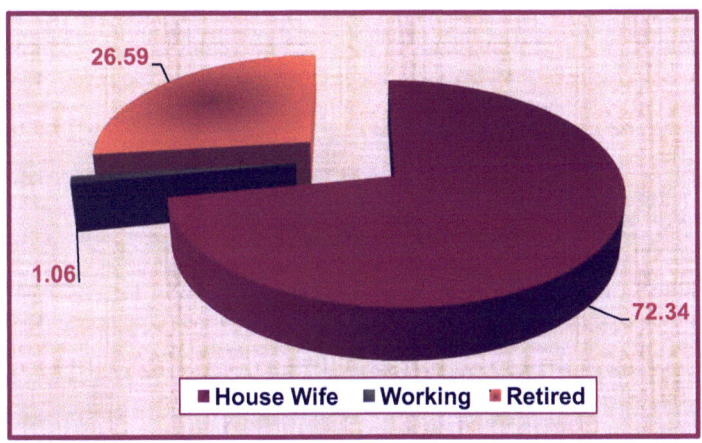

Figure 25: Percentage Distribution of the Silver Workers according to the Marital Status of the Son

(N=314)

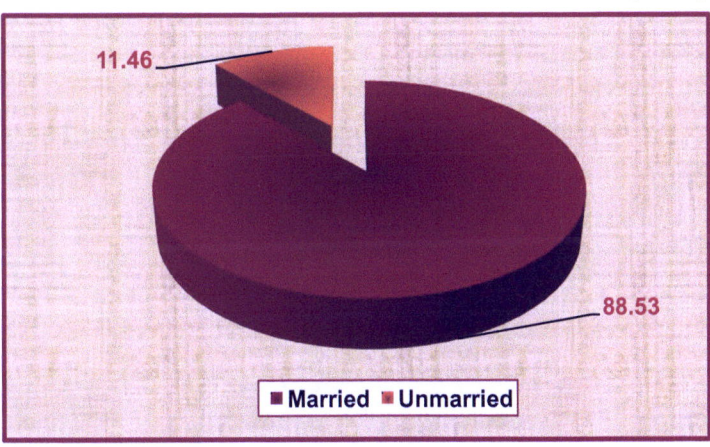

Figure 26: Percentage Distribution of the Silver Worker according to the Marital Status of Daughter

(N=206)

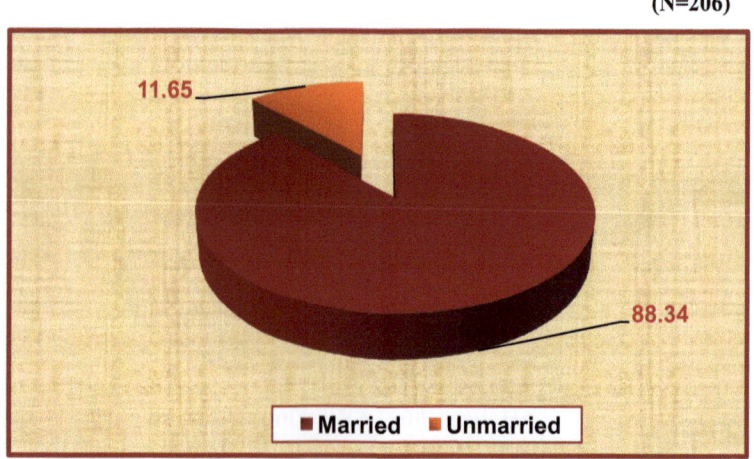

Figure 27: Percntage Distribution of the Silver Workers according to the Occupational Status of the Son

(N=314)

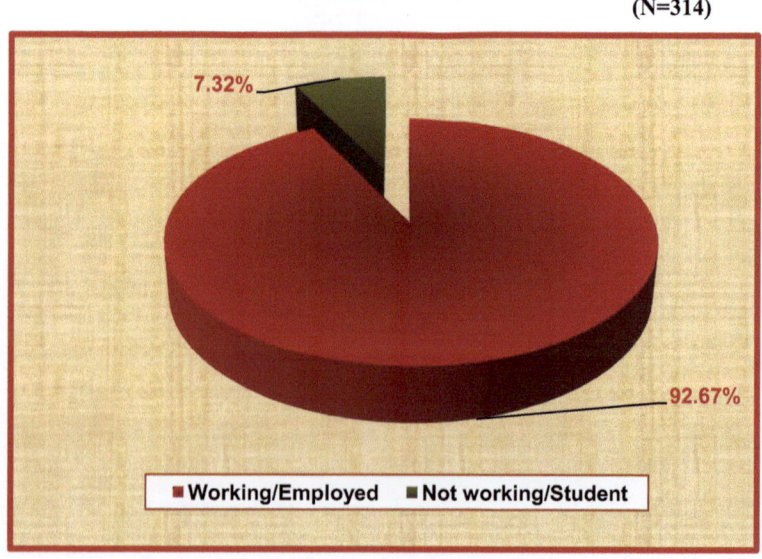

Figure 28: Percentage Distribution of the Silver Wokers according to the Occupational Status of the Daughters

(N=206)

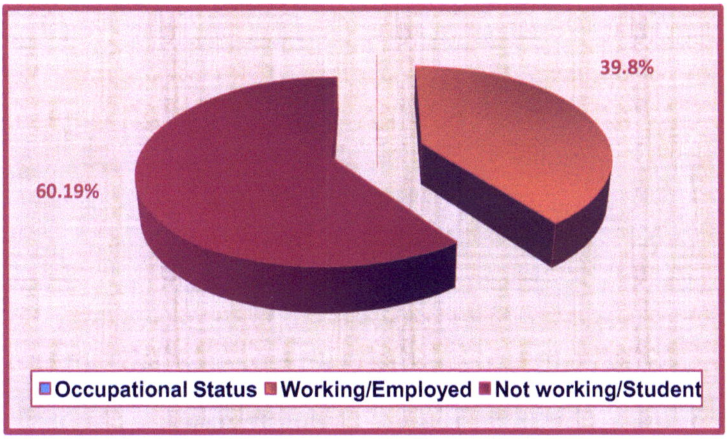

- 39.8%
- 60.19%
- ■ Occupational Status ■ Working/Employed ■ Not working/Student

Figure 29: Percentage Distribution of the Silver Wokers according to the Occupational Status of the Occupational Status of Daughter in Law

(N=278)

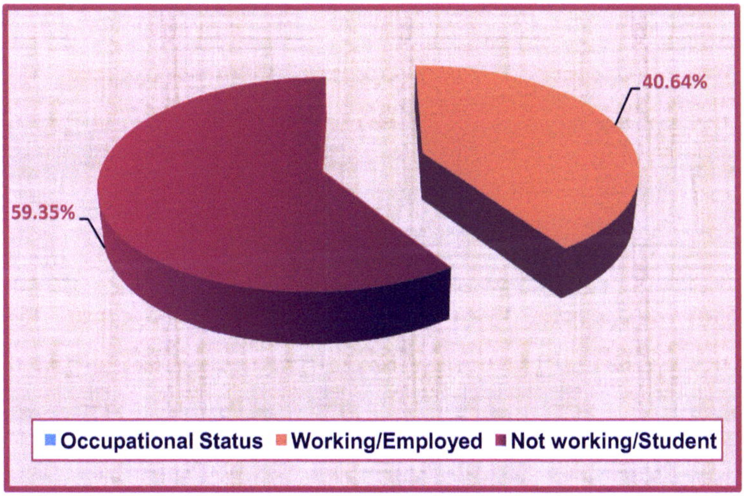

- 40.64%
- 59.35%
- ■ Occupational Status ■ Working/Employed ■ Not working/Student

Figure 30: Percentage Distribution of the Silver Workers according their Sources of Income

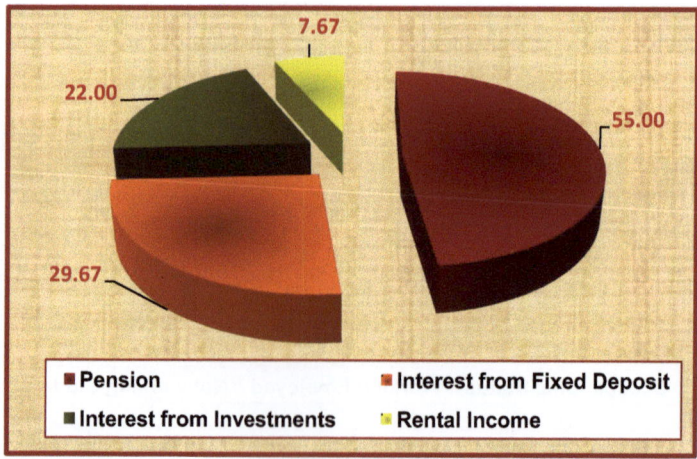

4.1.2 SILVER WORKERS AND THEIR PRESENT OCCUPATION

In previous section information about the personality of the silver workers is obtained from the data concerning the personal profile and comfort levels their social and economical condition, it would be useful to focus on their job profiles. While this section will look into the diversity in jobs after retirement where some workers who retire embark on a second full-time career, others work highly flexible hours and only when it suits them. In addressing this diversity, we will examine different aspects of the job, such as the nature of employment, the type of work, and earnings. We will also look at the quality of the job as perceived by persons engaged in jobs after retirement and compare this with the perceived quality in their former career jobs. We focus on flexibility, workload and job challenge.

Table 24: Percentage Distribution of the Silver Workers According to the Gap of time between the year of Retirement and the year of Joining Present Job

(N=300)

Gaps	F	%
No Gap (Same year)	123	41.00
Small Gap (Within 1 to 3 years)	142	47.33
Moderate Gap (Within 4 to 6 years)	28	9.33
More Gap (Beyond 6 years)	7	2.33

Table 24 and Figure 31 reflects on the profile of present job. To begin with the gap of time between retirement and the present employment, it shows that 41 percentages of the silver workers had got the present job within a year of the retirement. Little less than fifty percent (47.33%) of them got a job in a time span of 1 to 3 years. While nearly one tenth of the silver workers (9.33%) were employed in the present job in moderate gap. Lesser percent of them (2.33%) took more than six years to join the present job. It shows that high percentages of the silver workers started working in a new job within a year of their retirement.

To begin with, the first point that may be reviewed would be the time of their reemployment or the time gap between their retirement and new employment after retirement. As the data reveal, several of the silver workers had their search for jobs to end soon after the retirement and got a new job during the same year, so for them, the waiting was not very long, or it might be the reasons that they wanted to get back to work soon after retirement. For about half of them, the search for job prolonged little longer and ended with new employment in a small gap of one to three years. This reveals that for such silver workers it might have been difficult to search jobs soon after retirement. It is understood that the waiting was torturing to them. Or the other reason of joining work after this much gap can be a they wanted to spend some quality time with their family, or they were in search of work that was much according to their expectation.

A small number of them had a moderate gap of four to six years after their retirement when they got the present job. One can understand the extent of anxiety and depression he/she had to suffer during the time of waiting ,if this waiting was because of not finding the work .There is an American saying "Waiting is a torture" and it became the reality for a few of the silver workers who had a relatively longer waiting for job after retirement. One would, in fact, feel sympathy for such silver workers. We may understood that delay in getting new employment might have occurred on the consideration like low level of education and skills, lacking skills and capability for the job, unfavourable trends on job markets and the like or it can be the other way round like lack of jobs available for them according to their expertise, skills and education, as well in the city they live and according to their expectations, or because of age discrimination in the job market. The reasons behind joining jobs after long gap can be because they wanted to spend some quality time with their family before joining the next job after retirements as well as they were not in financial pressure to take up job just after retirement. However it passes a message that a silver workers with adequate knowledge skill and experience does not have to wait longer for new employment. Such people are always in demand as it said "there is always a room at top and the bottom is always overcrowded" .It also reveals that there are employers who give an opportunity to the silver workers to work post retirement and that is being proved from the results of the present study as many of them took up the jobs in very less gap after their retirement which proves that are employers who understands and value the experience and knowledge that silver workers possess and they know that by recruiting them they will have lot of advantage

Table 25: Percentage Distribution of the Silver Workers According to Organization they are working in after Retirement

(N=300)

Working Organization	F	%
Different	228	76.00
Same	72	24.00

Table 25 and Figure 32 revealed seventy six percentages of the silver workers joined different organization for the new jobs and less percent (24%) joined same organization as before retirement. This shows that there are organizations, companies, corporate who gives an opportunity to silver workers to continue working even after retirement.

From the data obtained through the survey about the present occupation of the silver workers, it is revealed that high majority of them were re-employed in different organizations and only about one fourth of them were appointed in their own organization. It explains that when a silver worker had to adjust in a place with new work environment and jobs to be performed, of course, with different expectations from the other side it might become a bit strenuous causing some kind of undue botheration on the silver workers. It naturally takes away from him/her ease of working, such a condition particularly at an age when there can be little of compromise and more of rigidity of human nature.

It can also be revealed from the findings that there are very few organizations, companies corporate, business houses who gives an opportunity to silver workers to continue working in the same organization after retirement, others have to struggle to find out jobs in different organization which becomes difficult, but with all the difficulties and obstacles also silver workers do find jobs and works in new environment ,with new people adjust themselves in every ways which show their willingness to continue working after retirement . At the same time to compromise and to work in new environment can be because of the financial crunch. In such situation and with many obstacles, the findings of the study revealed that silver workers took the new job as a challenge.

Table 26: Percentage Distribution of the Silver Workers According to their Employment Status

(N=300)

Employment Status	F	%
Temporary	119	39.67
Contract Basis	84	28.00
Permanent	52	17.33
Consultancy	45	15.00

Table 26 and Figure 33 shows that almost forty percentages (39.67%) of the silver workers were working on temporary basis and little less than thirty percent of them (28%) were working on contract basis. About eighteen percent of the silver workers were working on permanent basis and 15 percent of them were rendering the consultancy services. It shows that higher numbers of silver workers were working on temporary basis.

Employment status matters much to as or robs away workers ease and peace of mind. It is a general experience that when a person is employed on a permanent ground he/she feels sense of stability and security with assurance of steady source of income. For a working person in the present time of lot economic upheavals and high soaring prices, a permanent job would be most aspired arrangement for income. In this light, if an elderly person is employed after retirement in temporary or contract basis he/she is destined to difficult conditions of life. The data reveal that such was the destiny for more than two–third percent of them. For remaining one-third the condition was relatively better with permanent employment or a status of consultancy. It is understood that good education, level of skill and experience would make such status of employment possible for a person. So the overall picture of the psychology of the silver worker project anxiety, tension botheration feeling of insecurity, unsteadiness and a kind of fear of probable retrenchment from jobs any time. The findings also revealed that that there are very less organization who recruit the silver workers on permanent basis after retirement, which might cause insecurity for silver workers, as they always have to work under pressure and they might develop a feeling of insecurity of losing the job.

Table 27: Percentage Distribution of the Silver Workers According to the Type of Organization

(N=300)

Type of Organization	F	%
Private Organizations like Hospitals, Educational Institutes, Service Industries, Business houses, Corporate, Banks, Agencies, Firms	297	99.00
Government like Educational Institutions	3	1.00

Table 27 and Figure 34 revealed that a very high majority (99%) of the silver workers were working in private organizations and only one percent of the silver workers were reemployed in government educational institutions .Among those working in private organizations, 22 percentages of them were working in firms, 15 percent in corporate offices and little less than 10 percentages (7.67%) were working in agencies. Almost 5 percent (4.67%) of them were working in business house. Thus it shows that high percentages of the silver workers were working after retirement in non-government/private sectors after retirement.

The data obtained about the type organizations which the silver workers are employed after retirement .It can be revealed from above table that only three of them were employed at government organizations and all of them were educational institutions. A very huge majority of almost 294 silver workers were employed at private organisations that included hospitals, schools, private banks and colleges, corporate, business houses, firms. It can also be revealed that private organization recruit the silver workers or give them a chance to continue working in the same organization after retirement, such positions and opportunities should be created by government organizations too as the finding shows that in comparison to private organization there are very less government organization who recruit silver workers after retirement..

Table 28: Percentage Distribution of the Silver Workers According to the Type of Work they are doing

(N=300)

Type of Work	F	%
Full Time	184	61.33
Part Time	116	38.67

Table 28 and Figure 35 shows that the majority of silver workers (61.33%) were employed on full time basis, whereas little less than forty percent of them were employed on part time basis. It shows that high percent of the silver workers preferred to work on the full time basis.

It was further revealed that majority (sixty percent) of the silver workers were employed on full time jobs and about forty percent of them had part time jobs. Such a situation again reflects on the resultant financial comfort for majority of them and the resultant financial constraints for the minority. In cases like those who had permanent jobs on full time basis prior to retirement, being employed on part time basis would be a matter of dissatisfaction and discomfort.

Table 29: Percentage Distribution of the Silver Workers According to their Present Designation

(N=300)

Designation	F	%
Class I	27	9.00
Class II	190	63.33
Class III	71	23.67
Class IV	12	4.00

Table 29 and Figure 36 shows that less than one tenth (9%) of the silver workers were employed as class I officers. Majority (63.33%) of silver workers were employed in the designation of the class II officers and little more than one fifth (23.67%) were working as the class III officers. While 4 percent of them were working on class IV designation.

From the above table feeling recorded in the matter of designation on which the silver workers work after retirement. If we compare the relevant data regarding the jobs prior to and after retirement, we may notice that a good number of them who were working on the class I designation are employed after retirement on the class II designation and a few of them are lucky to get same designation.

Designation is mark of recognition of work that a worker had performed in the benefit of organization. It is a kind of reward for his/her commitment to work and dedication to his/her profession, designation implies confidence, power and some kind of ego on the part of a worker who holds. After holding higher designation throughout career if a person is employed after retirement on a lower designation, he/she may feel deeply hurt at lack of recognition to his/her knowledge, efficiency and experience by his/her new employer. But finding him/her in helpless condition after retirement he/she is unable to speak out his/her dissatisfaction, but forced to suppress it. To the contrary results of the study revealed that in spite of holding higher designations before retirement many of the silver workers accepted the jobs with lower designation after retirement which shows their willingness to work and nature of adjustment which is good sign. This shows that silver workers were giving more importance to the work offered to them rather than the designation.

Table 30: Percentage Distribution of the Silver Workers According to Their Type of Designation

(N=300)

Type of Designation	F	%
Different	216	72.00
Same	84	28.00

Table 30 and Figure 37 reveals that seventy two percent (72%) of the silver workers were not reemployed with the same designation as before retirement .Whereas 28 percent of them were however appointed on the same designation that they had before the retirement. It reveals that higher percentages of the silver workers did not have to compromise with their designations which they used to hold before the retirement.

Table 31: Percentage Distribution of the Silver Workers According to their Present Salary and Type of Salary

(N=300)

Salary (In Rupees)						Type of Salary					
Lower Salary (Less than 17,000 Rupees)		Moderate Salary (17,000 Rupees)		Higher Salary (More than 17,000 Rupees)		Fixed		Consolidated		On the basis of work	
F	%	F	%	F	%	F	%	F	%	F	%
145	48.33	22	7.33	133	44.33	227	75.67	52	17.33	21	7.00

Table 31 and Figure 38 reveals those little less than 50 percentages (48.33%) of the silver workers were getting lower salaries. While less than one tenth (7.33) of them were getting moderate salaries. Almost forty five percentages of them were paid higher salaries receiving higher salary in their present jobs.

The table further indicates that majority of (75.67%) of the silver workers were paid fixed salaries and little less than one fifth of them were paid consolidated salaries. The remaining 7 percentages of them were paid salaries on the basis of work they do. It clearly shows that higher percentages of silver workers were getting fixed amount as the salaries for the post retirement employment.

In the matter of salary and this feeling may stay close to the reality that a person faces in life after retirement. It may further be intensified with anxiety and tension caused with financial constraints that one may faces. The relevant data reveal that the silver workers were paid salaries of the types like fixed, consolidated and on the basis of work. None of them were appointed on a graded scale of salary. In view of the amount of salary majority of them were paid salary higher than 17000 rupees and lower than it. A small number of them were paid the salary of rupees 17000 per month. The amount of the salary would reflect that they would afford moderate standard of living. When the present salary goes in addition to the present income from pension, interest from investments etc, it would be good enough for decent life. Findings of the study also revealed that silver workers did not rejected the jobs due to lower salaries , but they accepted it which shows that they were not doing the present jobs due to financial crunch, or they did not had baggage of attitude, they had compromising nature which is very much required to sustain in job market.

Table 32: Percentage Distribution of the Silver Workers According to Duties Performed by them Prior to Retirement and in their Present Job

(N=300)

Duties	Prior to Retirement		In Present Job	
	F	%	F	%
Executive/Managerial /Administrative	217	72.33	235	78.33
Technical	71	23.76	53	17.67
Clerical /Sales	12	4.00	12	4.00

Table 32 anf Figure 40, 41 show that high majority (72.33%) of silver workers performed executive /managerial/administrative duties as the part of their job before retirement. Whereas little more than one fifth percentages of them reported that they were performing technical duties and remaining 4 percentages of them used to perform clerical or sales duties in their job.

The table further shows that comparatively higher majority (78.33%) of the silver workers were performing executive /managerial or administrative duties for their present job. Whereas eighteen percent of them were performing technical duties. The remaining 4 percent of them continued with clerical or sales duties in their present jobs.

Making comparisons is a common tendency for a person who is reemployed. The silver workers fall into this category when they are employed after retirement. Reflecting on this tendency, the data reveal a mixed picture for the most of the duties the silver workers were performing. Prior to retirement, 217 of them performed executive, managerial or administrative duties, while the number was higher for such silver workers. For technical jobs, the number went down from 71 to 53 of them and for clerical/sales jobs the number remained unchanged.

Table 33: Percentage Distribution of the Silver Workers According to the Type of Duties Performed as the part of Present Job

(N=300)

Type of Duties	F	%
Different than before Retirement	177	59.00
Same as before Retirement	123	41.00

Table 33 and Figure 42 shows that in comparison to their pre retirement jobs, little less than sixty percentages (59%) of silver workers were performing different duties, whereas 41 percentages of them were performing same duties. It further indicates that the silver workers could perceive some kind of transition after retirement. This indicated that silver workers perceive the transition to retirement as clear cut in life. It can be a sign of a change of the role after the retirement. The silver workers appeared to feel that they would not get the similar kind of work after retirement.

The second point of comparison is type of duties they performed in the present job. Majority of the silver worker informed that they were supposed to do different work than the duties they had performed before retirement. More than forty percent of them felt relieved that they were employed for similar kind of work after retirement. In this sense, the comfort level among more of them was relatively lower and for some of them it remained good enough. It can be revealed from the findings that in spite of having different kind of duties they took up the job as a challenge, this shows that they were having the readiness to learn new skills required for the job. It also shows that employers also recruited such silver workers who were not having specific experiences but were ready to take up the job and learn new skills. It is very important for the silver workers to be open minded and to accept the changes, they should have the readiness to learn new skill and undergo the training if required, if they really want to work post retirement and data of the study shows that there are silver workers who were ready to learn, which show a positive sign on the part of silver workers, it shows their willingness to work

Table 34: Percentage Distribution of the Silver Workers According to their Working Hours Per Day

(N=300)

Working Hours	F	%
2 to 4 hours	107	35.67
8 hours	175	58.33
More than 8 hours	18	6.00

Table 34 and Figure 43 displays the data to indicate that almost 36 percentages (35.67%) of the silver workers were working between 2 to 4 hours in a day. Nearly sixty percentages (58.33%) of them were working for 8 hours in a day and remaining few percentages of the silver workers were working for more than 8 hours per day.

When inquired about the duration that they were supposed to work in the new employment, the data record that good majority of them were supposed to work for eight hours a day and about one third of them had to work for 2 to 4 hours which means part time jobs. Only eighteen of them had to work for more than eight hours which may indicate some kind of compulsion or exploitation in the present job. It can also be the other way that in spite of working after retirement many of the silver workers opted to work for full time. This shows that they still have that much physical and mental capacity to work for longer hours and they are not tired of being employed or to work for many hours. This also insists us to think that are they doing this job willingly for these long hours? Or is it just out of compulsion as they are not able to get jobs with fewer hours they have taken this job. Or is there any kind of pressure from family like ignorance, financial pressure, due to which they prefer to remain out with the reason of work

Table 35: Percentage Distribution of the Silver Workers According to the Distance of their Workplace

(N=300)

Distance of Workplace	F	%
Short Distance (1 to 6 Kms)	183	61.00
Long Distance (6 to 20 Kms)	117	39.00

Table 35 and Figure 44 shows that majority (61%) of the silver workers used to travel for 1 to 6 kilometres to reach their workplaces. Whereas nearly forty percent of them had to travel for about 6 to 20 kilometres. The table reveals that majority of the silver workers preferred to opt for job/work at places nearer to their residence.

The silver workers were also asked about how much they have to travel to reach the places of work. The data reveal in the proportion of 60-40 percent that the majority of them have to travel a short distance of 1 to 6 kilometres from their residences and the minority of them have to travel long distance of more than 6 kilometres to 20 kilometres. It reflects that for most of them, reaching the places of work was not much strenuous.

Table 36: Percentage Distribution of the Silver Workers According to the People who helped them in getting Present Job/Work

(N=300)

Helped in Getting Job	F	%
Self Initiative (Active Search/News Advertisements/ Websites/Internet Browsing)	101	33.67
Colleagues	98	32.67
Friends	63	21.00
Family Members	33	11.00
Relatives	5	1.67

The silver workers were asked about how they procured the present job. What they narrated unfolded interesting facts about their search of jobs after retirement. All the silver workers (100%) said that the present job was their first job after the retirement. As the table 36 and Figure 45 reveals one third of the silver workers (33.67%) got the jobs with their own initiatives and little less than that percentage (32.67%) of silver workers got the present job with help of their colleagues. Whereas one fifth percent of them got the jobs with their friends help. 11 percentages of them were helped by their families for the present job. Very less (1.67%) percent of the silver workers admitted that they got the present jobs with the help of their relatives.

The story is radically different from a story of a fresh candidate's search for a job. In fact, searching for a job is not an easy going activity specifically when job markets are tight huge supply against limited openings for jobs and the expectations too very much. The result is unemployment for many aspiring young candidates causing depression in them. The story of the silver workers search for jobs after retiring too remained difficult as reported by majority of the silver workers. For a small number of them, the search did not remain much difficult. These findings throw the light on the struggle that a silver worker had to go through in spite of having so many years of experience and knowledge they find it difficult to search jobs.

Table 37: Overall Intensity Indices and Percentage wise Distribution of the Silver Workers According to the Problems they faced in Searching Jobs after Retirement

(N=300)

Problems	Intesity Indices
Lack of advertisements for jobs	2.53
Lack of jobs suiting to their expertise/abilities	2.47
Lack of organizations who would be ready to recruit silver workers	2.46
Lack of jobs to suit to the according to qualifications	2.32
Lack of jobs to suit their past experience	2.24
Lack of jobs offering the same designation	2.18
Lack of jobs in the city they live	2.04
Lack of jobs with salary similar to what they were getting earlier	1.96

Table 37 is significantly reflecting on the overall intensity indices addressing problems that the silver workers faced while searching jobs after retirement. The indices which ranged from 2.53 to 1.96.It indicate high and medium level of agreement on the mentioned items referring to problems that the silver workers confronted, while searching jobs.

According to what is projected through the above table, there was high level of agreement among the silver workers on the problems that they confronted while searching jobs after retirement are specified below:

- Lack of advertisements for jobs
- Lack of jobs suiting to their expertise/abilities
- Lack of organizations who would be ready to recruit silver workers
- Lack of jobs to suit to the qualifications

The table further projects that there prevailed medium level of agreement among the silver workers on the following specific problems while searching jobs after retirement.

- Lack of jobs to suit their past experience
- Lack of jobs offering the same designation
- Lack of jobs in the city they live
- Lack of jobs with salary similar to what they were getting

The silver workers were asked about how they obtained information about the present jobs. Almost one third of them informed that they knew about the present jobs. They tried on their own initiative to search for the jobs in number of ways like searching through jobs advertisements, surfing relevant websites, browsing the internet and the like. This shows their search remained very active and it reflects the extent of exposure to job markets and positive approach to compute application to explore even the electronic media for the purpose. About half of the silver workers admitted that they learnt about the present jobs from their colleagues and friends and a small number of them were helped by their families and friends to get the present jobs. The status reflects that a good number of them searched the present job on their own or they got the help form their colleagues.

It is understood that getting a job and agreeing to what was available to them would also be bit problematic. The reasons would be difference between what one used to be getting and what would be getting, which means difference between expectation and actual gain. As it reveals from their responses, the problems that they confronted varied from greater to lesser extent and the variation is indicated in form of intensity indices too.

As it reveals from the data presented that silver workers faced problems to greater extent in matters like finding advertisement for jobs and finding jobs suitable to their skills and capabilities. Further, a few organizations showed inclination to employ silver workers. Further, for those holding post graduate degrees, it was a big problem to get jobs suiting to their qualification and they had to be ready to compromise and take up jobs of lower calibre. Such compromise is expected for silver workers who desire to work after retirement.

The silver workers further admitted that they faced problems to some extent in matters like getting jobs suitable to their experience, similar designations offered to them, jobs locally available in the same city they live in and jobs with similar salaries .Such problems were expected in relation with employment after retirement and the silver workers were supposed to agree to the offers made to them if they really desired to work after retirement. This findings revealed number of problems that the silver workers faced while searching jobs after retirement. It is clearly understood that the problems occur because of lack of job opportunities, lack of government and private organization who recruit silver workers after retirement, lack of job advertisements, this all things should taken into consideration to make work for silver workers smooth and comfortable after retirement..

The table indicates it was not easy for the silver workers to search for and get suitable job after the retirement to suit their experiences, status, location and reward. It seemed that they had to compromise to some extent on these matters.

Table 38: Percentage Distribution of the Silver Workers According to Procuring the Present Job

(N=300)

Procuring Job	F	%
Difficult	221	73.67
Easy	79	26.33

In the light of above table 38 and Figure 46 indicates that majority of the silver workers (73.67%) faced difficulties in getting the present jobs and just one fifth percent of them (26.33%) got the present jobs bit easily. It makes it clear that it finding jobs after the retirement posed problems for the silver workers

Table 39: Percentage Distribution of the Silver Workers According to Social Security Benefits that they receive from their Present Job

(N=300)

Social Security Benefits	F	%
Receive	220	73.33
Do not Receive	80	26.67

Table 39 and Figure 47 shows that the majority of silver workers (73.33%) were receiving social security benefits from their present employment and nearly twenty seven percent of them (26.67%) said they do not receive social security benefits from the present jobs. Thus, for majority of them the benefits of social security was made available to them by their present employer.

In the context, social security would be significant expectation for each working person. Since such person lacks back up of property in form of land buildings or wealth he expects that his employers would help him/her to arrange for some provision for future through floating for them schemes of provident funds, medical benefits, house rent allowance, city compensatory allowance, conveyance allowance, leave travel, benefits and also benefits of normal leave, sick leaves, privilege leave etc. The government regulations for employment make it obligatory for employers that they avail these benefits to their employers. When inquired a good majority of three fourth of the silver workers informed with sense of relief that social security benefits were made available to them and the fourth part of them did not avail social security benefits on the present jobs.

Table 40: Percentage Distribution of the Silver Workers According to their Reasons for Working on the Present Job

(N=300)

Reasons	F	%
Money	220	73.33
Self respect	220	73.33
To earn good reputation in society	186	62.00
Opportunity to do quality work	167	55.67
Respect in family	158	52.67
Opportunity to use education	151	50.33
Friendly work environment	138	46.00
Opportunity to develop new skills	132	44.00
Freedom to share views	129	43.00
Good health benefits	127	42.33
Flexibility in work timings	124	41.33
Respect from co-workers	117	39.00
Good pension plan	60	20.00

One question may hover in anyone's mind why the silver worker thought in their advance age to work. Table 40 and Figure 48 shows the reasons that prompted the silver workers to work after retirement. Money and self respect were perceived as the most important reasons for silver workers (73.33%) to work on present job. While 62 percent of them earning good reputation in society remained the consideration. Fifty five percent of them expected an opportunity to perform quality work. They were followed by those who hoped respect in family (52.67%) and looked for more opportunities to use education (50.33%).Further the other reasons that prompted the silver workers for the present jobs included those like, friendly work environment (46%), getting opportunity to develop new skills (44%) , freedom to share views (43%), earning good health benefits(42.33%), enjoying flexibility in work timings (41.33%) ,earning respect from co-workers (39%) and availing good pension plans (20%) as their reasons for doing present job. The overall projection indicates that for silver workers reasons like money and self respect remained the priority for working after retirement.

The reasons that emerged from the responses of the silver workers bring forth interest considerations on their past. Economic reasons and personal reasons remained top priority among good majority of them. Considerations related to social respect and reputation and those of quality and education remained secondary priority to them. Other considerations like friendly work environment, skill development, sharing views, health benefits, flexible work schedule and expecting respect from co-workers received kind of preferences from some of them. Pension plan remained low priority to them as they were perhaps aware that for a person once retired would not be so important to think.

Table 41: Percentage Distribution of the Silver Workers According to their Expectations to Work after Retirement

(N=300)

Work after Retirement	F	%
Expected	255	85.00
Did not Expect	45	15.00

Table 41 and Figure 49 shows on the attitude of the silver workers to work after the retirement that very high majority of silver workers (85%) reported that even prior to their retirement; they had expected that they would work after retirement. Only 15 percent of them did not expect to work after retirement. This reveals that high majority of the silver workers had expectations and plan to work after the retirement even before the retirement.

Table 42: Percentage Distribution of the Silver Workers According to Work they expected to do after Retirement

(N=300)

Current Work	F	%
As expected	243	81.00
Not as expected	57	19.00

Table 42 and Figure 50 specify that very high percentages of the silver workers (81%) were currently doing the work as per their expectation. Whereas only 19 percent of them stated that the present jobs were not up to their expectations. It indicates that high percentages of silver workers were satisfied with their present jobs and some of them had to do some kind of compromise for the present jobs.

Expectation is basic human instinct and no one can escape it. As long as a person lives and works his/her expectation is closely knit to what he/she does. It is popularly believed that an expectation is kinetic energy that pushes a person to work and it gives him/her direction too. It is with expectation that a person keeps hope for desirable results. In worldly sense, expectation is a booster to energy to work. Further, expectation may arise for a person's needs and intensity of one's needs determine intensity of his/her expectations. This may be true about the silver workers, because when they decide to work after retirement it might be because of needs and their intensity that prompt them to work even after retirement. When asked, a very high majority of them admitted that they expected to work after retirement and for a very small number of them it was beyond their expectations, as the situation turned for them abruptly. They were further asked about their expectations of the present work as to, was it to their expectations? Again a high majority of them said that they got a work up to their expectations and seemed to be bit satisfied with the present job. For some of them, the work was against their expectations and they had to compromise on this point. As they knew it was not so easy to get jobs after retirement.

Table 43: Percentage Distribution of the Silver Workers According to the Lacunas noticed in the Present Job as compared to the Previous Jobs before Retirement

(N=300)

Lacunas in Present Job	F	%
Work ethics and system of working	128	42.67
Work environment	54	18.00
Work timings	42	14.00
Old colleagues/friends at workplace	40	13.33
Respect given to the employees by the co-workers and employers	36	12.00

Table 43 and Figure 51 shows nearly 43 percentages of the silver workers reported that they miss work ethics and system of working in the present jobs while comparing it with their job before retirement. While 18 percent of them stated that they missed the working environment in their present jobs. Whereas 14 percent of them reported to miss the work timings and almost equal percent of them reported that (13.33%) they missed earlier colleagues/friends at new workplace. Whereas 12 percent of silver workers felt a bit sensitive about missing the respect given to an employee by co-workers and employers .The table clearly reveals a kind of regret and dissatisfaction faced by the silver workers about the subjective apprehension in the new work environment

It does not happen always that a person's expectations are fully met and he/she is fully satisfied always. Such things are rare in human life. In case like silver workers, one may not hope that their expectations are fully realized. As they compared their present situation with the situations prior to the retirement, they were bound to find some kind of lacunas in the situations of the present jobs. They admitted about them in their responses. Several of them specified lacunas of work ethics and system of working. Some of them mentioned about lacunas in work environment at places of work. Some complained about lacunas of timing of work and some mentioned about old colleagues and friends at workplaces. Some of them even spoke about lacunas in respect that they received from their co-workers and employers.

Table 44: Percentage Distribution of the Silver Workers According to Passion for the Present Work

(N=300)

Extent	F	%
Great Extent	176	58.67
Some Extent	79	26.33
Less Extent	45	15.00

Table 44 reveals that almost 60 percent (58.67%) of silver workers showed passion for the present work. Little more than 25 percent of them showed passion in some extent. Very less 15 percent of them showed lesser extent of passion for the present work. The table indicates that though in second innings the silver workers showed relatively good passion for work and still they do their work with same passion as they did it before retirement.

Further, the data reveal surprising fact about passion for work that silver workers mentioned in view of their present job. According to it, a good majority of them felt great passion for present work, may it be out of compulsion or preferences. About one fourth of them showed some passion for the present work and a small number were found less passionate about work. It indicates that majority of them believed in performing jobs with good or at least some interest. They seemed to understand the situation they were facing in grown up age and what remained for them to compromise willingly or unwillingly. It sounds to be practical attitude on their part. Further, good number of them expressed that the present work was very important to them. Giving reasons for it, they admitted that the present work rendered to them good financial support, kept them active and fit and earned them social respect to some extent so they showed great passion for it.

Table 45: Percentage Distribution of the Silver Workers According to the Current Retirement Benefits Received

(N=300)

Retirement Benefits	F	%
Pension	165	55.00
Health Benefits	122	40.67
Security Benefits	13	4.33

Table 45 and Figure 52 shows that in new employment little more than half of silver workers (55%) were receiving benefits of pension and 40.67 percent of them were receiving health benefits. A very few percent of them said that they were receiving security benefits.

Table 46: Percentage Distribution of the Silver Workers According Importance of their Present Work

(N=300)

Present Work	F	%
Very Important	136	45.33
Equally Important	93	31.00
Less Important	71	23.67

Table 46 and Figure 53 reveals that high percentages of silver workers (45.33%) reported that their present work was very important. While 31 percentages of them reported that their work in present is equally important as their work in past .Less percent of them (23.67%) reported that their present work assignment is not so important. This shows that majority of the silver workers attached equal importance to their present work in view of their work before retirement.

Table 47: Percentage Distribution of the Silver Workers According to Age they think appropriate for their Second Retirement (age when they will be financially able to Retire from full/part time Work for pay)

(N=300)

Age of Re-Retirement	F	%
Want to continue working till health permits (it's important to remain active.)	104	34.67
Working post retirement till an employer allows to share knowledge and experiences and not for financial gains.	86	28.67
Never want to retire as the earning is not enough	62	20.67
By the age of 70 years	37	12.33
By the age of 65 years	11	3.67

Table 47 and Figure 54 shows that nearly 35 percentages (34.67%) of the silver workers stated that they would like to continue working till health permits as to kill time it's important for them to remain active. While almost 30 percent (28.67%) of them shared that they were working post retirement basically to share their knowledge and experience with others and not for financial gains. So they wish to continue working till there would employers allow them. Further it was revealed that one fifth percent (20.67%) expressed that since their earning was not enough they will continue working. While some of them (12.33%) stated that they would like to work up to 70 years of age and few (3.67%) said that they would prefer to work up to 65 years of age. It clearly shows that regardless of age and financial needs and gains high percent of the silver workers stressed the reasons like to remain healthy and active while deciding to continue work.

When there is matter related to employment, matters related to retirement do matter to capture one's mind. They include basically an age when a person would cease to be working and the benefits he would be liable to in view of his job and its tenure. The matter was raised to the silver workers in view of their second inning of working following the first retirement. Their responses are presented through the data according to which about one third of them expressed desire to work as long as their health permits, because it keeps them active. Some one-fourth of them preferred to leave it to their employers. Discretion and said as long as the employers would consider them valuable for their knowledge and experience they would feel like working. Money was not that important for them, but the fact that their knowledge and experience are respected would give them great satisfaction with sense that they would be able to contribute some part from them to growth and development of the human society. Some twenty percent of them showed desire never to be retired. The reason behind this might that they had so much of motivation to continue working, that they did not wanted to re-retire A very small number of them specified the age of retirement as 70 years(12.33%) and 65 years (3.67%) and ground if declining health in that phase of life

Table 48: Percentage Distribution of the Silver Workers According to the Extent of Appreciation they receive for the Present Work

(N=300)

Extent of Appreciation	F	%
Great Extent	67	22.33
Some Extent	104	34.67
Less Extent	129	43.00

Table 48 shows that nearly 23 percent (22.33%) of silver workers reported that they received appreciation for their present job on great extent. While almost 35 percent (34.67%) of them said that they received appreciation to some extent. High percent (43%) of them mentioned that they received lesser extent of appreciation for their present work. This clearly indicates that the silver workers were not satisfied with the amount of appreciation they were received for their work after the retirement.

Attached to gains or benefits is a point of appreciation of jobs by employers. Are employers appreciation is well reflected in gain or benefits released in favour of silver workers? The matter was revealed in the data presented. According to it, sixty seven silver workers expressed satisfaction about the employer's appreciation on greater extent and about one-third of them felt satisfied at receiving the employer appreciation to some extent. Good number of them gave out a tone of regret that they were appreciated by the employers on lesser extent. Thus it was indicated that for good majority of them the work was not appreciated and there prevailed among them a general feeling of dissatisfaction.

Table 49: Percentage Distribution of the Silver Workers According to the Extent they fulfil the Demands of Present Work

(N=300)

Demands of Work	F	%
Great Extent	176	58.67
Some Extent	88	29.33
Less Extent	36	12.00

Table 49 shows that almost 60 percent (58.67%) of the silver workers reported that they fulfil the demands of the present work to the greater extent and nearly 30 percent (29.33%) of them reported that they fulfil the demands to some extent. A very less percent of them (12%) reported to fulfil the demands of work to lesser extent. Such projection indicates self satisfaction on the part of majority of the silver workers.

Against it the survey revealed through the data that on greater extent majority of the silver workers fulfilled the demands in their present jobs. Some of them showed average performance and a small number of them could not fulfil the demands on reasonable grounds. The two picture project a scene that majority of the silver worker tried to perform the work in a better way so that the demands were fulfilled in appropriate manner, yet the employers failed to recognize their efficiency and dedication to the work.

Figure 31: Percentage Distribution of the Silver Workers according to the Gap between Retirement Year and Year of Joining Present Job

(N=300)

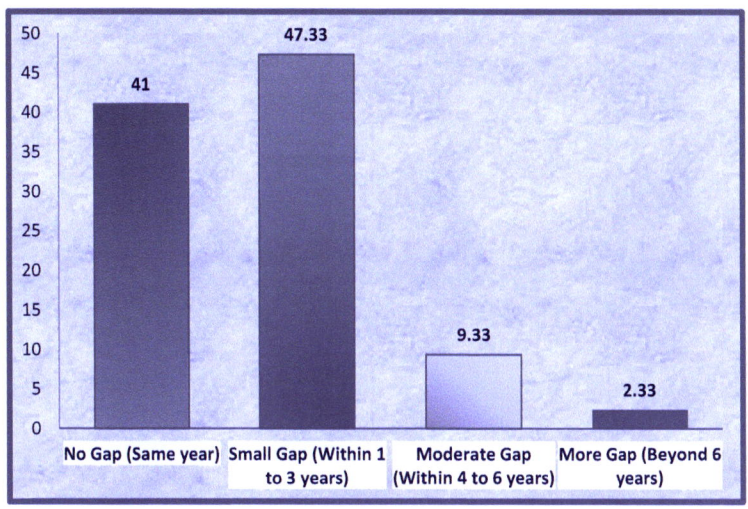

Figure 32: Percentage Wise Distribution of the Silver Workers According to Organization they are working in after Retirement

(N=300)

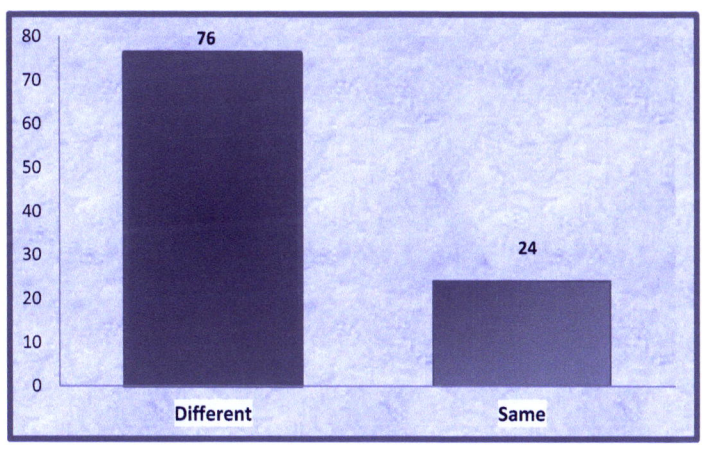

Figure 33: Percentage Distribution of the Silver Workers according to the Employment Status

(N=300)

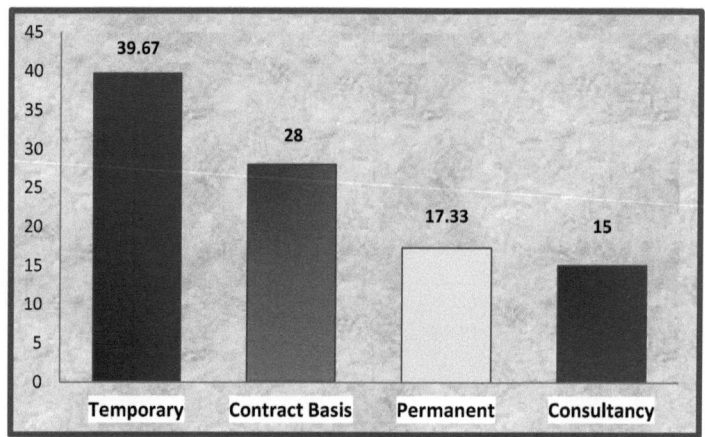

Figure 34: Percentage Distribution of the Silver Workers according to the Type of Organization

(N=300)

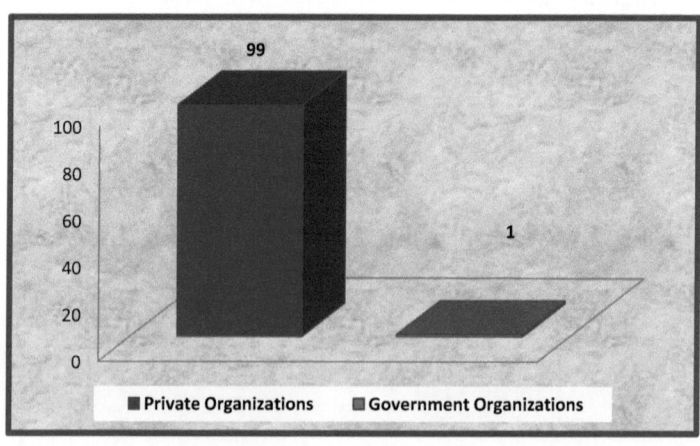

Figure 35: Percentage Distribution of the Silver Workers according to the Type of Work

(N=300)

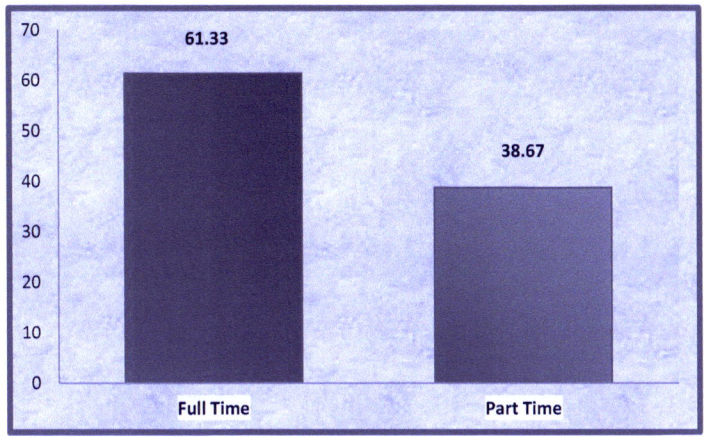

Figure 36: Percentage Distribution of the Silver Workers according to the Present Designation

(N=300)

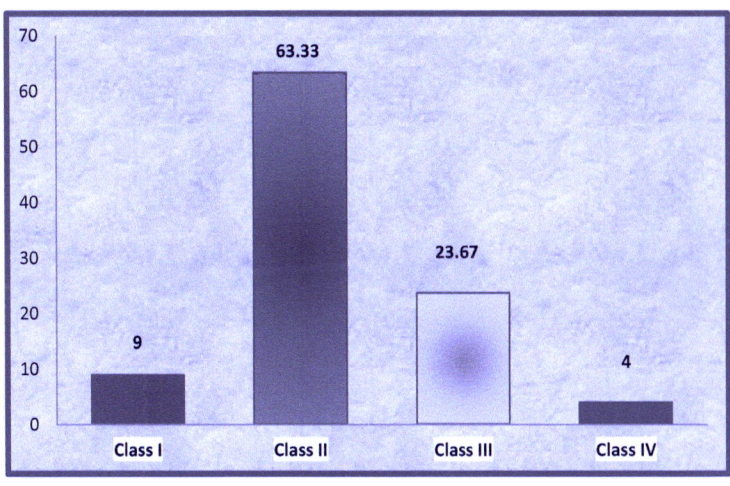

Figure 37: Percentage Distribution of the Silver Workers according to the Type of Designation

(N=300)

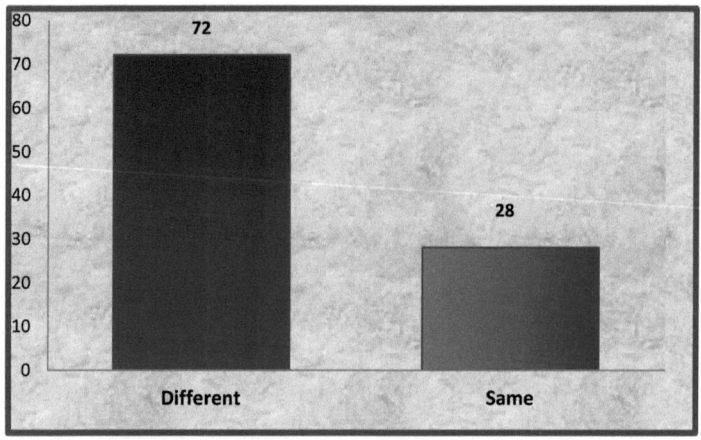

Figure 38: Percentage Distribution of the Silver Workers according to the Present Salary

(N=300)

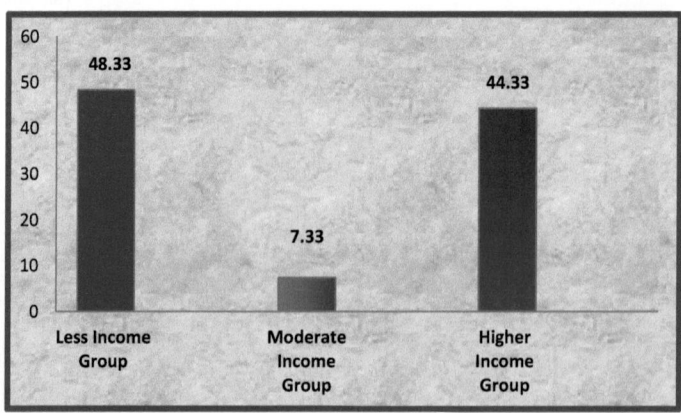

Figure 39: Percentage Distribution of the Silver Workers according to the Type of Salary

(N=300)

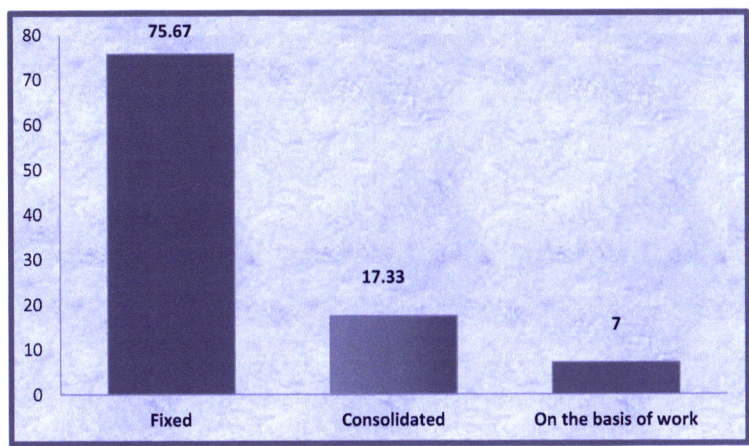

Figure 40: Percentage Distribution of the Silver Workers according to the Duties Performed before Retirement

(N=300)

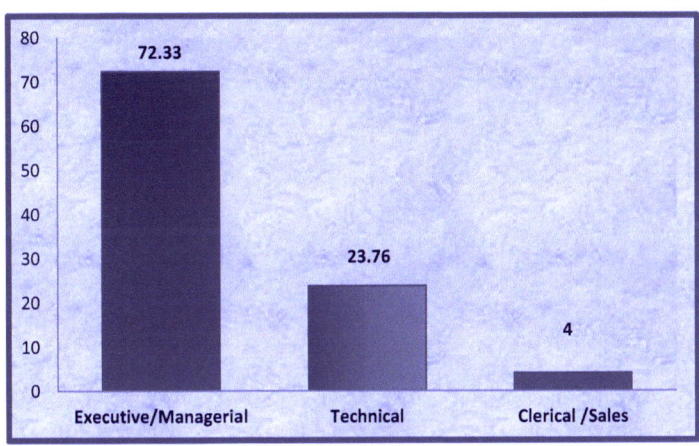

Figure 41: Percentage Distribution of the Silver Workers according to the Type of Duties Performed in Present Job

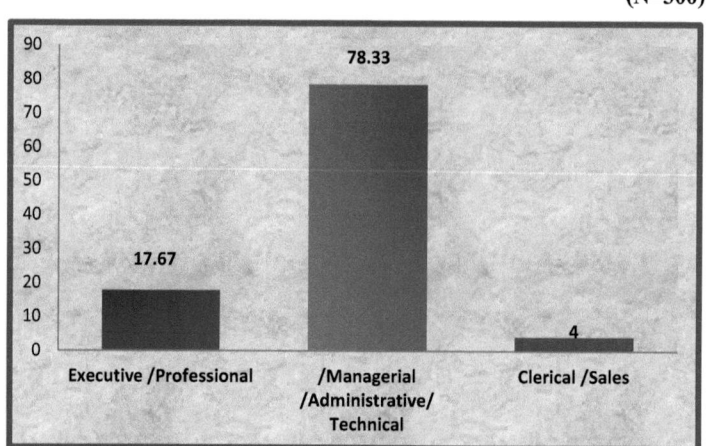

Figure 42: Percentage Distribution of the Silver Workers according to the Type of Duties Performed as Part of Present Job Wise

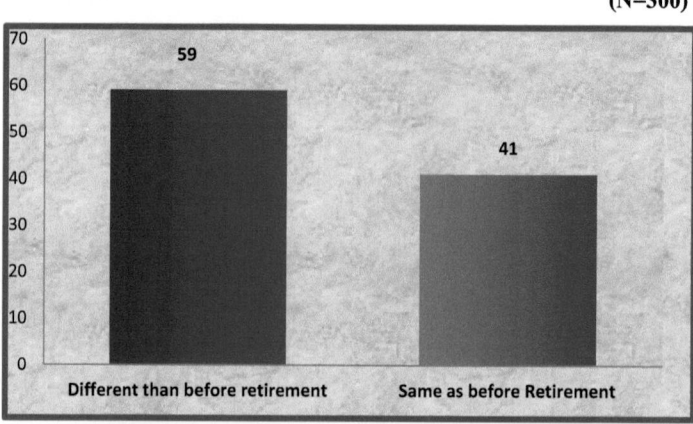

Figure 43: Percentage Distribution of the Silver Workers according to the Working Hours

(N=300)

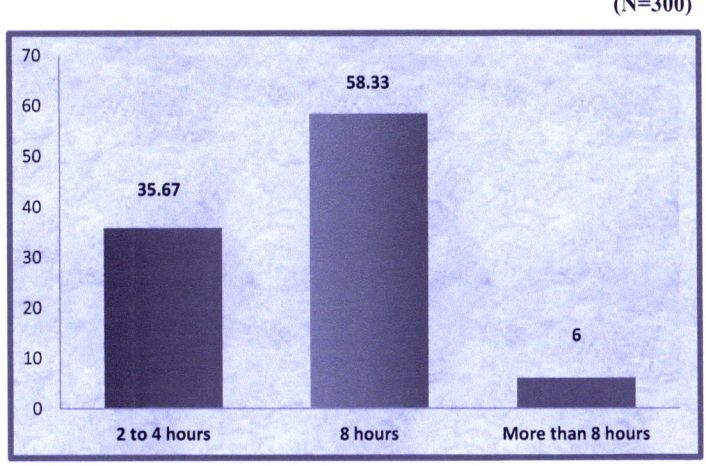

Figure 44: Percentage Distribution of the Silver Workers according to the Distance of Work

(N=300)

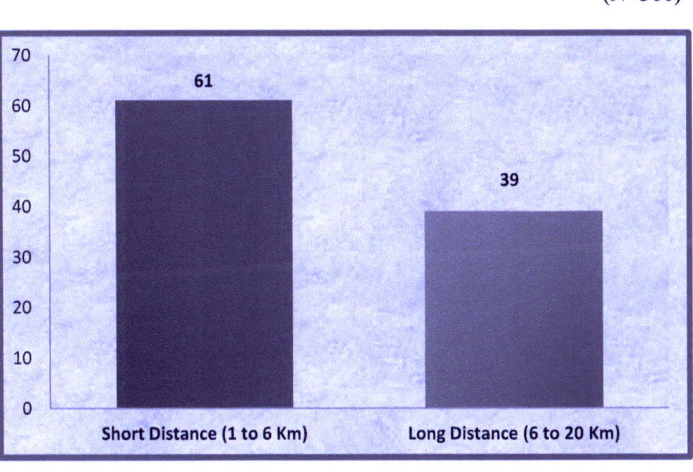

Figure 45: Percentage Distribution of the Silver Workers according to the Persons who helped in Getting Present Job

(N=300)

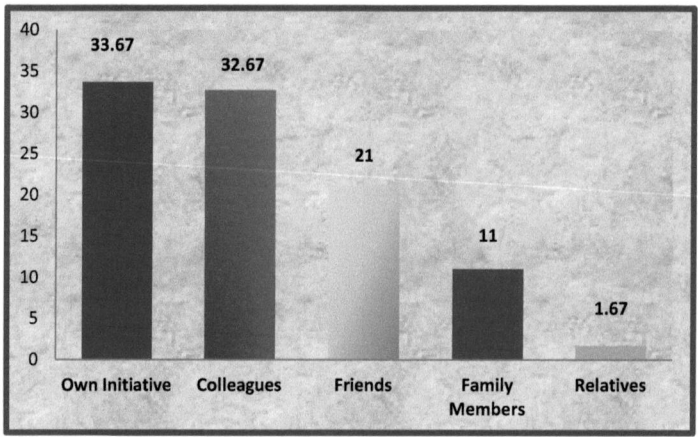

Figure 46: Procuring present job Wise Percentage Distribution of the Silver Workers

(N=300)

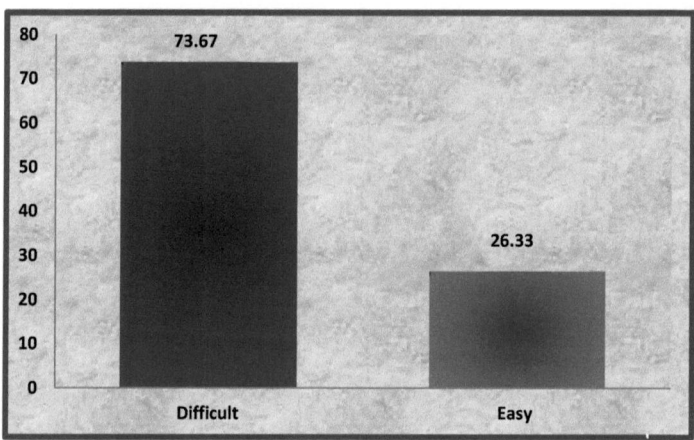

Figure 47: Percentage Distribution of the Silver Workers according to the Social Security Benefits

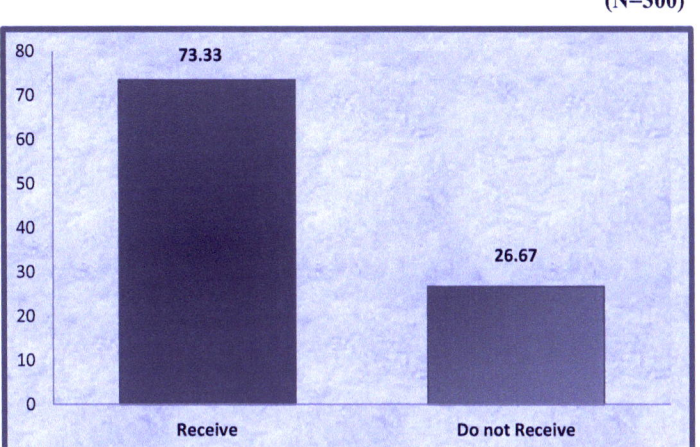

Figure 48: Reasons of Working on Present Job Wise Percentage Distribution of the Silver Workers

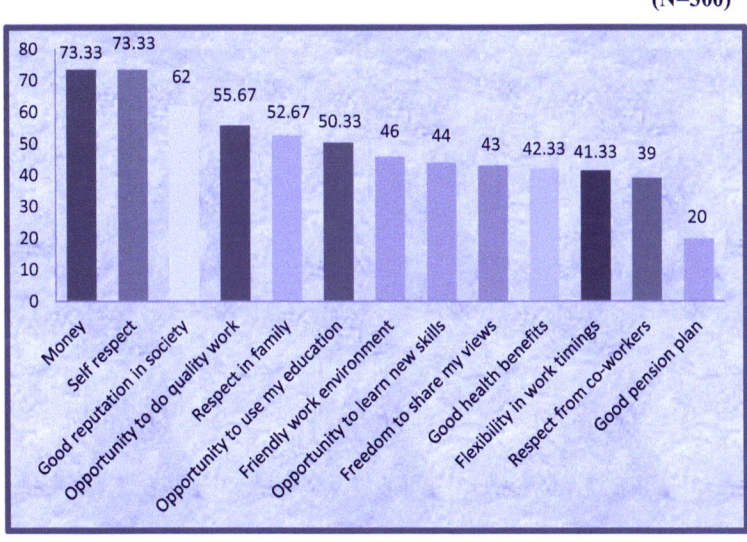

Figure 49: Percentage Distribution of the Silver Workers according to the Expectations to Work after Retirement

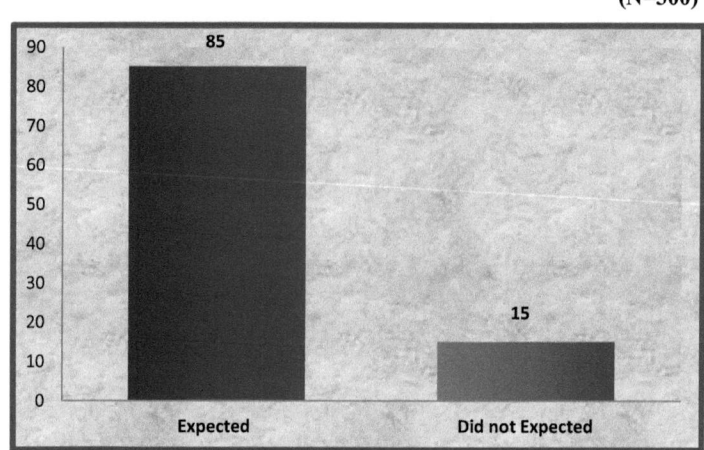

Figure 50: Percentage Distribution of the Silver Workers according to the work they expected to do after Retirement

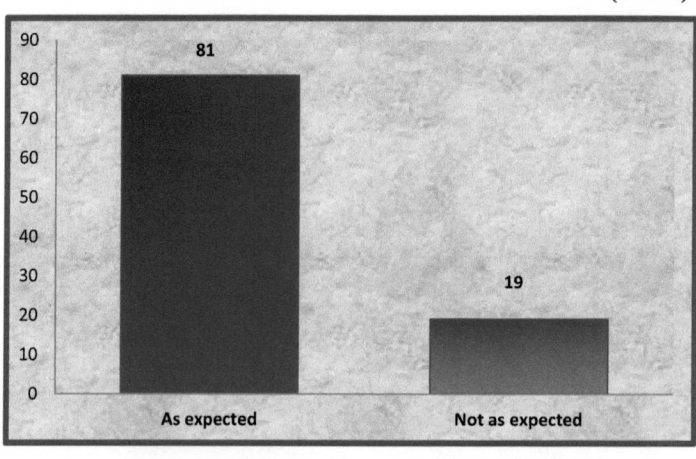

Figure 51: Percentage Distribution of the Silver Workers according to the Lacunas in the Present Job as Compared to the Previous jobs before Retirement

(N=300)

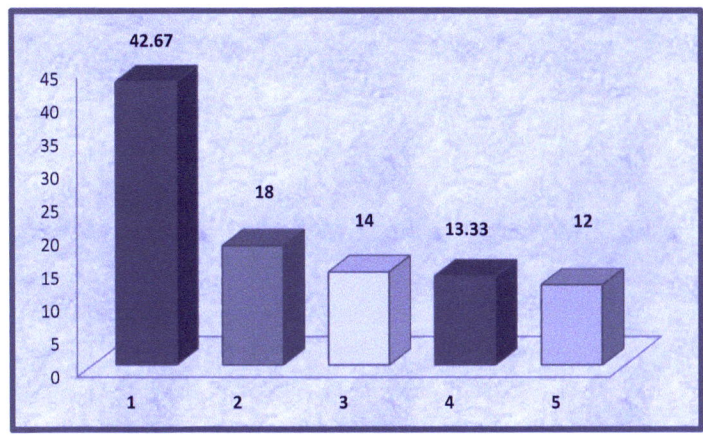

1. - Work ethics and system of working
2. - Work environment
3. - Work timings
4. - Old collgues/ friends at workplace
5. - Respect given to the employees bu the co-workers and employers

Figure 52: Percentage Distribution of the Silver Workers according to the Retirement Benefits

(N=300)

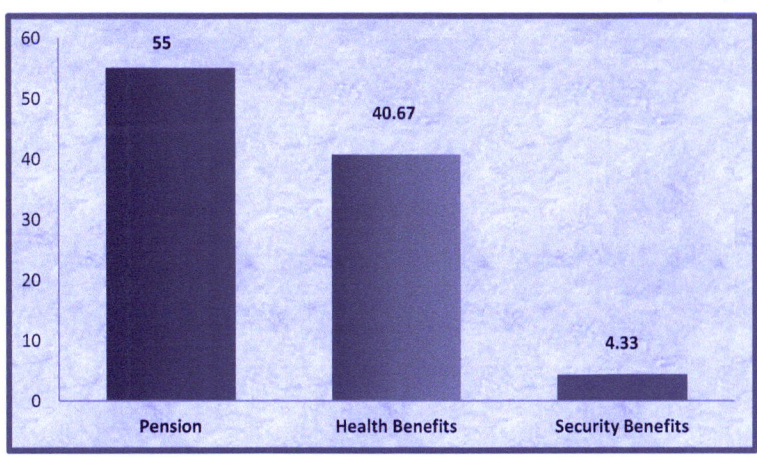

Figure 53: Percentage Distribution of the Silver Workers according to the Importance of Present work

(N=300)

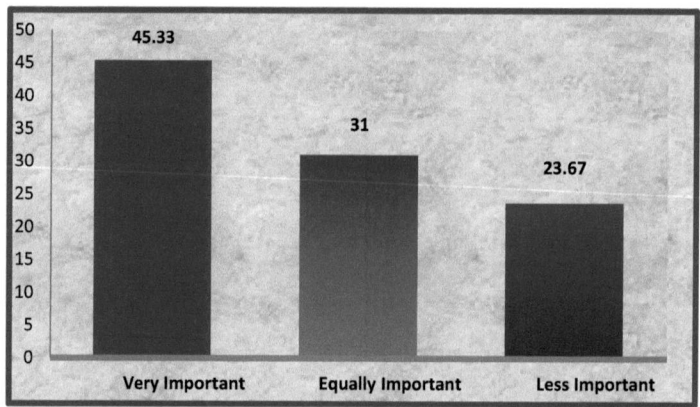

Figure 54: Percentage Distribution of the Silver Workers according to the Age of Re-retirement

(N=300)

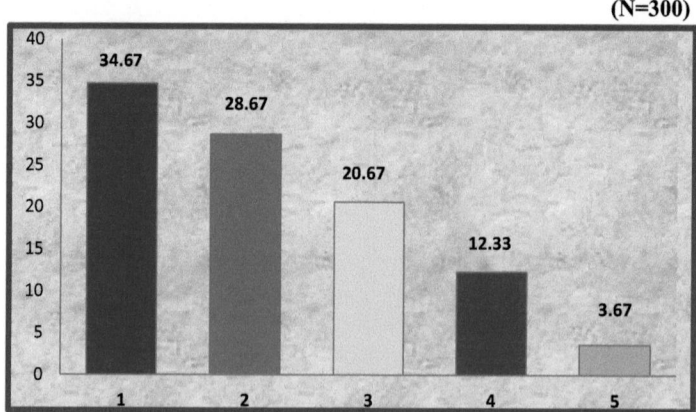

1- Want to continue Working till Health permits as to kill time its important to remain active
2- Working post retirement to share knowledge and experiences and not for financial gains so wanted to continue working till employers allows.
3- Never want to retire as earnings are not enough
4- By the age of 70 years
5- By the age of 65 years

4.1.3 WORK HISTORY

In the light of what the silver workers were doing in the present work and the way they were appreciated for their performance, it would be interesting to throw a glance at the history of performance prior to retirement. As mentioned earlier, human nature tends to compare the present experience with the past experience and derive conclusions to give out reactions .this tendency is commonly found in elderly person. Hence, it would be interesting and also useful to assess the responses and reactions of the silver workers in the conditions they were confronting in the last jobs.

Table 50: Percentage Distribution of the Silver Workers According to their Past Designation

(N=300)

Designation	F	%
Class I	136	45.33
Class II	121	40.33
Class III	31	10.33
Class IV	12	4.00

Table 50 and figure 55 represents that nearly 46 percentages of silver workers worked on class I designation before the retirement. Little less than that (40.33%) percent of them worked on class II designations. One tenth (10.33%) percent of the silver workers worked on class III designations and a very few of them (4%) worked on class IV designations. This clearly shows that majority of the silver workers were having class I designation before the retirement.

The data reveal that prior to retirement in the first job good number of the silver workers used to hold the class I designations and several of them were appointed in the class II designations. So it might give a reason for dissatisfaction for the present condition of work.

Table 51: Percentage Distribution of Silver Workers according to Work of Experience Pre- Retirement

(N=300)

Work Duration	F	%
Short Duration (less than 32 years)	82	27.33
Average Duration (32 years)	156	52.00
Long Duration (more than 32 years)	62	20.67

Table 51 and Figure 56 shows that little less than thirty percent (27.33%) of them had worked for short duration. Whereas 52 percent of them did the previous jobs for an average duration and one fifth percent of them had worked for a long duration in job before retirement. It reveals that majority of silver workers had worked for an average duration before retirement.

Further, the tenure of the first job for majority of them was the usual duration of 32 years. Any of them worked for the first job for a shorter duration of less than 32 years and several of them worked for longer duration. It is noticed that the longer one works in one job more confident he/she would feel for the job performed. As a result, he/she would carry relative air and arrogance for possessing more experience. Such thinking would cause problems to them when they are placed in lower ranks. It might be true about the silver working employed in the present jobs after retirement.

Table 52: Percentage Distribution of the Silver Workers According to their Past Salary

(N=300)

Salary	F	%
Moderate Salary (Less than 26,000 Rupees)	167	55.67
Higher Salary (More than 26,000 Rupees)	133	44.33

Table 52 and Figure 57 reveals that 55.67 percent of the silver workers received moderate salary. Almost 45 percent of them (44.33%) received higher amount prior to the retirement as the salary. Thus the silver workers can be put into two almost equal categories in view of the salary for the first job

Table 53: Percentage Distribution of the Silver Workers According to their Type of Salary

(N=300)

Type of Salary	F	%
Fixed	289	96.33
Consolidated	8	2.67
On the basis of work	3	1.00

It is surprising to note that as table 53 and figure 58 represents that a very high majority (96.33%) of the silver workers used to be paid fixed monthly salary every month. Very few percent of them (2.67%) used to be paid consolidated salary and one percent of them got salary on the basis of the work.

Most of them were employed on fixed salaries, whereas a few of them used to be paid salaries on consolidated basis, on the basis of the work performed. Thus, the type of salary for the present jobs was almost the similar, but the amount was somewhat less. It might be a cause for their dissatisfaction with feeling that even their knowledge and long experience was not considered in their new appointments. They would have expectations for higher salaries. But the fact remains the present job was a second job for them and it would not attract similar appreciation. Their knowledge and long experience would be found as getting lower weightage against younger candidates possessing fresh blood, more computer skills. They are more exposed to the recent world of fast development and against them the silver workers would prove slow going and falling back in recent technologies. Such are the realities that elderly workers need to understand and prepare their minds what comes to them. The need to learn the new technologies if they want to survive in the job markets post retirement as well as they need to learn and compromise and accept the work opportunities that come in their way.

Table 54: Percentage Distribution of the Silver Workers According to their Employment Status

(N=300)

Employment Status	F	%
Permanent	289	96.33
Temporary	8	2.67
Contract Basis	3	1.00

Table 54 and Figure 59 shows the status of the first jobs; very high percentages of the silver workers (96.33%) were employed on permanent basis before the retirement. Whereas very few percent of them were employed on temporary basis (2.67%). Only one percent of them were employed on contract basis.

The employment status was another point to mark their work history. Most of the silver workers were appointed on permanent basis and on full time basis. It remained a matter of security in their first jobs. Further, majority of them were employed in government organizations and less number were working in private, business houses. It too might give them a point to complaint.

Table 55: Percentage Distribution of the Silver Workers According to the Type of Work

(N=300)

Type of Work	F	%
Full time	294	98.00
Part time	6	2.00

Table 55 and Figure 60 shows high percentages (98%) of the silver workers were employed on full time basis and the remaining 2 percent of them were working on part time basis.

Table 56: Percentage Distribution of the Silver Workers According to the Type of Organizations

(N=300)

Type of Organizations	F	%
Government	165	55.00
Private Organizations like Corporate, Business Houses, Agencies ,Firms	135	45.00

Table 56 and Figure 61 indicates that 55 percent of the silver workers were employed in government organizations and forty five percent of them were working in private organizations. (Among them, less than the one third percent of the silver workers worked in corporate and nearly 8 percent of them were employed by non government organizations. While 7 percent of them worked in business houses, nearly two percent of them were working in agencies and only 0.33 percent of them were working in firms)

Table 57: Percentage Distribution of the Silver Workers According Importance of their Work in Past

(N=300)

Work in Past	F	%
Very Important	198	66.00
Equally Important	93	31.00
Less Important	9	3.00

Table 57 and Figure 62 shows that high percent (66%) of the silver workers considered their work in the past as very important. While 31 percent of them said that their work in past as equally important to their work in present .Very less percent of them (3%) mentioned that their work in past was less important .This clearly indicates that most silver workers has given high importance to their work in the past as well in present

The data on the work history reveals a point about attitude that silver workers held for their past jobs. Good majority of them believed that their work in the past held for them lot of importance and so they would attach high value to it. This kind of thinking would imply some kind of discontent for the level of the present work. About one third of them seemed to attach equal importance to their work in the past and it allowed them some sense of satisfaction for the present work. A few of them considered their previous wok less important and so they appeared o be more satisfied and luckier with the present jobs.

In this way, the profile of the present work the work history of the work prior to retirement project for the silver workers mixed pictures causing in them mixed feelings of satisfaction on some favourable condition and regret for the conditions that go against their expectations. It reflects human nature and attitude at such grown up age that a person reaches passing through good struggles, tensions and family obligations. They face conditions that may not be upto their expectations when they actual wish that things go smooth and get them peace of mind. But one has to accept the reality that thing in life would not be always favourable and comfortable and it demands to cultivate positive mind and compromise with the situation. That is the way, a person can make him/her happier, satisfied and calm in the prevalent conditions.

Figure 55: Percentage Distribution of the Silver Workers according to the Past Designation

(N=300)

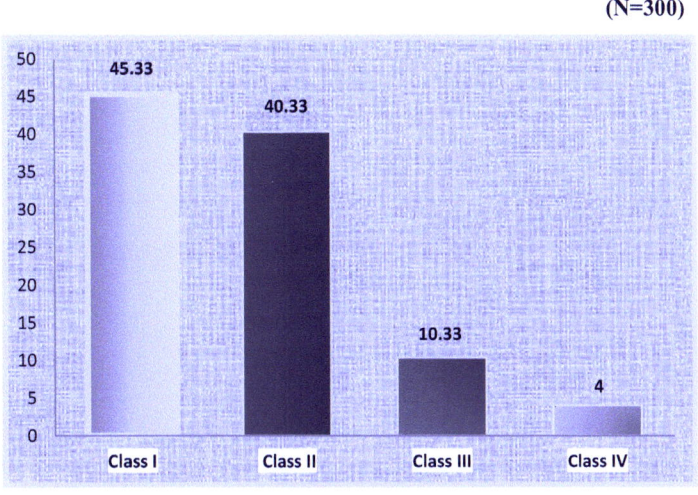

Figure 56: Percentage Distribution of the Silver Workers according to the Work Experience of Pre-Retirement

(N=300)

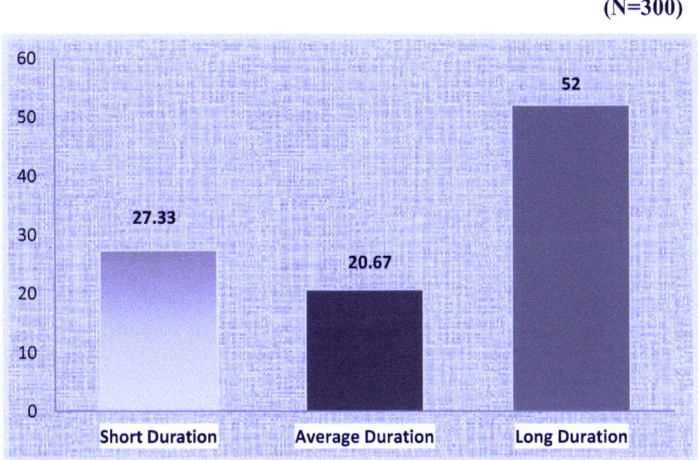

Figure 57: Percentage Distribution of the Silver Workers according to their Past Salary

(N=300)

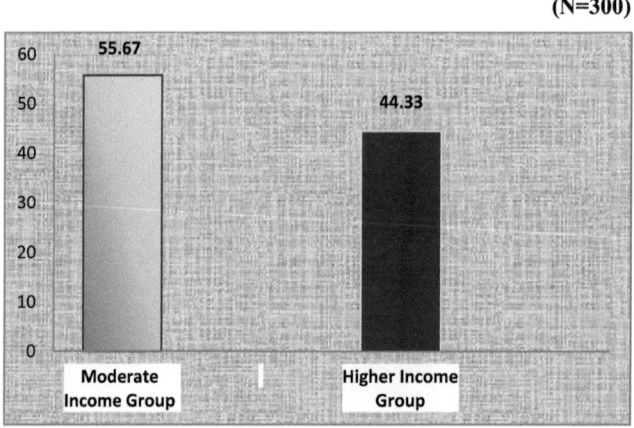

Figure 58 : Percentage Distribution of the Silver Workers according to theType of Salary

(N=300)

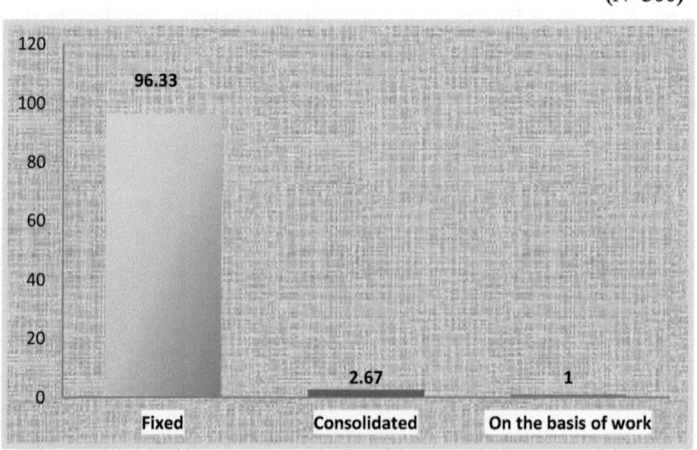

Figure 59: Percentage Distribution of the Silver Workers according ot the Employment Status

(N=300)

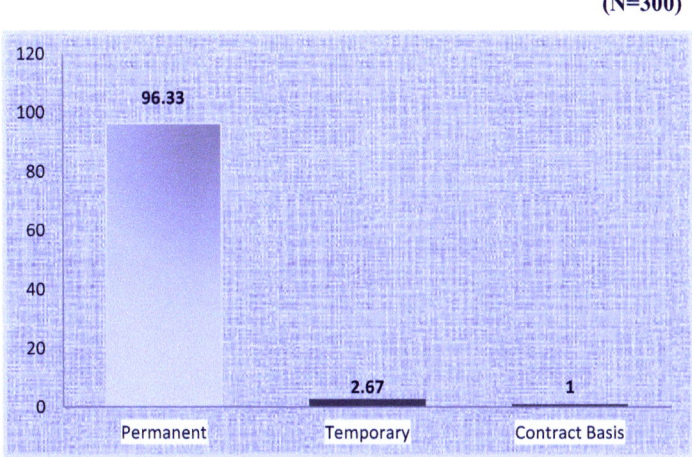

Figure 60: Percentage Distribution of the Silver Workers according to the Type of Work Wise

(N=300)

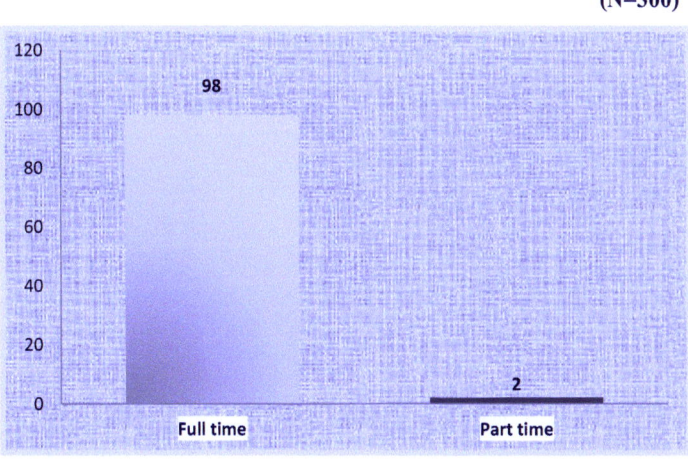

Figure 61: Percentage Distribution of the Silver Workers according to the Type of Organization

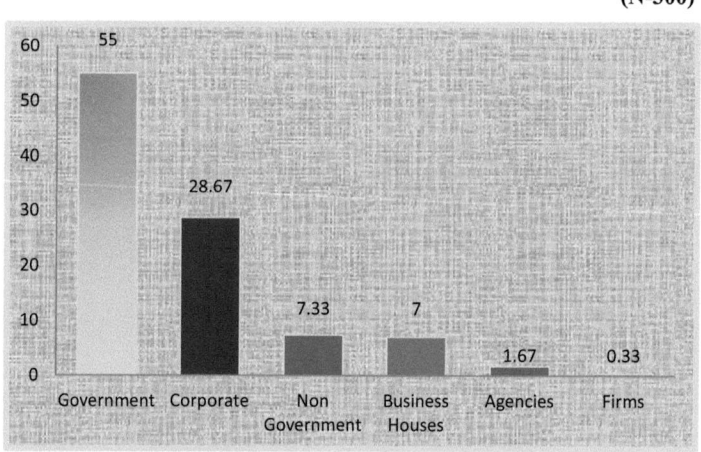

Figure 62: Percentage Distribution of the Silver Workers according to the Work in Past

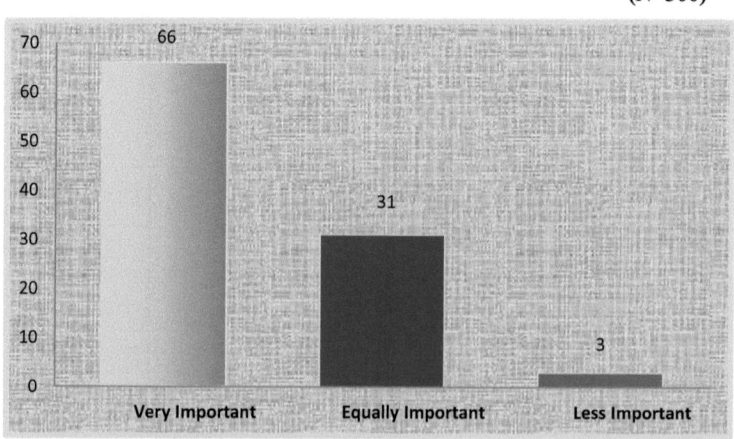

4.1.4 HEALTH STATUS

Table 58: Percentage Distribution of the Silver Workers According to their Health Status

(N=300)

Health Status	F	%
Healthy	193	64.33
Somewhat Healthy	102	34.00
Less Healthy	5	1.76

Table 58 and Figure 63 reveal that almost 65 percentages (64.33%) of the silver workers were healthy. Whereas 34 percentages of silver workers were somewhat healthy and very less percentage (1.76%) were identified as less healthy. This table clearly shows that majority of silver workers were having less number of health problems which may affect their work status

Figure 63: Percentage Distribution of the Silver Workers according to their Health Status

(N=300)

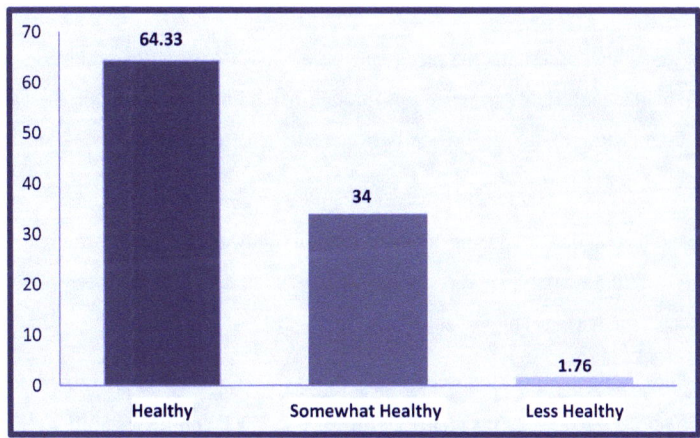

4.2 Overall and Aspects Wise Reasons of Silver Workers to Work after Retirement

As it indicate at the outset of the present chapter that the interpretation of the findings revealed through the data collected would be presented in the parts like interpreting the quantitative and qualitative data in view of the two perspectives like that of the silver workers and the employers who agree to employ them. Thus, if form perspectives on the issues related to the silver workers .The discussion conducted so far take care of a past of the first angle of the perspective as to explain the comfort level among the silver workers in view of their decisions to work after retirement. The interpretations if the data on hand evolves a realistic picture. But in order to confirm the reading of the data it has to be read further with an analytical eye to verify how far it conforms to the objectives set for the present study and the null hypothesis drawn in their relation.

Looking to this need on analysis of the data was carried out through a twofold technique namely

a) t-test and f-test
b) Intensity Indices

The first technique ascertains the difference between reasons and variables. So in the second part the analysis was carried out through t-test and f-test to obtain the t-ration and f-ratio in view of the difference between the selected reasons and the selected variables.

The second technique explains through the intensity indices an extent of the reasons in view of different variables. The second technique works out an analysis of the difference of the reasons and variables.

The reasons for people wanting to continue employment after reaching retirement age have not yet been clearly delineated. Terms for continued employment after reaching retirement age such as "bridge employment" and "silver work" have become established (*Shultz* 2003; *Deller et al.* 2007). Work after retirement is understood as the transitional phase between leaving one's previous full-time job and full retirement. This can be a phase, for example, in which a person works part time/full time or undertakes a new type of work this are so called silver workers or active retirees. There are a large number of factors that influence retirement decisions. Based on *Wang et al.* (2008) and *Wang/Schultz* (2010), we differentiate between four groups of influencing factors (cf. *Gobeski/Beehr* 2009; *Deller/Maxin* 2010; *van Dam et al.* 2009):

- Financial Reasons
- Social and Familial Reasons
- Work related Reasons
- Personal Reasons

Therefore in this section we will deal in more detail with the question what were the reasons for silver workers to work beyond regular retirement. We will look into this question from two perspectives. First approach entails presenting the results analysed through intensity indices in which we analyse employment after retirement based on a variety of reasons. Second approach to gaining a better insight into what drives silver workers to start afresh after retirement entails examining through t-test and f-test, the reasons that silver workers gave themselves for doing so. This information can shed more light on the question of whether their decision is driven primarily by financial or extrinsic reasons or whether intrinsic reasons such as the nature of the job play a more important role.

Whereas the drawback of this approach is that the silver workers may give socially desirable answers, the advantage is that the reasons may tie in better with the silver workers own experiences. In the survey it was made a distinction between four major reasons for entering employment after retirement and respondents were asked to indicate which reason was most important in their particular case. The purpose of this analysis is to ascertain an extent of intensity of particular reasons in view of the silver workers decision to work after retirement. Based on these two analysis, null hypothesis drawn in view of the objectives are confirmed to obtain definite picture in the issue to interpret the analytical readings

Table 59: Overall Extent Aspects and Percentage wise distribution of the Reasons of the Silver Workers to Work after Retirement

(N=300)

Reasons	Extent of Reasons			I.I
	More Number of Reasons	Moderate Number of Reasons	Less number of Reasons	
Overall	34.33	38.33	27.67	1.97
Social and Familial Reasons	6.33	61.33	33.33	2.29
Financial Reasons	17.67	51.00	24.33	2.26
Personal Reasons	16.67	47.00	36.67	1.60
Work related Reasons	36.67	19.00	45.00	1.32

It can be seen from table 59 that according to the intensity indices, overall and extent wise, there were moderate to less number of reasons for silver workers to work after retirement. It can be further revealed that higher percentage of the silver workers reported that compared to other reasons there were more of social and familial reasons for them to work after retirement. Little more than the half percentage (57%) of them reported to the moderate level that there were more number of financial reasons that compelled the silver workers to work after retirement. The silver workers who mentioned that there were more of personal reasons (47%) and very few of them reported work related reasons (19%) for them to work after retirement.

It can be concluded from the findings that for silver workers social and familial were more important factors for making them work after retirement. They were not working for themselves or for work related reasons

According to the index, the social and familial reasons recorded higher extent of intensity and the financial reason recorded moderate extent of intensity, the personal reasons and work related reasons recorded lower extent of intensity .This explains that in the Indian context for the silver workers based in city of Vadodara (Gujarat) social and familial and financial reasons mattered more when they decide to work after retirement. This reading projects exactly an opposite picture to the one that is projected in the study of the Geneva Association on "Silver Workers" in Germany. In the European context, the personal reasons and work related reasons attract higher considerations, whereas in the Indian contexts social and familial and financial reasons are given higher considerations.

Table 60: Overall Extent of the Reasons of the Silver Workers to Work after Retirement in Relation to the Selected Variables

(N=300)

Variables	N	Reasons to Work Post Retirement		
		More	Moderate	Less
1. Age				
Young –Old	116	52.21	22.62	25.19
Old	184	39.67	49.89	10.42
2. Educational Qualification				
High Level of Education	254	60.02	22.00	17.07
Moderate Level of Education	31	48.59	45.32	6.05
Low Level of Education	15	13.33	20.00	66.67
3. Past Designation				
Class I	136	48.52	45.58	5.88
Class II	121	64.46	30.57	4.95
Class III	31	48.38	38.07	13.30
Class IV	12	58.33	33.34	8.33
4. Present Salary				
Less Salary	145	69.16	21.21	10.06
Moderate Salary	22	18.18	40.90	40.09
High Salary	133	17.51	43.03	3.89
5. Health Status				
Healthy	192	48.95	28.12	22.91
Somewhat Healthy	103	37.86	32.03	30.09
Less Healthy	5	20.00	40.00	40.00
6. Type of Family				
Living Alone	7	28.57	42.85	28.56
Living with Spouse	104	19.23	50.00	30.76
Living with Family	189	34.39	43.91	21.68

The overall reasons of silver workers to work after retirement refer to all kinds of general matters. The table 60 reflects that higher percentages of the silver workers belonging to following categories of variables reported about moderate number of reasons to work after retirement.

- Silver workers belonging to old age group
- Silver workers possessing high level of education.
- Silver Workers belonging to the class II designation
- Silver workers earning high salary
- Silver workers who were less healthy
- Silver workers living with their families

Table 61: Extent of Social and Familial Reasons of Silver Workers to Work after Retirement in Relation to the Selected Variables

(N=300)

Variables	N	Social and Familial Reasons of Working after Retirement		
		More	Moderate	Less
1. Age				
Young – Old	116	40.51	33.62	25.85
Old	184	39.67	29.89	30.42
2. Educational Qualification				
High Level of Education	254	42.12	29.92	27.43
Moderate Level of Education	31	25.80	35.48	38.07
Low Level of Education	15	13.03	46.67	40.00
3. Past Designation				
Class I	136	42.64	31.61	25.07
Class II	121	31.40	44.62	23.96
Class III	31	12.90	38.70	48.38
Class IV	12	16.67	58.33	25.00
4. Present Salary				
Less Salary	145	36.55	33.79	29.64
Moderate Salary	22	13.63	31.81	54.54
High Salary	133	45.11	28.57	26.31
4. Health Status				
Healthy	192	22.91	48.95	28.12
Somewhat Healthy	103	37.86	32.03	30.09
Less Healthy	5	20.00	40.00	40.00
5. Type of Family				
Living Alone	189	44.44	29.62	25.91
Living with Spouse	104	2.88	30.76	66.34
Living with Family	7	14.28	14.28	71.42

Social and familial reasons prompting the silver workers to work after retirement draw glaring attention and apprehensions from all the corners of human society. The table 61 reveals that higher percentage of the silver workers belonging to the following categories of variables confronted more of social and familial reasons to work after retirement.

- Amongst the category of age silver workers belonging to young-old age group had moderate number of social and familial reason to work after retirement and silver workers belonging to old age group had less number of social and familial reasons to work after retirement.
- Silver workers possessing high level of education had less number of social and familial reasons to work after retirement .whereas silver workers possessing moderate level of education had more reasons to work.
- Silver workers belonging to the class I, II and IV designation had less social and familial reasons to work. Whereas silver workers having class III had moderate social and familial reason to work after retirement.
- Silver workers earning high and less salaries had less reason
- Silver workers who were healthy had less social and familial reason tow work after retirement.
- Silver workers living alone had high number of social and familial reason to work after retirement .whereas silver workers living with family had less number of social and familial reason to work after retirement

Table 62: Extent of Financial Reasons of Silver Workers to Work after Retirement in Relation to the Selected Variables

(N=300)

Variables	N	Financial Reasons of Working after Retirement		
		More	Moderate	Less
1. Age				
Young –Old	116	19.82	37.93	42.23
Old	184	7.60	4.90	87.30
2. Educational Qualification				
High Level of Education	254	11.02	25.59	63.38
Moderate Level of Education	31	16.12	64.51	18.54
Low Level of Education	15	20.00	40.00	39.97
3. Past Designation				
Class I	136	7.35	23.52	68.21
Class II	121	31.40	19.83	48.75
Class III	31	22.58	41.93	35.47
Class IV	12	16.67	33.33	50.00
7. Present Salary				
Less Salary	145	26.89	42.06	31.21
Moderate Salary	22	18.18	40.90	40.09
High Salary	133	7.51	23.03	69.16
8. Health Status				
Healthy	192	6.20	33.89	60.04
Somewhat Healthy	103	23.30	41.74	34.94
Less Healthy	5	20.00	40.00	40.00
9. Type of Family				
Living Alone	7	28.57	29.00	42.39
Living with Spouse	104	19.23	50.00	30.76
Living with Family	189	34.39	43.91	21.68

Table 62 reveals project that higher percentage of the silver workers belonging to the following categories of variables confronted less number of financial reasons to work after retirement.

- Amongst category of age very high percent of old had less number of financial reason to work after retirement

- In the category of education majority of silver workers having moderate level of education had moderate number of reasons to work whereas equal percent of silver worker having high level of education had less number of financial reasons to work after retirement.
- Amongst category of designation class I silver workers had less finicail reasons to work after retirement
- In the category of present salary silver workers having high salary had less number of financial reasons to work after retirement
- Amongst health status silver workers who were health had less financial reasons to work after retirement
- Type of family wise silver workers living alone had less number of financial reason to work after retirement

Table 63: Extent of Personal Reasons of Silver Workers to Work after Retirement in Relation to the Selected Variables

(N=300)

Variables	N	Personal Reasons of Working after Retirement		
		More	Moderate	Less
1. Age				
Young –Old	116	3.44	48.27	48.27
Old	184	7.60	48.36	44.02
2. Educational Qualification				
High Level of Education	254	7.08	41.73	51.17
Moderate Level of Education	31	12.90	45.16	41.92
Low Level of Education	15	20.00	60.00	20.00
3. Past Designation				
Class I	136	52.20	8.82	38.96
Class II	121	23.96	39.66	36.35
Class III	31	12.90	54.61	32.25
Class IV	12	41.67	25.00	33.34
4. Present Salary				
Less Salary	145	5.51	48.27	46.19
Moderate Salary	22	54.54	36.36	9.08
High Salary	133	6.76	47.36	45.86
5. Health Status				
Healthy	192	49.74	6.73	43.65
Somewhat Healthy	103	4.90	49.01	46.07
Less Healthy	5	20.00	20.00	60.00
6. Type of Family				
Living Alone	189	5.82	54.49	39.67
Living with Spouse	104	47.11	39.42	13.46
Living with Family	7	57.14	14.28	28.56

Table 63 reveals that higher percentage of the silver workers belonging to the following categories of variables had moderate number of personal reasons to work after retirement.

- Silver workers belonging to young old age group had moderate or less number of personal reason to work after retirement
- Silver workers possessing Moderate and Low level of education had less number of personal reasons to work after retirement.
- Silver workers belonging to the class I had more number of personal reason to work after retirement and class III designations
- Silver workers earning high and less salaries
- Silver workers who were somewhat healthy

Table 64: Extent of Work Related Reasons of Silver Workers to Work after Retirement in Relation to the Selected Variables

(N=300)

Variables	N	Work Related Reasons of Working after Retirement		
		More	Moderate	Less
1. Age				
Young –Old	116	5.17	19.82	74.99
Old	184	4.89	25.54	70.11
2. Educational Qualification				
High Level of Education	254	22.00	60.02	17.07
Moderate Level of Education	31	6.05	45.32	48.59
Low Level of Education	15	13.33	20.00	66.67
3. Past Designation				
Class I	136	5.88	45.58	48.52
Class II	121	4.95	64.46	30.57
Class III	31	13.90	48.38	38.07
Class IV	12	8.33	58.33	33.34
4. Present Salary				
Less Salary	145	6.20	14.48	79.03
Moderate Salary	22	9.09	77.27	13.63
High Salary	133	4.51	58.64	36.84
5. Health Status				
Healthy	192	20.31	61.45	17.77
Somewhat Healthy	103	25.24	53.39	21.44
Less Healthy	5	20.0	20.00	60.00
6. Type of Family				
Living Alone	189	7.40	22.22	70.36
Living with Spouse	104	1.92	25.00	73.07
Living with Family	7	28.57	14.28	57.13

Work related reasons reflect more on willingness rather than compulsion on the part of the silver workers. The table 64 reveals that higher percentage of the silver workers

belonging to the following categories of variables had less number of work related reasons to work after retirement.
- Silver workers belonging to young-old and old age group
- Silver workers possessing high and moderate and low level of education.
- Silver workers belonging to the class I designations
- Silver Workers earning less salary
- Silver workers who were less healthy
- Silver workers living alone, living with spouse and living with family

4.3 Differences in the Overall Reasons of Silver Workers to Work after Retirement in Relation to the Selected Variables

Earlier we discussed the extent of reasons of silver workers to work after retirement in relation to the selected variables. It would be now interesting to know if it varies in relation to the variables selected for the study. This would unfold another fact of the study .Extent of reasons of the silver workers to work after retirement differed significantly with respect to the variables like educational qualification and health status. The survey revealed interesting and useful findings to help the analysis of the reasons.

The findings related of the differences in the reasons of silver workers to work after retirement in relation to the selected variables are described below:

DIFFERENCES IN THE OVERALL REASONS OF SILVER WORKERS TO WORK AFTER RETIREMENT IN RELATION TO THE SELECTED VARIABLES

Table 65: t-Ratio Showing the Difference in the Reasons of Silver Workers to Work after retirement in Relation to their Age

(N=300)

Variable	Categories	N	Mean	S.D	t-value
Age	Young-Old	116	54.28	14.858	.138 NS
	Old	184	54.05	13.244	

NS=Not Significant

It can be seen from the table 65 that in relation to their age there was no significant difference in reasons of silver workers to work after retirement. It indicates that the age wise difference does not exist with respect to the reasons of their work after retirement. Thus, the null hypothesis stating that there will be no significant difference in the reasons of silver workers to work after retirement in relation to their age was accepted.

In relation to their age there was no significant difference in reasons of silver workers to work after retirement. It indicates that the age wise difference does not exist with respect to the reasons of their work after retirement. It means that the reason to work after retirement does not differ according to the variation in age. This clearly shows that age was not the reasons nor it was barrier for them to work after retirement.

Table 66: Analysis of Variance (ANOVA) Indicating Reasons of Silver Workers to Work after Retirement in Relation to their Educational Qualification

(N=300)

Variables	Source of Variance	DF	Sum of Squares	Mean Square	F-Value	Sig.
Educational Qualification	Between Groups	2	1449.514	724.757	4.732**	.009
	Within Groups	297	45487.883	153.158		
	Total	299	46937.397			

**F Significant at 0.01 levels, F-tab, 0.01 level df 2/299 = 4.68

Table 66 reveals that there was significant difference in the reasons of silver workers to work in relation to their educational qualification. In order to know which group of the reasons differed significantly the data were further analysed through t-test.

Table 67: t-Ratio Showing the Difference in the Reasons of Silver Workers to Work after retirement in Relation to their Educational Qualification

(N=300)

Educational Qualification	X	SD	High Level of Education	Moderate Level of Education	Low Level of Education
High Level of Education	96.59	12.743		1.251	2.843**
Moderate Level of Education	93.61	10.141			2.081*
Low Level Education	89.07	9.699			

**Significant at 0.01 level and * Significant at 0.05 level

It can be seen from the table 67 that the difference appeared in reasons to work post retirement existed between silver workers who were having high level of education and low level of education. Similarly, the difference in the reasons existed for the silver workers who possessed moderate level of education and low level of education. It can be revealed that the silver workers having moderate level of education had more reasons to work than those having lower level of education. Likewise, the silver workers having higher level of education had more reasons to work than those having lower level of education.

Thus, the null hypothesis stated that no significant difference was noticed in the reasons of silver workers to work after retirement in relation to their educational qualification was not accepted.

There was significant difference in the reasons of silver workers to work in relation to their educational qualification. The difference appeared in reasons of the silver workers existed between silver workers who were having high level of education and low level of education. Similarly, the difference in the reasons existed for the silver workers who possessed moderate level of education and low level of education. It can be revealed that the silver workers having moderate level of education had more reasons to work than those having lower level of education. Likewise, the silver workers having higher level of education had more reasons to work than those having lower level of education. In a US survey from the year 2000 it was observed that persons with a higher level of education demonstrate a much higher probability of wanting to continue to work in "bridge employment" than persons with a lower level of education (von Bonsdorff et al. 2009).

These findings clearly suggest that the silver workers having higher level of education were more inclined to work after retirement than their counter parts. Further, it was also revealed that silver workers having moderate level of education were more inclined to work after retirement in comparison to those holding lower level of education. This result clearly shows that silver workers having high level of education were more inclined to work after retirement; the reason behind it can be that they wanted to share their knowledge with others. As for them financial reasons could not be the major reason to work post retirement. Human capital is a key factor in explaining labor force choices and opportunities. In general, chances in the labour market are greater for individuals that have greater access to human capital (Becker 2009). The amount of human capital in terms of education and experience may also influence the degree to which re-entering the workforce after retirement is an attractive option as well as the older adult's chances of finding work (Ruhm 1990).

People having higher level of education showed higher interest in working post retirement than those having moderate level of education which also indicates that silver workers having moderate level of education were not that much inclined to work post retirement, the reason behind that can be the lack of education, or lack of confidence or they might be they were having the fear or inferiority complex of working with younger generation as in today's world education play a vital role and in they might lack in terms of education .As the silver workers with higher level of education has more knowledge to share they have that confidence in them to deal and work with younger generation and as they have achieved so much of education they had the feeling to work after retirement. When it comes to the silver workers holding low level of education the findings reveals that there was difference in the reasons of the silver workers who were having moderate level of education and those having low level of education. This might be the situation because the silver workers having moderate level of education might have different sets of reasons to work after retirement in comparison to those having low educational level. As people holding low level of education might be working because of financial crunch. They might be working after retirement out of choice, or say necessity to earn money.

Table 68: Analysis of Variance (ANOVA) Showing Difference between Reasons of Silver Workers to Work after Retirement in Relation to their Last Designation

(N=300)

Variables	Source of Variance	DF	Sum of Squares	Mean Square	F-Value	Sig.
Last Designation	Between Groups	3	489.433	163.144	.847 NS	.469
	Within Groups	296	57001.964	192.574		
	Total	299	57491.397			

NS=Not Significant

Table 68 shows that reasons of silver workers to work after retirement in relation to their last designation did not differ significantly. Thus, the null hypothesis, stating that there will be no significant difference in reasons of silver workers to work after retirement in relation to their last designation, was accepted.

Further it was revealed from the findings that reasons of silver workers to work after retirement in relation to their last designation did not differ significantly. Occupational status is especially important to the topic of bridge employment because individuals of differing levels of occupational prestige tend to have different attitudes towards work. Statistics Canada (2006) finds professionals to be the most likely to return to work after retirement, followed by managers, and then by technicians. Similarly, Maestas (2010) claims that professionals and managers are more likely to undergo a partial retirement or to return to the labour force after a first retirement than are labourers, operators, and those who work in the service sector. Studies have shown that levels of continued work late in life are high among men who were employed in higher status occupations marked by greater amounts of complexity. On the other hand, those who were employed in low status jobs marked by low levels of autonomy, monotonous work, and high levels of danger and physical demand tend to have undergone an earlier retirement (Raymo et al. 2010).

Table 69: Analysis of Variance (ANNOVA) Showing Difference between Reasons of Silver Workers to Work after Retirement in Relation to their Present Salary

(N=300)

Variables	Sources of Variance	DF	Sum of Squares	Mean Square	F-Value	Sig.
Present Salary	Between Groups	2	753.403	376.702	1.972 NS	.141
	Within Groups	297	56737.993	191.037		
	Total	299	57491.397			

NS=Not Significant

Table 69 reveals that the reasons of silver workers to work after retirement in relation to their economic status did not differ significantly. Thus, the null hypothesis, stating that there will be no significant difference in reasons of silver workers to work after retirement in relation to their present salary was accepted.

It was revealed that the reasons of silver workers to work after retirement in relation to their present salary did not differ significantly. According to *Dorbritz* and *Micheel* (2010) higher income does not lead to consideration of continued employment. This would concur with the argument that employees with lower income are more likely to feel the need to continue to work even beyond retirement age (*Beehr* 1986; *Feldman* 1994; *Opaschowski* 2008).

Table 70: Analysis of Variance (ANOVA) Showing Difference between Reasons of Silver Workers to Work after Retirement in Relation to their Health Status

(N=300)

Variables	Source of Variance	DF	Sum of Squares	Mean Square	F-Value	Sig.
Health Status	Between Groups	2	1301.595	650.797	4.235*	.015
	Within Groups	297	45635.802	153.656		
	Total	299				

F * Significant at 0.05 level, F-tab, 0.05 level df 2/299 =3.03

Table 70 reveals that there was significant difference in the reasons of silver workers to work in relation to their health status. In order to know among which group of the reasons differed significantly the data were further analysed through the t-test.

Table 71: t-Ratio Showing the Difference in the Reasons of Silver Workers to Work after retirement in Relation to their Health Status

(N=300)

Health Status	X	SD	Healthy	Somewhat Healthy	Less Healthy
Healthy	96.84	12.520		1.528	2.593**
Somewhat Healthy	94.52	12.258			2.11*
Less Healthy	82.20	9.654			

**Significant at 0.01 level and * Significant at 0.05 level

It can be seen from the table 71 above that the mean scores on the reasons of the healthy silver workers were significantly higher than their counterparts. It indicates that the healthy silver workers had more reasons to work after retirement than those silver workers who were somewhat healthy or less healthy.

Thus, the null hypothesis, stating that there will be no significant difference in the reasons of silver workers to work after retirement in relation to their health status, was not accepted.

Many research studies have shown the positive relationship between education and health (Cutler and Lleras-Muney 2006; Goldman and Smith 2011). In fact, over the past quarter century, the importance of education to health has increased (Goldman and Smith 2011). As good health has consistently been shown in the literature to be associated with an increased likelihood of return to work after retirement (as is discussed below), this offers an indirect means through which higher levels of education might be associated with a higher probability that one will take up post-retirement work. As it can be revealed from the findings that there was significant difference in the reasons of silver workers to work in relation to their health status. The mean scores on the reasons of the healthy silver workers were significantly higher than their counterparts. It indicates that the healthy silver workers had more reasons to work after retirement than those silver workers who were somewhat healthy or less healthy. This shows that being in good state of health can be one of the reasons for them to work after retirement, as by working they can keep themselves active and mentally fit.

Table 72: Analysis of Variance (ANOVA) Showing Difference in Reasons of Silver Workers to Work after Retirement in Relation to their Type of Family

(N=300)

Variables	Source of Variance	DF	Sum of Squares	Mean Square	F-Value	Sig.
Type of Family	Between Groups	2	436.838	218.419	1.137 NS	.322
	Within Groups	297	57054.559	192.103		
	Total	299	57491.397			

NS=Not Significant

Table 72 shows that the reasons of silver workers to work after retirement in relation to their type of family did not differ significantly. Thus, the null hypothesis, stating that there will be no significant difference in reasons of silver workers to work after retirement in relation to type of family was accepted.

The reasons of silver workers to work after retirement in relation to their type of family did not differ significantly. It can be concluded that the motivations for work would not change for every person in similar way. For some, the motivational drive was economic gain never all the time and for many others economic motives would be preference next to a need to accomplish something meaningful in life their early sixties.

In this way, the interpretation of the quantitative data and the results of the analysis of the data explain objective perspective on the issue of the silver workers in view of their decision to work after retirement. But it presents only one side of the issue, it needs to be balanced with subjective dimension of the issue by reviewing and interpreting the perception of the silver workers on a matter of working after retirement. Hence, the next point of discussion pertains to the silver workers perception about their retirement

4.4 Item Wise Findings Regarding Reasons Prompting Silver Workers to Work after Retirement

The scale to judge the reasons of silver workers to work after retirement includes 36 items. Under each items, there were three options which indicated three intensity related to the reasons of silver workers to work after retirement. The items, for which more number of silver workers had marked, are specified below:

Table 73: Intensity Indices Showing Reasons to a great extent of the Silver Workers to Work after Retirement

(N=300)

Reasons	Intensity Indices
Become financially independent	2.58
To stay physically active	2.52
Cannot imagine life without work	2.51
To stay mentally active	2.50

Table 73 shows that silver workers reported following reasons to work post retirement to a great extent

- Financial independency
- To stay physically active
- Life without work

Table 74: Item Wise Intensity Indices showing the Social and Familial Reasons of Silver Workers to Work after Retirement

(N=300)

Items	Intensity Indices
The only earning member in the family	1.86
Long term care of dependents	1.80
Important financial responsibility towards family (like Children's Education, Marriage)	1.78
Support children financially	1.76
Attention and respect from family	1.69
Income for health care of the spouse	1.63
Pressure from family to work	1.42
Responsibility of children's education	1.35
Renovate house	1.30
To buy another property	1.28
Reinvest for capital growth	1.27

Table 74 focuses on the overall intensity indices concerning social and familial reasons of silver workers ranged from 1.86 to 1.27. . It means there were moderate to less number of reasons for silver workers to work after retirement. This can be seen from the table that silver workers had some extent and less extent of social and familial reasons to work after retirement were as follows

- The only earning member in the family
- Long term care of dependents
- Important financial responsibility towards family (like Children's Education, Marriage)
- Support children financially
- Income for health care of the spouse
- Attention and respect from family

Social and familial reasons to work after retirement to a less extent in regards to the following were as follows:
- Pressure from family to work
- Responsibility of children's education
- Renovate house
- To buy another property
- Reinvest for capital growth

In similar sense, the intensity indices concerning reasons related to social and familial reasons indicate of high concern from the silver workers. The plight of silver workers with regard to their need to reconcile work and family life has received scant attention. That is to say, though this age group has received extensive attention with regard to extending their participation in the paid labour market, the conflict between their work and family responsibilities has not received corresponding attention. This at a time when many socio-economic factors have changed the work and family needs for many groups of workers, including those at the older end of the age spectrum. Social factors, such as declining fertility rates, increased divorce rates and increases in single-headed households have become more common in the last 30 years. At the same time, economic factors, such as greater access to training and education and rural to urban or international migration, have changed the dynamics of the working life of people. The cumulative impact of these socio-economic changes is a profound change in family structure and life on the one side, and a change in work life on the other. This is particularly true for the current generation of silver workers, who were at the forefront of these socio-economic changes in many industrialized countries. In order to ensure that the equality rights of silver workers are respected, there is a need to fully understand what family responsibilities may not be accounted for at the moment.

According to the item wise intensity indices, the first four items indicates the first hand financial responsibilities of the silver workers for their families as the only earner, caring dependents and children liabilities. It received concern of very high intensity. The reasons like respect in family and healthcare of the spouses received moderate concern from them, whereas those like pressure from family, children's education and property related matters made them less anxious about financial arrangements. Thus, it gets clear that concern for family and society captured attention of the groups of silver workers while deciding to work after retirement. Giang and Pfau (2006) conducted a study on a gender perspective on elderly work in Vietnam.

Table 75: Item Wise Intensity Indices showing the Financial Reasons of Silver Workers to Work after Retirement

(N=300)

Items	Intensity Indices
Become financially independent	2.58
Spend money according to their own wish	1.96
To add to retirement savings	1.81
Pension was not Sufficient	1.68
Income from other sources is not enough	1.68
Heavy expenditure on medicines	1.50
Pay off mortgage	1.49
No pension money	1.44
No savings	1.14

Table 75 shows that overall intensity indices regarding financial reasons of the silver workers to work after retirement ranged from 2.58 to 1.14.finanical reasons were to some extent and less extent to work post retirement. Financial reasons to work post retirement were as follows:

- Spend money as they wish
- To add to retirement savings

Silver workers had less financial reasons to work after retirement were as follows:
- Heavy expenditure on medicines
- Pay off mortgage
- No pension money
- No savings

According to the intensity indices, it can be understood that a reason like "to become financially independent" received greater extent of consideration from the silver workers to decided to work after retirement. This shows that more of them decided to work after retirement to remain financially independent and not for financial crunch. The other reasons like "spend more money according to their own wish", "to add to retirement savings" and "pension was not sufficient and "income from other sources is not enough were few of the reason to which silver workers agreed to moderate extent. While reasons like "no pension money , "no savings" and "to pay off mortgages" were the reasons for which silver workers agreed to very less extent. This clearly shows that they were not in any kind of financial pressure due to which they have decided to work after retirement. But remarkably the difference indicated by the intensity as quiet minimum. The picture projected by the financial arrangements for survival in an old age after retirement. It speaks about an intensity of to be financially independent that prompted most of the silver workers to decide to work after retirement. Brown, Auman, Catsopues, Ellen and bond (2010).

Thus the majority of silver workers seem to have an adequate financial background. Only some look for additional income. Therefore it can be concluded that the financial aspects plays a minimal role in terms of doing job in retirement. The activity itself seems to be more important than payment. In some cases however, payment seems to serve as factor representing appreciation, underlining the value of the activity.

Table 76: Item Wise Intensity Indices showing the Personal Reasons of the Silver Workers to Work after Retirement

(N=300)

Items	Intensity Indices
To stay physically active	2.52
To stay mentally active	2.50
To be productive, useful and helpful	2.25
Feeling bored sitting idle	2.25
To be surrounded with people	2.05
To maintain lifestyle	1.93

To enjoy social interaction with colleagues	1.75
Desire to learn new skills	1.49
Alone in family	1.29

Table 76 shows that there were moderate to less number of personal reasons of silver workers to work after retirement. The above table shows that there were moderate numbers of personal reasons of silver workers to work after retirement with regards to following items:

- To enjoy social interaction with colleagues
- To maintain lifestyle
- To be around people
- Feeling bored sitting idle
- To stay physically active
- To stay mentally active
- To be productive, useful and helpful

It can be further revealed from the table that there was less number of personal reasons to work after retirement with regards to following items:

- Alone in family
- Desire to learn new skills

The above mentioned preceding groups of the reasons speak of financial and social and familial and work related reasons to prompt the silver workers to decide to work after retirement. As against them, the personal reasons indicate about a person's choice, willingness work related reasons and positive mindset about working after retirement. The group of work –related reason indicate one preference to stay active in later stage of life. Among these reasons, those like staying active received very high consideration from the silver workers. Those like, interest in job received good considerations from them .Those like stress free and less laborious working was given good consideration Thus, the intensity indices indicate that silver workers desire to stay active seems to be an essential reasons for work in retirement. Support for this was found in a study conducted by Delong (2006) on "The Paradox of the 'Working Retired' – Identifying Barriers to Increased Labor Force Participation for Elderly in the U.S." Elderly who were 66 to 70 year old, this shift in priorities was merely dramatic, with 72 percent of them who said like "want to stay active and engaged" as the most frequently mentioned reason for working. The second choice for them was "want the opportunity to do meaningful work" (47 percent) and third choice was like "enjoy social interaction with colleagues" (42 percent).

Clearly, personal reasons are central to the work decisions of people as they get older. Individuals differ in the ways they prefer to be active, and their family and health circumstances. Work, in some form or another, has always been a preferred activity for many healthy, older individuals. It provides opportunities to stay active, feel productive and interact with others. Many silver workers value maintaining oftentimes long and supportive relationships with work colleagues and being able to continue to learn and have new experiences through their work. In a recent survey conducted by Towers Perrin on behalf of AARP, 49 per cent of Canadian respondents indicated that they intend to work in retirement. Although the top reason was for extra money (45 per cent of responses), the other reasons mentioned most frequently were to stay mentally active (42 per cent), to stay productive (27 per cent), to stay physically active (26 per cent), and to have something interesting to do (25 per cent)

Table 77: Item Wise Intensity Indices showing the Work related Reasons of Silver Workers to Work after Retirement

(N=300)

Items	Intensity Indices
Cannot imagine life without work	2.51
Job is interesting	2.07
Opportunity to work which is not too stressful	1.93
Chance to work that is not too physically demanding	1.81
Opportunity to work on dream job	1.54
The pay offered was too good to refuse	1.50
Opportunity to learn new job skills	1.50

Table 77 shows that the overall intensity indices in relation to the work related reasons of the silver workers ranged from 2.51 to 1.50. It means that there were more to less number of work related reasons for silver workers to work after retirement. It can be seen from the table that silver workers had more numbers of reason to work after retirement as they could not "imagine life without work"

Silver workers had moderate number of work related reasons to work after retirement were as follows:

- Job is interesting
- Opportunity to work which is not too stressful
- Chance to work that is not too physically demanding
- Opportunity to work on dream job

Silver workers reported following reason to less extent "the pay offered was too good to refuse" and "Opportunity to learn new job skills

Some work- and organisation-related factors that have proven relevant for the decision to continue working refer to enterprise size, position, and income. The group of work related reasons indicate one preference to stay active in later stage of life. Among these reasons, those like staying active receive very high consideration from the silver workers. Thus the intensity indices indicate that the silver worker showed concern of high intensity for activeness and interest in work. According to the item wise intensity indices

4.5 Perceptions of the Silver Workers about their Retirement

Part of every human being's self-image is based on their age, whether it is their chronological or their "subjective age", or how old they feel. Accordingly, when people reach retirement age, these two perceptions can widely differ. Society may view an individual of 65 as "ready to be put out to pasture". A silver worker tends to view himself/herself as still an active, energetic and productive member of community. The negative stereotypes perpetuated in society work against them causing people to behave in differently towards the elderly. Harmful biases are so deeply ingrained in people's minds to hamper or discourage the silver workforce.

Man stands apart from all animals on the planet by faculty of thinking. Man possesses mind so thinking is natural to him. Whatever he sees, knows or experiences his mind ponders on. He tries to understand and know things that is, asking and getting answers to his questions. As a result, he gets understandings to his questions. As a result, he gets understandings and knowledge which work to shape his views on the world outside him. His view mark and qualifies his perception in the world. In this way, perception is natural human phenomenon. Perception is a way to see the world. It co-exists with human way of living. Thus living and thinking or perception co-exists is marked and qualified with human perception. In this sense, silver workers identify is marked and qualified with his perception on the reality surrounding him.

Reality for man is what he lives and how he lives. As he lives life he is bound to think on his life in the current. Silver workers live the second innings of human life that begins after his retirement from his first employment. So they naturally think on a current stage of life. They may call it a new "stage of life" that brings to them different experiences. So it would be interesting t6o review the silver workers perception on their retirement.

As man grows in age he forms an image about his self. It is self image that keeps changing in different stages and age of life. As a child, he has one kind of self image and a s a youth another. Likewise, as a married person, a grown up person and in senior age he holds a different kind of self image. An old man too holds a typical self image and when he decides to work after retirement his self image would acquire qualitative change. Silver workers self image what he thinks about him, what others in family, co-workers at work places would think about him. It may surface his complexes, public view about him and typical mindset reacting against public view.

Societal perceptions of old age and older persons are based partly on the social and economic position of older persons, and ageist stereotypes abound in both developed and developing countries. This also dictates how older persons are viewed and treated, even when societal agreement for material support of older persons is strong.

Surveys on perceptions of old age and older persons in developing countries are lacking. One exception is a survey undertaken by the HSBC Bank on attitudes towards ageing and retirement, which includes countries with emerging economies such as Brazil, China, India and Mexico. The survey points to changing and differing perceptions between countries of what constitutes old age. In developed countries, retirement is increasingly viewed as a new beginning in life and "old age" is linked to the decline of a person's physical and mental abilities.

The silver workers perceptions forms subjective edge on the reality in the sense of what they feel and how they response or react. It may also bring in views, biases and stigma that prevail about these individuals. The silver workers perceptions may appreciate positive thinking about them and even react sharply to negative stereotype, damaging biases and stigmatized notions that are ingrained in peoples mind and perpetuate in society to hamper and discourage the silver work force to work after retirement. In these sense silver workers perceptions serves a mirror to reflect on the reality in view of the silver workers decision to work after retirement. Hence an analysis would help to explain what retirement means to them and what purpose would be served by their working after retirement the analysis may begin with reviewing the data obtained on the silver workers perception on retirement. The analysis of present study would bring in all such typical dimensions as they surface in the silver workers perception in their current stage on life of the working elderly.

So it would be useful to review decisions of the silver workers to work after retirement. It is worth analyzing this concept a little closer, before we arrive there, to make sure it's a place we want to go. What is the purpose and meaning of "retirement" to silver workers.

Table 78: Percentages wise Distribution of Overall Perceptions of the Silver about Retirement

(N=300)

Perceptions	F	%
Most Favourable	90	30.00
Favourable	97	32.33
Less Favourable	113	37.67

Table 78 and the related graph represent the status of the perceptions of the silver workers about retirement. Majority of them had less favourable perceptions about retirement. Whereas one third of them expressed favourable perceptions about retirement and thirty percentages of them had most favourable perceptions about retirement

First the silver workers perceptions about retirement was reviewed reflected the percentage was more or less, equally distributed in three opinions like "most favourable", "favourable" and "less favourable" closely viewing , relatively some more of the silver workers viewed their retirement as less favourable. It implies that they perceived some problem in their life after retirement to afflict their minds and these problems may prompt them to continue further after retirement.

Table 79: Percentage Distribution of the Silver Workers According to the Considerations in Deciding the Time to Retire

(N=300)

Considerations	F	%
Achieve certain amount of money for retirement	151	50.33
Accomplish certain career/job related retirement goals	100	33.33
When children start earning	82	27.33
When eligible for retirement health benefits	44	14.67

In their second innings, the silver workers would feel like working until they fulfil certain targets or goals. They think of retirement as certain considerations the table 79 reflects that half (50.33%) of the silver workers were more likely to retire after achieving certain amount as provision for the future retirement money. Following them by little more than one third (33.33%) of the silver workers considered in accomplishing certain career/job related goals as an important factor to decide time to retire. Further silver workers stated that they would retire when children would start earning (27.33%) and some other would be ready to retire when they would be eligible for post retirement health benefits (14.67%).The table shows that financial stability was the major consideration for silver workers to decide about when to retire .Majority of them wanted to have retirement savings.

Silver workers perceptions pertained to retirement as to when to retire, how to pass on the post retirement life and if a retired person desired to work after retirement who would help them to prepare for it. When to retire can be crucial question for a person beyond fifty years of age. As such an age of retirement is fixed by the government at which an employee's has to retire from a job. He/she is given post retirement benefits too in the form of pension, gratuity, and contribution to P.F. Almost half of the silver workers perceived that once they have enough provision for future they would think to retire. Some one third of them looked for professional career related or job based accomplishment in its regards. Some one fourth of them expected to be relieved of their liabilities to their children before retirement's small group of them thought of retirement on health grounds. Thus, it can be seen that one's decision to retire form job relied on a major part on economic considerations.

Table 80: Percentage Distribution of the Silver Workers According to their Preparation for Retirement

(N=300)

Preparation	F	%
Discussing with friends	193	64.33
Reading books	58	19.33
Attending lectures	49	16.33

Table 80 shows that majority of the silver workers (64.33%) discussed with friends how to prepare them for retirement; whereas little less than one fifth (19.33%) prepared themselves for retirement by reading books. Nearly 17 percentages of them (16.33%) prepared themselves by listening to talks and lectures. The table shows that majority of silver workers prepared themselves for retirement by discussing the matter with their friends.

Table 81: Percentage Distribution of the Silver Workers According to Personnel's primarily responsible for preparing the Workers for Retirement

(N=300)

Personnel's	F	%
All of the below	121	40.33
Employers	101	33.67
Co-Workers	86	28.67
Government	77	25.67

Table 81 reflects on who prepared the silver workers for retirement. Nearly forty one percentages (40.33%) of the silver workers believed that all the three employers, co-workers and the government were responsible for preparing them for retirement. Little more than one third percent of them (33.67%) believed that employers were responsible for preparing silver workers for retirement. While nearly thirty percent (28.67%) believed that co-workers were responsible for it and almost 26 percent of them (25.67%) believed that the government is responsible for preparing the silver workers for retirement. This shows that majority of silver workers expect that employers, government and co-workers all of them together should take an initiative to prepare silver workers for retirement.

Table 82: Percentage Distribution of the Silver Workers According to the Circumstances that they thought could be the Reasons for the Inadequate Retirement Savings of their Fellow Workers

(N=300)

Reasons	F	%
Lack of proper planning	260	86.67
Heavy medical bills used up their savings	106	35.33
Expecting others to look out financially for them	103	34.33

Table 82 specifies that little more than 85 percentages (86.67%) of the silver workers reported that the reason for inadequate retirement savings would be lack of proper planning. Silver workers further stated that heavy medical bills used up their savings (35.33%). Almost equal percentages (34.33%) of them reported that expecting others to look out financially for them as the reasons for inadequate retirement savings. The table reveals that the silver workers were aware about the importance of retirement savings and so very high majority of them believed that lack of retirement planning could be the major reasons that had left their fellow workers with inadequate retirement savings.

4.6 Item Wise Findings Regarding Perceptions of the Silver Workers about Retirement

The scale to judge the perceptions of silver workers about retirement includes 46 items. For each item, there were three options which indicate three intensity indices related to the perceptions of silver workers about retirement. The items that more number of silver workers reported are specified below:

Table 83: Item Wise Intensity Indices showing the Favourable Perceptions of Silver Workers about Retirement

(N=300)

Items	Intensity Indices
An opportunity to share knowledge and experience	2.56
Working after retirement because they enjoy working	2.53
A stage of more maturity	2.24
More respect in society	2.24
A stage to serve family	2.20
A stage of freedom from work pressures	2.16
A stage to fulfil dreams and aspirations that remained unfulfilled earlier	2.10
An opportunity to contribute to the society	2.03
A stage to enjoy with grandchildren	2.01
A stage with more control over personal time	1.99
A stage to relax	1.96
Getting more attention from family	1.94
A stage to have fun	1.92
A stage to travel	1.89
A stage with less financial responsibility	1.89
A stage with less family responsibilities	1.86
A stage to get involved in religious activities	1.84

Table 83 indicates the item wise intensity indices of the silver workers are related to their perceptions about retirement that ranged from 2.56 to 1.86. It can be seen from the above table that the silver workers agreed on having great extent of favourable agreement on perceptions about retirement with regards to the following matters:

- An opportunity to share knowledge and experience

  Further it can be revealed from the table that the silver workers expressed some extent of agreement on following matters:

- Accommodating in post-retirement lifestyle is difficult
- Coping with long hours with partner without children
- Worrying about retiring
- Learning new skills to survive in the post retirement life
- Managing surplus time at my disposal
- A stage of more maturity
- More respect in society
- A stage to serve family
- A stage of freedom from work pressures
- A stage to fulfil dreams and aspirations that remained unfulfilled earlier
- Establishing new routine
- An opportunity to contribute to the society
- A stage to enjoy with grandchildren
- A stage with more control over personal time
- A stage to relax
- Getting more attention from the family
- A stage to have fun
- A stage to travel
- A stage with less financial responsibility
- A stage with less family responsibilities
- A stage to get involved in religious activities

Table 84: Item Wise Intensity Indices showing the Unfavourable Perceptions of Silver Workers about Retirement

(N=300)

Items	Intensity Indices
Cursed stage of life	2.72
Feeling unwanted in society	2.68
Loosing interest in life	2.67
Loosing charm of looks	2.65
Problems of ageing and imminent death	2.65
Prone to disease	2.64
Starting of old age	2.59
A period of misery	2.59
Less fun in life	2.58
Feeling of insecurity	2.57
Decline in social life	2.57
Having fear of being dejected or left out by family members	2.55
Sense of worthlessness	2.55
Fear of isolation	2.55
Sense of worthlessness	2.55
Physically unable to do household work	2.54
Managing irregular or non-payment of retirement benefits	2.53
A slide to dependency	2.51
Developing feeling of inferiority complex	2.49
Unable to face people with confidence	2.48
Deteriorating health	2.44
Working in order to get by financially	2.35
Managing new and low social status	2.35
Accommodating in post-retirement lifestyle is difficult	2.34
Coping with long hours with partner without children	2.33
Worrying about retiring	2.32
Learning new skill to survive in the post retirement life	2.27

Managing surplus time at my disposal	2.26
Establishing new routine	2.06

Table 84 indicates the item wise intensity indices of the silver workers are related to their perceptions about retirement that ranged from 2.72 to 2.06. It can be seen from the above table that the silver workers agreed on having great extent of favourable agreement on perceptions about retirement with regards to the following matters:

- Cursed stage of life
- Feeling unwanted in society
- Loosing interest in life
- Loosing charm of looks
- Problems of ageing and imminent death
- Prone to disease
- Starting of old age
- A period of misery
- Less fun in life
- Feeling of insecurity
- Decline in social life
- Developing feelings of inferiority complex
- Unable to face people with confidence
- Feeling too young to retire
- Deteriorating health
- Working in order to get by financially
- Having the fear of being dejected or left out by family members
- Sense of worthlessness
- Fear of isolation
- Sense of worthlessness
- Physically unable to do household work
- Managing irregular or non-payment of retirement benefit
- Working after retirement because they enjoy working
- A slide to dependency

- Managing new and low social status

The item wise indices reflect on the extent of intensity of perceptions for the silver workers as they expressed their views on a stage of retirement. It is popularly view over the world as a "new stage of life" on diverse considerations. As indicated early, in this stage of life a shift is marked from active life to passive life. If one wishes to involve in activities they are linked with leisure time "as an attractive way of leisure time" as a US findings by Weiss (2005) reveals. The German perspective considers it a stage of self confidence and self interest with motivation free of monetary considerations. The Indian view projects rather um pleasing side if this new stage of life as it renders from the data presented. Silver workers reflections on a stage of retirement calling it "a cursed stage of life" with feeling of neglect, lack of interest without charm and prone to sickness , feeling of insecurity and fear of ageing and eventual death. All kinds of feelings capture their minds and affect their thinking and expressions. It implies that in this stage of life some kind of negativity arouses and grows to affect a person psychologically. Matters related to a person's utility in society, his/her value in society, insecurity, decline in health conditions, economic constraints, social recognition respect on family, enthusiasm and enjoyment with new thinking and creation, affect a person's psychology adversely and this is true about majority of the silver workers. However, on a lesser intensity some of them view this stage of life as a stage of maturity, earning respect in family and society, an opportunity to serve society, allowing most of personal space and choice to involve in activities of one's choice, enjoying freedom to travel, relieving from family responsibilities and enjoying allowing more involvement in religious and creative works for self development.

4.7 Preparation for Retirement

Table 85: Percentage Distribution of the Silver Workers According to their Stages of Planning Finance

(N=300)

Stages of Planning	F	%
Much earlier to Retirement	181	60.33
At the time of Retirement	101	33.67
After Retirement	18	6.00

It would be significant to know which stage in life the silver workers thought for planning the finance. The table 85 reflects that majority (60.33%) of silver workers started to plan finance much earlier to retirement. Little more than one third of them (33.67%) stated that they planned for finance a time of retirement. A very few of them (6%) thought of planning for finance after retirement

Table 86: Percentage Distribution of the Silver Workers According to the Specific Age when they started to Plan for Finance

(N=300)

Age (In Years)	F	%
51 years and Below	153	51.00
Above 51 years	147	49.00

Table 86 shows that little more than half percentages (51%) of the silver workers started to plan for finance at the age of 51 or below. Whereas nearly fifty percentages (49%) of them started to plan for finance after an age of 51 years .The table shows that majority of the silver workers started to plan for retirement savings much before retirement.

The second point that was reviewed was finance .In Indian context in which the outflow of money ever exceeds the inflow of money and one ever finds his/her income short of meeting his/her needs he/se ever faces problems with two ends of income and expenditure to meet. So planning finance becomes a crucial need particularly for a man in an age beyond retirement. A review of the silver workers perceptions on a matter of planning finance can be read through the data presented in the table 72. As the table represents, majority of the silver workers perceived that planning of finance has to be made much earlier in life, much earlier to retirement. Some of them thought of planning finance when they retire from the first employment and few of them thought of doing it after retirement. Thus, most of the silver workers were aware of importance of money and that proper planning of finance at the right time would make their life easy and comfortable. Right decision at right point of time always help a person decision to decide whether he/she would need to work after retirement..

In a matter of planning finance, a person's count very much when he/she finds him/her always pressed with managing expenditure against income. The data indicates that though majority of the silver workers perceived that planning of finance has to be done much earlier in life half of them could do it by an age of 51 years and half of them could do it after it. You may think in one direction and harsh reality drags you in the opposite direction.

Table 87: Overall Intensity Indices and Percentage Wise Distribution of the Silver Workers According to the Stages of Life that they enjoyed the most

(N=300)

Stages of Life	Intensity Indices
Brahmacharya (Student stage of life)	2.56
Grahasta (Family stage of life)	2.49
Vanprastha (Indicates departure from material possession)	1.91
Sanyasa or renunciation(The person leaves society to spend the remaining part of his life in meditation and contemplation of God in solitude	1.87

A stage of life that silver workers enjoyed the most would have some kind of perceptions of the silver workers in the present. The table 87 shows that overall intensity indices regarding stages of life silver workers enjoyed the most ranged from

2.56 to 1.87.It means that there was great extent to some extent of agreement about enjoying stages of life.

In view of stages of life enjoyed, majority of the silver workers (67%) reflected that they enjoyed the Brahmacharya (Student stage of life) most. Nearly 63 percent (62.33%) of them who reported that they enjoyed most the Grahasta (Family stage of life).Almost 41 percent of the silver workers were positive about enjoying Vanprastha most (Indicates departure from material possession).Nearly 36 percent of them agreed to some extent that though they have not yet reach a stage in life when they would enjoy, it may be the Sanyasa or renunciation (The person leaves society to spend the remaining part of his life in meditation and contemplation of God in solitude. The table clearly reveals that silver workers enjoyed the student stage of life more in comparison to other stages of life.

Pleasure or enjoyment is believed to be an important expectation in human life. One strives ever to be happy and enjoy life. As the silver workers perceptions in this regards are represented through the percentage and the intensity indices, it is understood that a good majority of them perceived that they enjoyed life with good intensity when they were merely boys or youth and lived students life (the brahmacharya).Some majority of them agreed to enjoy life after marriage (the gruhastha) and their family served them a vital source of enjoyment. Some of the silver workers agreed that they enjoyed life in a later stage when they withdraw from maternal life and handed over family responsibilities to their sons and daughters, whereas a small group of the silver workers admitted that they enjoyed real life when they renounced the world almost and most of time involved them in spiritual practices (the sanyasa).the percentage that indicates the intensity of enjoyment of life reveals showed high intensity during the bramcharya and the gruhastha stages of life and intensity to some extent during the vanprastha and to low extent during sanyasa stages of life.

Table 88: Percentage Distribution of the Silver Workers According to the Need of money During Retirement Age

(N=300)

Need of Money	F	%
Need more money	199	66.33
Do not need more money	101	33.67

Needing money in life is perpetual dilemma that influences intensity of need to work after retirement. To a silver worker, it would be more taxing to affect quality of life. The table 88 reflects that 66.33 percent of the silver workers reported that they need more money during the retirement age. Whereas little less than thirty five percentages of them (33.67%) stated that they do not need more money during the retirement age. Thus majority of silver workers said that they would need more money after retirement.

Money remains a vital source of enjoyment and happiness in life. In the modern context, money proves inevitable to make one comfortable at least by available facilities of housing, clothing .living arrangements .living conditions, communication and travel. Money enhances man's life by raising his comfort level. In this regards, a goof majority of the silver workers perceived that they would need more money and about one third of them thought they would not need any money and would rather be satisfied with the present income. It might be because they had made sufficient provisions for life after retirement during their first employment and so prefer to pass life quietly without involving in monetary activities. When this group of the silver workers decided to work after retirement the considerations would be other than the economic and they would be either social, work related or personal preferences. For the major group, it may be understood that the consideration would be on a major part economic and on a minor part societal or familial.

Table 89: Percentage Distribution of the Silver Workers According to the Purpose to Need Money during the Retirement Age

(N=300)

Purposes	F	%
Health emergencies	171	57.00
House maintenance	159	53.00
Domestic services	102	34.00
Tour and travels	71	23.67
Leisure entertainment	59	19.67
Old age homes	17	5.67

Money is needed for various purposes in life. For the silver workers money is essential to fulfil various crucial purposes specifying the purposes the table 89 shows that health emergencies emerged as the most crucial aspect (57%) for the silver workers in terms of spending more money in retirement. It was followed by other needs like house maintenance (53%), domestic services (34%), tour and travels (23.67%) leisure and entertainment (19.67%) on which the silver workers were ready to spend more money during retirement. A very less percentage of them (5.67%) reported that they were ready to spend more money in retirement on old age homes. This table clearly shows that majority of silver workers were ready to spend money on health emergencies and least percentages of them were ready to spend on old age homes.

What relate to money is the purpose and the priority to spend on money. On reviewing the silver workers perception on these two matters, a majority of them said they would need in case health emergencies and another major group put forth a purpose of house maintenance. A small group gave a purpose of managing domestic services. Another small group needed money for tours and travels on social or entertainment purpose. Some of them wanted to spend money on leisure entertainment. A very small group of the silver workers reported that they think that they might need money to take shelter in old age homes in their later life. These indicate the expenditures that one had to incur in order to keep up life family house and society that cannot be evaded. But if choice is given, the silver workers came out with their priorities on which they would spend money. A very high majority recognised their family liabilities. A good majority expressed a wish to keep some money for their children/grand children. A small group of them put forth old age condition and said they would need money for special assistance in conditions of dependency. Another small group gave a reason of partners death and said they would need money to sustain in such conditions. In this way, the silver workers perceptions revealed a variety of purpose and priorities and majority of them related it to their old age conditions .there might be fear related to old age because of which they have decided to save money

Table 90: Percentage Distribution of the Silver Workers According to the Preparedness to Spend More Money during Retirement

(N=300)

Spend More Money	F	%
Deteriorating Heath	246	82.00
Being burden on children	217	72.33
Being able to leave some money for children/grandchildren	182	60.67
Not Being able to take care of self	103	34.33
Death of partner	83	27.67

Table 90 shows that high majority of the silver workers (82%) reported that deteriorating health would be a major factor for which they were prepared to spend more money. While (72.33%) of them reported that they were prepared to spend more money in the case they would be of being burden on their children. A good number of silver workers felt that they should leave behind some money for their children (60.67%). Some of them also stated that they were ready to spend more money in case of not being able to take care of self (34.33%). The remaining percent of them (27.67%) believed to spend more money in case of death of partner. This table reveals that high majority of the silver workers did not wanted to be financial burden on their children as well as they wanted to leave some money for their children and grandchildren

A craze of socializing is natural instinct with all human beings. Particularly, when he/she feels lonely and bored he/she the thinks of friends with whom he can share pleasures and pain. He/she knows that his/her pleasures would doubled if he/she shares it with friends and also sharing pains would cut it down to get him/her some solace. It becomes the truth with persons aging beyond retirement. Once a person retires from an active life with hectic schedule from morning till evening he feels a kind of vacuum in life. Because he does not tire and feels fatigued with work or overwork he/she may not get good sleep even at night with too much of rest and nothing to do he develops a kind of boredom that slowly and gradually get converted into some kind of depression to capture minds. In such conditions it is important to decide how to prepare for retirement.

The expectation that a silver worker, after decades of work, will go casually and without thought as to what retirement entails is a product of a bygone era. Retirement from work, though expected in many industrialized countries, can provoke some anxiety for silver workers who may try to put off facing the adjustments that will have to be made in their lives. Regardless of the age when silver workers retire from work, they may need to come to terms with this situation before they leave work. This can be facilitated by providing them with information they may need to cope with their new status. Information that has been found to be useful in this process includes facts regarding post-retirement income (assessing what financial resources may be available so that the worker can enjoy decent retired life), the possibility of undertaking gainful activity during pension years, health-care information (including how to prevent premature ageing), information on the availability of cultural and voluntary activities and on where preparations for retirement are best made (at work or home).findings of the study reveals that one fourth of the silver workers perceived that can be a good help to them for the purpose, where about forty percent of them perceived that all the government, employers and co-workers can extent helping hands in different capacities to prepare the workers for their retirement. These people can help them to open their minds to what they expect in a new situation of post retirement employment and they would also help to shape viable suggestions for collective efforts to shape elderly workers as productive employees in the second innings of their working life.

4.8 Influence of Work on Silver Workers

It is assumed that although the silver workers show a high degree of motivation to work nonetheless different factors play role against them. Generally a person's motivation evolves and changes over course of time and it is stimulated with more experiences and appreciation. The present section focuses specifically on the factors that influenced the silver workers to work after retirement.

Encouraging greater silver worker participation in the labour force requires an understanding of the factors that can influence the work decisions of individuals as they get older. This section discusses some of the key factors that can have a bearing on the decisions of silver workers about their involvement in work. These include personal preferences and circumstances, employment policies and practices, knowledge and skills, and financial considerations. The silver workers belonged to persons in elderly age, which as their perceptions about retirement are reviewed earlier, seemed to be much afflicted with nothing to do, that is, passive state of life. Hence, they decided to work even after retirement. The consideration may be any of the specified, but the fact remains that work influenced their life after retirement. As most of them exhibited a high degree of motivation for work it would be interesting to review an extent of influence work exerted on them. Majority of them agreed that they carried a high level of influence of work, whereas about one third of them had moderate level of influence of work. A few of them admitted that work had influence on them at a low level. A scale of judging was drawn on the reasons that prompted the silver workers to work after retirement. For the purpose, the intensity indices was calculated item wise to uneducated on extent of their intensity on the silver workers. The items determined for the purpose were 24 pertaining to different reasons for influence of work. They ranged from the social like earning, attention, respect and recognition in society; to the personal like enhancing confidence, maintaining physical and mental fitness; to the social responsibility like contributing through interaction with people. It also related to one's responsibility to his family and personal satisfaction. It also related to health situation, skill development and some kind of complex.

Table 91: Percentages Wise Distribution of Overall Influence of Work on Silver Workers

(N=300)

Influence of Work	F	%
High level of Influence	184	61.33
Moderate Level of Influence	107	35.67
Low Level of Influence	9	3.00

Table 91 and related graph focuses on the extent of work on the silver workers (61.33%) carried high level of influence of their work. Almost 36 percent had moderate level of influence of work on them. A very few percent (3%) of them had low level of influence of work.

Table 92: Extent of Influence of Work on the Silver Workers in Relation to the Selected Variables

(N=300)

Table 92 reveals that higher percentage of the silver workers from the following

Variables	N	Influence of Work		
		High	Moderate	Low
1. Age				
Young –Old	116	44.82	37.06	18.10
Old	184	26.63	51.08	22.28
2. Type of Work				
Full time	184	21.19	52.17	26.63
Part time	116	17.24	58.62	24.86
3. Present Designation				
Class I	27	59.25	14.81	25.92
Class II	190	38.42	50.52	11.05
Class III	71	22.53	57.74	19.71
Class IV	12	16.67	33.03	50.00
4. Health Status				
Healthy	192	42.48	30.56	26.94
Somewhat Healthy	103	16.50	70.87	12.62
Less Healthy	5	20.00	20.00	60.00

categories of variables had influence of work on them to moderate level to work after retirement.

- Silver workers in old age group
- Silver workers doing part time jobs
- Silver workers having class III designations
- Silver workers who were somewhat healthy

4.9 Differences in the Influence of Work on Silver Workers in Relation to the Selected Variables

Earlier we discussed influence of silver workers to work after retirement. It would be now interesting to know if it varies in relation to the variables selected for the study. This would unfold another fact of the study

It may be noted that no significant differences were found in the extent of influencing factors exerted in relation to the variables like age, type of work, present designation, and health status. The survey revealed interesting and useful findings to help the analysis of the influence.

The finding related to the differences in influence of work on the silver workers in relation to the selected variables are presented below

DIFFERENCES IN INFLUENCE OF WORK ON THE SILVER WORKERS IN RELATION TO THE SELECTED VARIABLES

Table 93: t-Ratio Showing the Difference in the Influence of Work on Silver Workers in Relation to Age

(N=300)

Variables	Source of Variance	N	Mean	SD	t-value
Age	Young-Old	116	48.71	4.782	.786
	Old	184	48.27	4.694	NS

NS=Not Significant

Table 93 shows that influence of work on the silver workers in relation to their age did not differ significantly. Thus, the null hypothesis stating that there will be no significant difference in influence of work on the silver workers at workplace in relation to their age was accepted.

The results of various studies show no noteworthy difference between different age groups with regard to motivation. But this also means that elderly are not less motivated than younger workers. Basically, empirical studies reveal that the work motivation of older employees is high (Rabl 2010; Kooji et al. 2010). Also, no studies have been able to provide evidence confirming the generally negative age stereotypes (Stamov Rossnagel 2009; Grube/Hertel 2008). However, there are indications from studies that the factors behind motivation differ between age groups (Rhodes 1983; Lord 2002; Kanfer/Ackermann 2004; Lord/Farrington 2006; Rabl 2010; Stamov Rossnagel 2009; Kooij et al. 2010). Similarly no significant difference was found in relation to the influence and type of work, this finding reveals that type of work does not influence the decision of the silver workers to work after retirement either they are working part time or full time.

Table 94: t-Ratio Showing the Difference in the Influence on Silver Workers in Relation to their Type of Work

(N=300)

Variables	Source of Variance	N	Mean	SD	t-value
Type of Work	Full Time	184	48.35	4.840	.357
	Part Time	116	48.58	4.553	NS

NS=Not Significant

Table 94 reveals that influence of work on the silver workers in relation to their type of work did not differ significantly. Thus, the null hypothesis, stating that there will be no significant difference in influence of work on the silver workers at workplace in relation to their type of work was accepted.

Table 95: Analysis of Variance (ANOVA) Showing Difference in Influence of work on Silver Workers in Relation to their Present Designations

(N=300)

Variables	Source of Variance	DF	Sum of Squares	Mean Square	F-Value	Sig.
Present Designation	Between Groups	3	93.911	31.304	1.408 NS	.241
	Within Groups	296	6581.885	22.236		
	Total	299	6675.797			

NS=Not Significant

It can be seen from the table 95 that influence of work on the silver workers in relation to their present designations did not differ significantly. Thus, the null hypothesis, stating that there will be no significant difference in the influence of work on silver workers at workplaces in relation to their present designations was accepted.

Table 96: Analysis of Variance (ANOVA) Showing Difference in Influence of Work on the Silver Workers in Relation to their Health Status

(N=300)

Variables	Source of Variance	DF	Sum of Squares	Mean Square	F-Value	Sig.
Health Status	Between Groups	2	14.405	7.202	.321 NS	.726
	Within Groups	297	6661.392	22.429		
	Total	299	6675.797			

NS=Not Significant

It can be read from table 96 that the influence of work on the silver workers in relation to their health status did not differ significantly. Thus, the null hypothesis stating that there will be no significant difference in the influence of work on silver workers at workplaces in relation to their health status was accepted

4.10 Item wise Findings Regarding Influence of Work on Silver Workers

The scale to judge the reasons of silver workers to work after retirement included 24 items. For each item three options were mentioned that indicated three intensity indices regarding influence of work on the silver workers. The items for which more number of the silver workers marked, are specified below:

Table 97: Item Wise Intensity Indices Showing Influence of Work on Silver Workers

(N=300)

Items	Intensity Indices
Due to Work	
Got respect and attention in a family	2.62
Got recognition in society	2.62
Could face people with confidence	2.60
Remain physically active	2.55
Remain mentally active	2.55
Able to contribute my experience to the society	2.49
Able to interact with people	2.41
No dependence on children	2.34
Able save money	2.08
Able support children financially	2.02
Could spend time with family	2.01
Could accomplish certain career or job related goals	1.99
Unable get enough leisure time	1.95
Economic status has improved	1.95
Received health benefits and wellness supports	1.93
Able spend for leisure/entertainment activities	1.57
Being able to take care of spouse	1.50
Able to spend more for health related needs	1.47
Got an opportunity to work on new technologies such as computer, mobile, i-pad	1.47
Feeling insulted to work under younger generation	1.45
Feeling overburdened with responsibilities	1.41
Feeling more stressed after working for the whole week	1.41
Facing more health problems	1.41
Health does not permit to work for long hours	1.41

Table 97 reflects that the intensity indices regarding influence of work on silver workers ranged from 2.62 to 1.41.It means that due to work there was great extent of influence of work on silver workers with regards to

- To remain mentally active
- To face people with confidence
- To remain physically active
- To get recognition in society
- To get respect and attention from my family

Further it is revealed from the above table that the silver workers had moderate level of influence of work with regards to :

- To contribute my experience to the society
- To have interaction with people
- Do not have to depend on their children for financial requirements
- To save money
- To support children financially
- To spend time with family
- To accomplish certain career or job related goals
- Do not get enough leisure time
- To receive health benefits and wellness supports
- Economic status has improved
- To spend for leisure/entertainment activities
- To remain mentally active
- To remain physically active
- To face people with confidence
- To get respect and attention in a family
- To get recognition in society

  Further it can be seen from the above table that the silver workers had low level of influence in the following matters:
- To spend more for health needs
- To work on new technologies such as computer, mobile, i-pad

- Feeling insulted to work under younger generation
- Being overburdened with responsibilities
- Feeling more stressed after working for the whole week
- Facing more health problems
- Health does not permit to work for long hours

4.11 Problems Confronted by Silver Workers due to Work and Workplace

In a new and strange situation, problems are bound to confront a person and he has to find out solution to them to convert them into opportunities. The silver workers enter a new stage of working life in which he would find things new, strange and different to cope and manage. Naturally they would perceive them as problems. The data related to this fact reveal that several of them perceived more problems at workplaces and one third of them perceived moderate problems. Just about one fourth of them faced fewer problems at workplaces. Viewing the problems in relation to the selected variables we get clearer picture projecting diversity of the extent of the problems like more, moderate and less.

As a result of their decision to take a job after retirement, the silver workers faced consequences (i.e., challenges and opportunities). Although they were reluctant to talk about any problems or barriers, each silver worker identified at least one obstacle that they had encountered or were currently encountering. These challenges encompassed legal issues (e.g., age discrimination); financial matters (e.g., pension restrictions); career factors (e.g., lack of skills); and personal limitations (e.g., physical problems). Rather than deliberating over these problems, the silver workers were more anxious to recount the many opportunities or benefits that their job after retirement had contributed to their life. They said that they felt better about themselves, lived a more balanced life, and liked the work they were doing. silver worker identified the following four categories of challenges: a) financial challenges (i.e., lack of financial information or planning, pension restrictions, lower salary); b) problems switching careers (i.e., no plans, limited skills or experience, retraining demands, outside forces, adjusting to different environments, accepting changes in status); c) the age factor (i.e., subtle age discrimination, direct age discrimination); and d) personal challenges (i.e., self limitations, relationships, time management, emotional aspects, physical problems).

Making the decision to seek a job after retirement yielded two kinds of consequences for these silver workers, which were challenges and opportunities. When they made the transition or when they worked in their jobs after retirement, they faced challenges. They were confronted with financial issues, the ordeal of switching careers, age concerns, and personal challenges. They ran into financial problems when they lacked the financial information or had not planned; were restricted by their pension, made less in salary, or had added expenses. Switching careers posed problems for participants when they started their transition without a plan, needed to return to school (i.e., retraining), lacked the appropriate skill set or work experience, sought jobs that were part of a negative economic trend, had to adjust to a different work environment, and/or had to accept a change of status. As silver workers, age was cited numerous times as a barrier including direct age discrimination and subtle age discrimination. Many silver workers faced personal-type challenges that dealt with their own self-limitations, relationships, time management, and transition fears or concerns.

Although these silver workers faced challenges along this transition journey, they also gained many benefits (opportunities). If they were learning and growing, making a difference to others, demonstrating their competency, and/or were feeling physically better, they felt better about themselves. They described a life with structure or depicted living a more balanced life because they had more time and flexibility, a purpose, an expanded support system, and/or financial assistance. By connecting with their long-term career and controlling their own work situation (control), and/or just liking what they were doing in their bridge job, they said they enjoyed their work.

If silver worker had no career plans, lacked skills or experience, faced negative outside forces (i.e., poor economy), or needed retraining, they encountered problems switching to a new job. Additionally, some silver worker found it troublesome adjusting to a new work environment or accepting a change in their work role. A few silver workers made work part of their retirement plan but many did not.

Table 98: Percentage Distribution of the Silver Workers according to the Problems they confronted due to Work and Workplace

(N=300)

Problems	F	%
More Problems	122	40.77
Moderate Problems	104	34.67
Less Problems	71	23.67

Table 98 and related graph reveals higher percentages (40.77%) of the silver workers cofronted more problems due to work and workPlace. Nearly thirty five percentages (34.67%) of them confronted moderate problems. While 23.67 percent of them said they confronted fewer problems at their workplaces

Table 99: Percentage Distribution of the Silver Workers According to the Problems confronted due to Work and Workplace in Relation to the Selected Variables

(N=300)

Variables	N	More %	Moderate %	Less %
1. Age				
Young – Old	116	12.06	31.89	56.03
Old	184	14.67	34.78	50.54
2. Educational Qualification				
High level of Education	254	13.38	30.31	56.29
Moderate Level of Education	31	12.90	61.29	25.79
Low level of Education	15	20.00	33.33	46.67
3. Present Salary				
Less Salary	145	26.89	37.24	35.85
Moderate Salary	22	33.08	40.09	26.12
High Salary	133	10.08	33.01	56.11
4. Health Status				
Healthy	192	2.60	4.16	93.22
Somewhat Healthy	103	10.67	25.24	64.06
Less Healthy	5	40.00	20.00	40.00
5. Present Designation				
Class I	27	33.62	40.74	25.92
Class II	190	38.42	35.78	25.78
Class III	71	8.45	19.71	71.82
Class IV	12	25.00	8.33	66.67
6. Perceptions about Retirement				
Favourable	187	23.00	6.00	71.00
Unfavourable	113	25.78	8.45	66.67

In relation to the selected variables the table 99 reveals that higher percent of the silver workers confronted due to work and workplace.

- Silver workers belonging to the Young-Old age group
- Silver workers possessing high level of education
- Silver workers earning high salary
- Silver workers who were healthy and somewhat healthy
- Silver workers belonging to class III and IV designations
- Silver workers having favourable perception about retirement

Table 100: Percentage Distribution of the Silver Workers According to the Treatment received at Workplaces

(N=300)

Unfair Treatment	F	%
While making decisions to hire personnel	175	58.33
While increasing salaries	154	51.33
While laying off employees	138	46.00
While assigning desirable work	98	32.67

The table 100 and the related graph indicate that nearly sixty percent (58.33%) of the silver workers complained that the elderly were treated unfairly by the employers at the time of making decisions to hire of personnel. Little more than 50 percent (51.33%) of them regretted that while determining increase in salaries the elderly were treated unfairly. While 46 percent of them received unfair treatment in matter of laying off employees and also while assigning desirable work (32.67%). The table clearly reflects that the silver workers do feel deeply hurt by age discrimination of the employers and that they were treated unfairly at the workplaces.

4.12 Differences in the Problems Confronted by the Silver Workers due to Work and Workplace in Relation to the Selected Variables

The findings related to problems faced by silver workers at their workplace in relation to the selected variables are stated below:

DIFFERENCES IN THE PROBLEMS CONFRONTED BY THE SILVER WORKERS AT THEIR WORKPLACE IN RELATION TO THE SELECTED VARIABLES

Table 101: t-Ratio Showing the Difference in the Problems Confronted by Silver Workers due to Work and WorkPlace in Relation to their Age

(N=300)

Variable	Age	N	Mean	SD	t-value
Age	Young-Old	116	34.08	14.399	1.146 NS
	Old	184	36.19	16.234	

NS=Not Significant

It can be seen from the table 101 that problems that silver workers confronted due to work and workplace in relation to their age did not differ significantly. Thus, the null hypothesis, stating that there will be no significant difference in problems of the silver workers at workplaces in relation to their age was accepted.

That silver workers confronted problems due to work and workplace in relation to their age did not differ significantly. This reveals that silver workers did not face any kind of problems while working after retirement due to age. Silver workers belonging to young old age group and old age group both were reported about not facing any problem while working after retirement due to age which shows that they were positive about working and they were considering age just the number not as the obstacle while working post retirement.

Table 102: Analysis of Variance (ANOVA) Showing Difference between Problems Confronted by Silver Workers due to Work and Workplace in Relation to their Educational Qualification

(N=300)

Variables	Source of Variance	DF	Sum of Squares	Mean Square	F-Value	Sig.
Educational Qualification	Between Groups	2	1607.127	803.563	3.372*	.036
	Within Groups	297	70783.060	238.327		
	Total	299	72390.187			

* F Significant at 0.05 level, F-tab, 0.05 level df 2/299 =3.03

Table 102 reflects that there was significant difference in the problems of silver workersdue to work and workplace in relation to the educational qualification. In order to know among group the problems at workplace differed significantly the data were further analysed through t-test.

Table 103: t-Ratio Showing the Difference in the Problems Confronted by Silver Workers due to Work and Workplace in Relation to their Educational Qualification

(N=300)

Educational Qualification	X	SD	High Level of Education	Moderate Level of Education	Low Level of Education
High Level of Education	34.39	15.246		2.032*	1.792
Moderate Level of Education	40.35	16.828			0.253
Low Level of Education	41.67	15.769			

* Significant at 0.05 level

It can be seen from the table 103 above that there was significant difference in the extent of problems confronted by silver workers due to work and workplace in relation to their level of education. Those having moderate level of education faced more problems than those having high level of education. Those having moderate level of education and high level of education differed significantly. Thus, the null hypothesis, stating that there will be no significant difference in the problems confronted by the silver workers due to work and workplace in relation to their educational qualification was not accepted.

There was significant difference in the extent of problems confronted by silver workers due to work and workplace in relation to their level of education. Those having moderate level of education faced more problems than those having high level of education. Those having moderate level of education and high level of education differed significantly. Thus it can be revealed that those having moderate or low level of education confronted problems while working after retirement in comparisons to those having higher level of education, this shows that education plays important role while the silver workers decide to work after retirement. With the advancements in the field of employment sector they need to have proper and adequate education to sustain in the field of job sector. It shows that lack of education was the reasons for the silver workers use to which they were facing problems while working after retirement.

Table 104: Analysis of Variance (ANOVA) Showing Difference between Problems Confronted by Silver Workers due to Work and Workplace in Relation to their Present Salary

(N=300)

Variables	Source of Variance	DF	Sum of Squares	Mean Square	F-Value	Sig.
Present Salary	Between Groups	2	2458.145	1229.073	5.220**	.006
	Within Groups	297	69932.041	235.461		
	Total	299	72390.187			

**F Significant at 0.01 levels, F-tab, 0.01 level df 2/299 =4.68

The table 104 shows that there was significant difference in the problems of the silver workers due to work and workplace in relation to their present income. In order to know for which group the problems at workplace differed significantly the data were further analysed through t-test.

Table 105: t-Ratio Showing the Difference in the Problems Confronted by Silver Workers due to Work and Workplace in Relation to their Present Salary

(N=300)

Present Salary	X	SD	Less Salary	Moderate Salary	High Salary
Less Salary	35.91	14.627		2.418*	1.475
Moderate Salary	44.50	20.678			3.049**
High Salary	33.28	15.112			

**Significant at 0.01 level and * Significant at 0.05 level

It can be seen from the table 105 that the mean scores on problems of silver workers belonging to the middle income group were significantly higher than their counterpart. It indicates that silver workers belonging to the middle income group tends to confront more problems at their workplace as compared to those belonging to higher the income group and the low income group. Thus, the null hypothesis, stating that there will be no significant difference in the problems confronted by the silver workersdue to work and workplace in relation to their present income was not accepted.

There was significant difference in the problems of the silver workers due to work and at workplace in relation to their present income. In order to know for which group the problems at workplace differed significantly the data were further analysed through t-test. The mean scores on problems of silver workers belonging to the middle income group were significantly higher than their counterpart. It indicates that silver workers belonging to the middle income group tends to face more problems at their workplace as compared to those belonging to higher the income group and the low income group. This reveals that silver workers who were belonging to middle income groups were facing more problems than those who were in higher income group, it might be because of financial crunch or the dissatisfaction at their end due to which they were facing problem related to their income.

Table 106: Analysis of Variance (ANOVA) Showing Difference between Problems Confronted by Silver Workers due to Work and Workplace in Relation to their Health Status

(N=300)

Variables	Source of Variance	DF	Sum of Squares	Mean Square	F-Value	Sig.
Health Status	Between Groups	2	556.986	278.493	1.151 NS	.318
	Within Groups	297	71833.201	241.863		
	Total	299	72390.187			

NS=Not Significant

It can be seen from the table 106 that overall problems confronted by the silver workers due to work and workplace in relation to their health status did not differ significantly. Thus, the null hypothesis stating that there will be no significant difference in the problems faced by the silver workers at workplaces in relation to their health status was accepted.

Overall problems confronted by the silver workers due to work and workplace in relation to their health status did not differ significantly. This clearly shows that they were physically and mentally fit and did not face any problem due to health while working after retirement. This give show a positive sign that they are in good state of health and so they were working post retirement.

Table 107: Analysis of Variance (ANOVA) Showing Difference between the Problems Confronted by Silver Workers due to Work and Workplace in Relation to their Present Designation

(N=300)

Variables	Source of Variance	DF	Sum of Squares	Mean Square	F-Value	Sig.
Present Designation	Between Groups	3	958.638	319.546	1.324 NS	.267
	Within Groups	296	71431.548	241.323		
	Total	299	72390.187			

NS=Not Significant

Table 107 reflects that problems confronted by the silver workers in relation to their present designation did not differ significantly. Thus, the null hypothesis, stating that there will be no significant difference in problems faced by the silver workers at workplaces in relation to their present designation was accepted.

Problems faced by the silver workers in relation to their present designation did not differ significantly. Thus, the null hypothesis, stating that there will be no significant difference in problems faced by the silver workers at workplaces in relation to their present designation was accepted. This clearly shows that silver workers did not face any problem in their present job due to their designation.

Table 108: t-Ratio Showing the Difference in the Problems Confronted by Silver Workers due to Work and Workplace in Relation to their Perceptions about Retirement

(N=300)

Variables	Source of Variance	N	Mean	SD	t-value
Perceptions about Retirement	Favourable	150	28.29	16.162	8.850**
	Unfavourable	150	42.46	11.114	

**Significant at 0.01 level, tab-2.34

Table 108 represents that that there was significant difference in the problems faced by the silver workers due to work and workplace in relation to their perceptions about old age. Thus, the null hypothesis stating that there will be no significant difference in the overall problems faced by the silver workers at workplace in relation to their perceptions about old age was not accepted. The reasons are that the silver workers who held unfavourable perceptions about old age faced more problems at workplaces compared to those having favourable perception.

There was significant difference in the problems confronted by the silver workers at workplaces in relation to their perceptions about old age. This reveals that those silver workers who were having unfavourable perceptions about retirement faced more problems at their workplace.

4.13 Item wise Findings Related to Problems Confronted by the Silver Workers due to Work and Workplace

The scale to judge the problems confronted by the silver workers due to work and workplace includes 25 items. For each item there were three options mentioned which indicated three intensity indices related to the problems confornted by silver workers due to work and workplace. The matter, for which more number of the silver workers had reported, are specified below:

Table 109: Item Wise Intensity Indices Showing the Problems Confronted by the Silver Workers due to Work and Workplace

(N=300)

Items	Intensity Indices
Opinions and experience are not valued	2.24
Being discriminated due to age	1.89
Co-workers are not willing to work with me	1.85
Co-workers are neglecting	1.85
Over burdened with work	1.78
Work environment is unsuitable	1.71
Remuneration is insufficient	1.70
Work is uninteresting	1.67
No flexibility in working hours	1.60
Work place is very far from residence	1.58
Lack of appreciation from employers	1.58
Co-workers do not respect	1.56
Lack of independence in terms of taking decision related to work	1.55
Lack of clearly defined roles and responsibilities	1.53
Job is physically demanding	1.42
Designation is not appropriate to experience	1.09

Table 109 shows that overall the intensity indices regarding problems that the silver workers confronted due to work and workplace ranged from 2.24 to 1.09. It means that problems faced by silver workers at their workplace due to work ranged from more to less on the above mentioned matters. It is revealed from the table that the silver workers were facing more problems at workplaces in relation two matters like anxiety and fear of losing job and working on new technologies like computers ,laptops, fax, E-mails to a great extent

It can be further seen from the above table that the silver workers faced following problems to some extent:

- Opinions and experience are not valued
- Being discriminated due to age
- Co-workers are not willing to work with me
- Co-workers are neglecting
- Over burdened with work
- Work environment is unsuitable
- Remuneration is insufficient
- Work is uninteresting
- Lack of flexibility related to working hours
- Work place is very far from residence
- Lack of appreciation from employers
- Co-workers do not respect
- Lack of independence in terms of taking decision related to work
- Lack of clearly defined roles and responsibilities

The silver workers faced less extent of problems with regards to the following matters:
- Physical demand at job
- Did not give Designation according to the experience

Table 110: Item Wise Intensity Indices Showing the Problems Confronted by the Silver Workers at Workplaces due to Self

(N=300)

Items	Intensity Indices
Anxiety and fear of losing job/work	2.60
Working on new technologies like computers ,laptops, fax, E-mails	2.52
Facing difficulty in travelling to work place	1.91
Unable to concentrate on work	1.74
Unable to face people with confidence	1.72
Tendency to compare the present and previous jobs	1.66
Feeling uncomfortable to work with younger generation	1.54
Lack of necessary skills or education	1.45
Finding office hours very long	1.05

Table 110 shows that overall the intensity indices regarding problems that the silver workers faced at workplaces due to work ranged from 2.60 to 1.05. It means that problems faced by silver workers at their workplace due to work ranged from more to less on the above mentioned matters.

It can be further seen from the above table that the silver workers faced following problems to some extent:

- Facing difficulty in travelling to work place
- Unable to concentrate while working
- Unable to face people with confidence
- Tendency to compare the present and previous jobs
- Feeling uncomfortable working with younger generation

The silver workers faced less extent of problems with regards to the following matters:

- Lack of necessary skills or education
- Finding office hours very long

4.14 Satisfaction of the Silver Workers related to Work and Workplace

Level of satisfaction is indicative of how happy a worker feels about work and workplace. It reflects the extent of appreciation that they receive for their work and efficiency from co-workers and employers.

Table 111: Percentage Distribution of the Silver Workers according to their Satisfaction related to Work and Workplace

(N=300)

Work Satisfaction	F	%
High Satisfaction	57	19.00
Moderate Satisfaction	136	45.33
Less Satisfaction	107	35.67

Table 111 shows that nineteen percent (45.33%) of the silver workers were highly satisfied with their work and workplace. While little less than forty six percent (45.33%) were moderately satisfied. Whereas almost thirty six percent (35.67%) of them were less satisfied

Satisfaction marks a sense of accomplishment for a worker in view of work and the related matters like monetary benefits of work and the related matters like monetary benefits, appreciation, recognition and self satisfaction through personal development of skills and knowledge, by , it a worker feels happy with sense of with. Considering this important aspect concerning more to the silver workers, the level of satisfaction among them was analysed through different related test. At the outset, the silver workers showing moderate satisfaction showed high percentage (45.33%) as compared to those showing less satisfaction (35.67%) and those sowing high satisfaction (19%). The scale indicated overall level of satisfaction among the silver workers ranged on most pt from moderate to low level. It implies that they perceived more problems and has more to suggest in relation to work and workplaces to which they are closely associated. To confirm this of the data obtained was further analysed in view of the selected variables

Table 112: Percentage Distribution of the Silver Workers According to their Satisfaction related to Work and Workplace in Relation to the Selected Variables

(N=300)

Variables	N	Satisfaction related to Work and Workplace		
		High	Moderate	Less
1. Type of Work				
Full time	184	45.65	28.80	25.53
Part time	116	16.37	14.65	68.96
2. Present Salary				
Less Salary	145	6.89	35.17	57.93
Moderate Salary	22	72.72	9.09	18.18
High Salary	133	43.60	30.07	26.31
3. Present Designation				
Class I	27	44.44	29.62	25.92
Class II	190	42.10	31.57	26.31
Class III	71	11.26	40.84	47.88
Class IV	12	16.66	8.33	75.00

Table 112 reveals higher percentage of the silver workers belonging to the following categories of variables admitted about less satisfaction with their present jobs.

- Silver workers doing part time job
- Silver workers earning less salary
- Silver workers belonging to the class III and class IV designations

First, the silver workers satisfaction was analysed in relation to the selected variable and the percentages distribution were obtained. According to the data, about the half of them engaged in the full time jobs expressed high satisfaction about work and workplace and about two third of them engaged in the part time jobs admitted about less satisfaction. As regards the present salary, about three fourth of them drawing moderate salaries expressed high satisfaction, but a good majority of them drawing low salaries complained about less satisfaction. Several of them drawing high salaries, however felt happy with high satisfaction

In view of the present designation, about three-fourth of the silver workers in the class V designations were less satisfied about half of them in class III designations too were less satisfied. It was only with those holding class and class II designations that about equal of several of them expressed bout high satisfaction .thus it can be understood that the silver workers engaged in full time jobs drawing moderate and high salaries and holding positions in the upper cadres felt happy about their work with high satisfaction.

Table 113: Percentage Distribution of what the Silver Workers thought about an Ideal Age of Retirement

(N=300)

Ideal Retirement Age	F	%
Never want to retire, as thought itself of getting retired makes a person mentally sick, till death a person should keep working	104	34.67
Never want to retire as earning is not enough	62	20.67
By the age of 65 years	11	3.67
By the age of 70 years	42	14.00
70 to 75 is ideal age to retire	58	19.33
By the age of 80 years	23	7.67

The silver workers were asked what they thought of an ideal age to retire from work based on what they expressed. The table 113 shows that when questioned about an ideal age of retirement nearly 35 percentages (34.67%) of them reported that they would never want to retire. They thought that retirement would make a person mentally sick, and so a person should keep working as long as he/she lives. Thus according to them there is no ideal age to retire .While one fifth percent of them (20.67%) expressed that they would never want to retire as their earning was not enough. Little less than 20 percent (19.33%) of the silver workers mentioned 70 to 75 years as an ideal age to retire. Further 14 percentages of them reported that they would like to continue work up to 70 years as according to them it would be an ideal age of retirement. Some of them (7.67%) believed that 80 years would be an ideal age for retirement and a few (3.67%) said that they would like to work until they would be 65 years old. It clearly shows that if silver workers were allowed they would like to work till they are physically and mentally fit and till their health permits them to work. They do not believe in any specific age as ideal age to retire until they are forced to retire. According to them thought of retirement makes them "mentally sick".

For further clarity open ended questioned were floated to them on the subject of an ideal age of retirement. The responses received can be reviewed through their percentage distribution. On calculated it is known that about one third of the silver workers were not in favour of retirement and considered it as a cause for mental sickness. So they showed preferences to keep working until death .About one fifth of them did not want retirement on economic grounds and perceived it as new stage of working life that can fetch them flow of income continuously all through the life. The remaining less than the half of them specified an idea; age of retirement life like 65 years, 70 years, or 75 years or even 80 years. These reflections indicate that they were sure about the level of energy, fitness and capability to work with productive results for more of 15 to 20 years after retirement after their requirement from the first employment. In 2005, HSBC a multi-national banking and service organization reported similar findings in their research study; they surveyed over 21,000 individuals and 6,000 employers in 20 countries and territories to capture global attitudes towards aging and retirement. The study, entitled The Future of Retirement, found a significant proportion of individuals would like to continue to work as they get older. Only 20 per cent indicated they would prefer to never work for pay again.

4.15 Differences in Satisfaction of the Silver Workers related to Work and Workplace in Relation to the Selected Variables

The findings related to the differences in satisfaction of the silver workers related to work and workplace in relation to the selected variables are specified below:

DIFFERENCES IN SATISFACTION OF THE SILVER WORKERS RELATED TO WORK AND WORKPLACE IN RELATION TO THE SELECTED VARIABLES

Table 114: t-Ratio Showing the Difference in the Overall Satisfaction related to Work and Workplace of Silver Workers in Relation to their Type of Work

(N=300)

Variable	Source of Variance	N	Mean	SD	t-value
Type of Work	Full Time	184	26.40	6.398	1.662
	Part Time	116	25.10	6.814	NS

NS=Not Significant

Table 114 shows that overall satisfaction of the silver workers in relation to their type of work did not differ significantly. Thus, the null hypothesis, stating that there will be no significant difference in overall satisfaction of silver workers at workplace in relation to their type of work was accepted.

It was revealed from the findings that overall satisfaction of the silver workers in relation to their type of work did not differ significantly. This indicates that silver workers were not having any kind of dissatisfactions with their type of work , it also give a positive sign and shows their intensity of willingness to work after retirement.

Table 115: Analysis of Variance (ANOVA) Showing Difference in Overall Satisfaction related to Work and Workplace on Silver Workers in Relation to Present Salary

(N=300)

Variable	Source of Variance	Sum of Squares	DF	Mean Square	F-Value	Sig.
Present Salary	Between Groups	292.833	2	146.417	3.436*	.033
	Within Groups	12656.963	297	42.616		
	Total	12949.797	299			

* F Significant at 0.05 level, F-tab, 0.05 level df 2/299 =3.03

Table 115 reflect on the fact related to the salary like that there was significant difference in the overall satisfaction of silver workers in relation to their present income. In order to know for which group satisfaction differed significantly the data were further analysed through t-test

The findings reflect on the fact related to the salary like that there was significant difference in the overall satisfaction of silver workers in relation to their present income. Overall satisfaction of silver workers belonging to middle income group was significantly higher than their counterparts. It indicates that silver workers belonging to middle income tends to be less satisfied with their workplaces compared to those belonging to higher income group and low income group.

Table 116: t-Ratio Showing the Difference in the Overall Satisfaction of Silver Workers related to Work and Workplace in Relation to their Present Salary

(N=300)

Present Salary	X	SD	Less Salary	Moderate Salary	High Salary
Less Salary	25.36	6.517		2.682**	0.722
Moderate Salary	29.27	6.460			2.225*
High Salary	25.92	6.551			

**Significant at 0.01 level and * Significant at 0.05 level

It can be seen from the table 116 that the mean scores on overall satisfaction of silver workers belonging to middle income group were significantly higher than their counterparts. It indicates that silver workers belonging to middle income tends to be less satisfied with their workplaces compared to those belonging to higher income group and low income group.

Thus, the null hypothesis stating that there will be no significant difference in overall satisfaction of silver workers with their workplaces in relation to their present income was not accepted.

Table 117: Analysis of Variance (ANOVA) Showing Difference in Overall Satisfaction of the silver workers related to Work and Workplace in Relation to their Present Designation

(N=300)

Variable	Source of Variance	Sum of Squares	DF	Mean Square	F-Value	Sig.
Present Designation	Between Groups	385.348	3	128.449	3.026*	.030
	Within Groups	12564.449	296	42.447		
	Total	12949.797	299			

* F Significant at 0.05 level, F-tab, 0.05 level df 2/299 =3.03

Table 117 reveals that there was significant difference in the overall satisfaction of the silver workers at workplace in relation to their present designation. In order to know for which group satisfaction differed significantly the data were further analysed through t-test.

Table 118: t-Ratio Showing the Difference in the Overall Satisfaction of Silver Workers related to Work and Workplace in Relation to their Present Designation

(N=300)

Income	X	SD	Class –I	Class-II	Class-III	Class-IV
Class –I	26.96	6.653		1.729	0.902	2.858**
Class-II	25.38	6.279			0.619	2.169*
Class-III	26.00	7.129				2.200*
Class-IV	21.42	2.151				

**Significant at 0.01 level and * Significant at 0.05 level

It can be seen from the table 118 that there was significant difference between level of the satisfaction of the silver workers belonging to the class I designation and class IV. Class I was more satisfied than class II, while class IV was least satisfied. Thus, the null hypothesis stating that there will be no significant difference in overall satisfaction of the silver workers with their workplaces in relation to their present income was not accepted.

There was significant difference between level of the satisfaction of the silver workers belonging to the class I designation and class IV. Class I was more satisfied than class II, while class IV was least satisfied. This reveals that silver workers were getting bothered by their present designation, those who were high higher designation were obviously satisfied, but those who were having lower e designation were not satisfied with their designation in the present job.

4.16 Item Wise Findings related to Satisfaction of the Silver Workers related to their Work and Workplace

Further, to confirm the intensity of overall satisfaction in different matters, the items were listed and the item wise intensity indices for each of them were calculated.

The scale to judge satisfaction of the silver workers related to their work and workplace included 12 items. For each item there were three options mentioned which indicated three intensity indices related to satisfaction of the silver workers relate to their work and workplace. The matter that more number of silver workers reported, are mentioned below

Table 119: Item Wise Intensity Indices Showing the Satisfaction of Silver Workers related to their Work and Workplace

(N=300)

Items	Intensity Indices
Colleagues are very friendly	2.49
Enjoying full freedom to do work	2.36
Salary for the nature of work done is enough	2.23
Feeling satisfied with the value system	2.21
Employees co operate with each other and there are no quarrels	2.20
Getting encouragement from employers to take own decisions in day to day work	2.18
Believe in the principles by which employer operates	2.14
Good opportunities for learning new job skills	2.14
Work offer challenges to advance their skills	2.12
There is good arrangement for settlement of disputes	2.08
Welfare facilities are good	1.86

It can be seen from the table 119 that for the specified matters the overall intensity indices ranged from 2.49 to 1.86. It means that there prevailed moderate satisfaction among the silver workers related to their work and workplace, colleagues and employers.

The above table further classifies that the silver workers held moderate satisfaction related to their work and workplace in following matters:

- Colleagues are very friendly
- Enjoying full freedom to own work
- Salary for the nature of work done is enough
- Feeling satisfied with the value system
- Employees co operate with each other and there are no quarrels
- Getting encouragement from employers to take own decisions in day to day work
- Believe in the principles by which employer operates
- Good opportunities for learning new job skills
- Work offer challenges to advance their skills
- There is good arrangement for settlement of disputes
- Welfare facilities are good

Matters like friendly attitude of colleagues and freedom to work gave satisfaction to the silver workers with high intensity. The matters like salary, value system, co-operation, encouragement from employers, principles and opportunities to learn new skills gave them moderate satisfaction. Likewise, those like challenges for new skills, settlement of disputes too gave them some satisfaction. The silver workers, however not much satisfied with welfare facilities at the workplaces .This scale of judgment explains which matters need more attention and improvement to enhance the level of satisfaction.

4.17 Suggestions by the Silver Workers

Table 120: Percentage Distribution of the Silver Workers according to their Suggestions for Specific Personnel Policy for Elderly Employees

(N=300)

Specific Personnel Policy	F	%
Needed	222	74.00
Do not need	78	26.00

Table 120 shows that high percentages of the silver workers (74%) expressed that there is a need for specific personnel policy for elderly employees. Only 26 percent of them said that they do not feel need for specific personnel policy. It clearly shows that the silver workers expected that specific personnel policies should be framed for them.

In view of the perception of the retirement, problems and satisfaction, the silver workers came out with suggestions for specific personnel policy for elderly employees by which many of their problems can be resolved and they can be assured about positive work environment for them at workplaces. A good majority of them appeared to be favourable to it and expressed that it is very much needed. About one forth of them seemed to be not so hopeful about it and said it was not needed. Based on the suggestion of those who favoured specific personnel policy for elderly employees, 'Need for Action' was specified on several matters. The most significant matter in their view was like supporting transfer of knowledge and experience at which their utility would count most to train and update younger workers with adequate skills and knowledge. It sounds very valuable suggestions. The matters related to attitude, evaluation and appreciation were also considered important. Exchange programme too attracted equal attention from them. The matters related to adjustments of work, further development and attending demands of work, further development and attending demands acquired good attention from them. The matter related to payment rewards, public policy and focus on younger people too attracted some attention from them. Some of them even aid 'no need for action'. However on most part the silver worker showed favourable attitude to positive changes at workplace through active steps.

Table 121: Percentage Distribution of the Silver Workers According to the Need for Action Concerning Engagement of Elder Employees

(N=300)

Need for Action	F	%
Support transfer of knowledge and experience	274	91.33
Change of attitude/valuation /appreciation	213	71.00
Exchange between young and old	193	64.33
Make work suitable to elders possible	176	58.67
Make further development possible	166	55.33
Attending demands in everyday work	150	50.00
Change payment regulations	149	49.67
Change public policies	142	47.33
Concentrate on younger people	120	40.00
No need for action	37	12.33

Table 121 shows that the silver workers felt the greatest need for action by the employers for support transfer of knowledge and experience (91.33%). High majority (71%) of them suggested about a change in attitude. While nearly 65 percentages (64.33%) of them suggested about allowing exchange between young and old workers. Another major point suggested were like making work for elderly possible (58.67%) and making further development possible (55.33%). Half (50%) of the silver workers felt that due attention should be paid to demands in everyday work and little less than half (49.67%) of them suggested about change in regulations. It was followed by a suggestion for change in public policies (47.33%). Further 40 percent of them suggested to concentrate on younger people. However a very less (12.33%) percent of them felt need for action on the part of organization. This table lays high emphasis on the silver workers suggestion on the need for action by employers towards support transfer of knowledge and experience and change in attitude. It means that the silver workers confronted problems of attitude while working after retirement and they expect that it should be duly resolved.

Table 122: Percentage Distribution of the Silver Workers Suggestions for the Important Services for Elder Employees

(N=300)

Important Services	F	%
Health care services	291	97.00
Reduced/flexible working hours	170	56.67
Counselling/support	157	52.33
Company pension scheme	149	49.67
Integration into company	135	45.00
Adapted demands and workplace design	117	39.00
Domestic supply	112	37.33
Contacts	103	34.33
Further education	52	17.33

Table 122 shows that high majority of the silver workers (97%) believed that a health care service was most important service. Reduced or flexible working hours was considered important by little more than 55 percent (56.67%) of them. Further nearly 53 percent of the silver workers (52.33%) attached importance to counselling and support. Then followed the company pension scheme was held important by almost half percent of them (49.67%) and 45 percent of silver workers called integration into company a important matter. Further the silver workers thought that adapted demands and workplace design (39%), domestic supply (37.33%), contacts (34.33%), and further education (17.33%) were important services.

The silver workers also suggested for important services for elderly employees. In view of the age and age related limitations of body and mind, they would expect some kind of special assistance through specific kind of support services and facilities provided to them at workplaces. The services that they expected in descending priorities were like: health care services with top priorities; flexibility in working hours with good priority; counselling, pension and demands and design, domestic supply and contact and further education with some more priority, demand and design domestic supply and contacts with some priority and further education with somewhat priority. The services of too and very priorities count for reasonable demands. Those with some more priority indicate their positive approach to a new work environment and those with somewhat priorities are usual demand natural with everyone.

Among the important services under the second set of suggestion, that of integration into company" sounds most of genuine. Concern for it prevails internationally among silver workers as it indicates to their neglect and negative social stereotypes that work against them at workplaces' to inflict on them pain of being excluded merely as "outsiders". The study of silver workers in Germany conducted by the Geneva Association too voices this concern in the sense that "organization can benefit from competencies" offered by retirees and so it of greatest interest to society and organization alike to integrate those who are prepared and happy to contribute (Herzog, House and Morgan 1991) quoted in the Geneva Association report that in case of "predicted lack of specialised staff" post retirement activity need to be prompted as " silver workers accumulated work experiences and knowledge will be valuable for filling the gap in skilled work force.

Table 123: Percentage Distribution According to the Facilities that Employer can Provide to the Silver Workers

(N=300)

Facilities	F	%
Opportunity to guide and teach young workers	230	76.67
Opportunity to work fewer hours	187	62.33
Enjoyable and stimulating work place	181	60.33
Ability to undertake less physically demanding work	163	54.33
Ability to continue earning an income	160	53.33
New kinds of work	151	50.33
Opportunity to learn new skills	54	18.00
Nothing	21	7.00

Table 123 reflects that high majority of the silver workers (76.67%) expressed an opinion that employers can provide opportunity to guide and teach young workers. It was followed by an opportunity to work fewer hours (62.33%). Majority of them (60.33%) believed that employers should provide enjoyable and stimulating work place. Further the silver workers expected facilities like an ability to undertake less physically demanding work (54.33%), an ability to continue earning income (53.33%), and new kinds of work (50.33%), while 18 percent of them wished for an opportunity to learn new skills and remaining 7 percent of them did not expect any facility.

This set of suggestions that the silver workers presented pertained to what employers can offer to their employees, specifically the elderly workers known popularly as "silver workers". In view of age and age related limitations, the silver workers would expect some kind of special favour from their employers in the form of facilities that can assure them special assistance in view of their physical and mental limitations. A good majority of them expected that their employer should provide them an opportunity to guide and teach young workers. Majority of them expected favours like to work fewer hours to provide enjoyable and stimulating work environment at workplaces, some relief from physical labour, continued earning and also new kind of work. Some of them expected from their employers an opportunity to learn new skills. A few of them held no expectation from their employers and preferred to be satisfied and adjusted to what prevailed and was provided at work places. On a major part, many of the silver workers expected their employers to consider their age and age related limitations to allow their age and age related limitations to allow some relief in work but at the same time, most of them expected that their employers should recognize their knowledge base, technical know-how, skill and long term work experiences and allow them to contribute to training of younger workers in the organizations. Thus, the silver workers would feel to enhance the base of knowledge and skills to benefit their organizations. It counts for a genuine gesture on their part.

This may in part explain recent survey data by the American Association of Retired People (AARP), which found that two-thirds of respondents in the United States have witnessed or experienced age discrimination at work (AARP, 2002). Perhaps because silver workers have experienced this situation more commonly in recent years, there may be heightened awareness of age discrimination. This may account for the results of the 57th Eurobarometer survey carried out in 15 European Union Member States, in which workers aged 45-64 years were found to be more likely to report discrimination when looking for work (Marsh and Sahin-Dikmen, 2003; Marsh and Sahin-Dikmen, 2002). Thus, diminishing the barriers to employment through age discrimination legislation can be integral to improving the conditions of work and employment for silver workers in the labour market.

The equality approach is grounded in respect for the rights and dignity of the individual. In this case, equality entails that all people, regardless of age, should have a set of alternatives from which to choose and thereby to pursue their own version of a good life or, as Armatya Sen has stated: "the ability – the substantive freedom – of people to lead the lives they have reason to value and to enhance the real choices they have" (Spencer and Fredman, 2003; Sen 1999). In order to effectively meet this definition, an equality approach for silver workers must operate on three levels. On one level, it must address the barrier of age discrimination by removing explicit barriers (direct discrimination) and implicit barriers (indirect discrimination), both of which can limit the range of choices for silver workers, as will be discussed in detail the next section. On another level, choice must be more than "what is on paper" in law. It must offer real chances to take advantage of available opportunities. For an equality approach to have noteworthy impact, proactive measures must be developed to ensure people have choices and can genuinely pursue them. This requires not only the removal of age barriers, but also skills training, the introduction of flexible work, decent wages and recognition of responsibilities outside the workplace, among others. The third level is that the primary focus is not necessarily to require greater numbers of silver workers to remain in the workforce or to allow businesses to benefit from the advantages of retaining them – although these are among its expected outcomes. Instead, it aims to achieve true equality of opportunity for silver workers through offering them a genuine choice between continuing to work or enjoying retirement after a lifetime of working, both in decent conditions (Spencer and Fredman, 2003)

Part 1- (B) Findings of the Qualitative Data

Silver workers are "open books of experiences," these are the books that too often go unread. Silver workers possess treasure of memory. They need and want to be listened to. They wish to share their experiences and wisdom with others. A process of relating their memories would be extremely rewarding for their well-being and also for their listeners.

Experiencing an old age is never an isolated phenomenon. The life experiences of older people are intricately intertwined with the history of their work, families, communities, nations as well as global trends. In this sense, plights an individual self is usually related to social self of the others. Understanding an individual's pains and happiness cannot be fully appreciated without having a deep sensitivity to the social self of the larger social structure. (Mills, 1959; Odin, 1996; Aboulafia, 2001) If there is any validity to these statements, it follows that causes of the personal troubles of the elders cannot be attributed solely to an individual elderly. The experiences of silver workers obtain through interviews are summarized in this chapter clears one point that the silver workers are not very keen to accept an idea that their personal concerns can be ascribed exclusively to their cultural differences or by labelling them "traditional", using already existing dominant and binary concepts of "modern" and "tradition". They rather see themselves as active participants in their aging process in various aspects

The interviews were scheduled with some of the silver workers. Out of the sample size of 300 selected silver workers, some 15 silver workers were selected and short listed for the purpose on the ground of quality of responsiveness to the questions put to them. The consideration for their selection was primarily how better they can talk, respond to queries, reflections on prevailing conditions, shape responses and voice their views and concern on their predicament in the prevailing labour markets. They were supposed to represent the feelings and concern of the selected silver workers and also of all silver workers at large to make a strong case for their inclusion and integration in to present labour market with due appreciation and respect for their abilities and capabilities to work productively even after retirement.

The profile of the silver workers selected for the purpose of interviews was considered on the ground of quality of representation that they can assure. The percentage distribution of their profile reflects this view in the sense that more of old silver workers were selected. Likewise since male usually an earning member in a family in the Indian context, their number remains very high. Since education counts significantly to be able t respond and react, the silver workers possessing high and moderate education were considered. Furthermore of the silver workers working in private sector, in the view of designation workers were belonging to the class II and Class III designations, lastly silver workers were working on full time basis.

Conducting personal interviews with the silver worker was considered useful for a purpose of ascribing validity to the findings projected through figure based facts. Looking to the sensitiveness of the subject of the present research, mere figure based findings would be inadequate to frame clear and balanced projection of the silver workers decision to work after retirement. Instead just leaving the silver workers as passive participation in the process of research, it was thought more appropriate to call for their active involvement and participation through interviews. Interviews would enable them speak , express and voice their inner feelings and concerns unheard so far and suppressed with a kind of apathy and indifference shown by people around them. They would feel involved and included in the process of research and feel kind of integration with the investigator. It would encourage them to open their hearts and let the investigator know what is lying inside. More significant point about it is from the point of research it would add subjective dimension to the findings to balance with the objective dimension projected through the figure based data, in this relation, when the silver workers are involved as active participants and what they reflect on the current conditions and situations would add a valuable dimension to the material for analysis to yield first hand observation , authentic views and opinions and more reliable direction to the present research to study the validity of the silver workers decision to work after retirement.

Considering utility and significance of the interview scheduled for the purpose of the present study, the questions were devised for the silver workers an asked to the representative 15 respondents selected from among the silver workers. A due care was taken to select points of inquiry and frame questions that would be enough evocative and concerning to arouse responses, reactions and reflections from the affected silver workers. The questions were focused on the areas like:

1. Right to work after retirement
2. Opinions of silver workers who work after retirement
3. Provision for silver workers at government organizations
4. Environment at workplaces for silver workers
5. Exploitation of silver workers by employers
6. Suggesting employers how to help silver workers
7. Creating opportunities for silver workers suggesting type of work that they can perform better.
8. How civic society can promote the elderly for active life after retirement.

Aim of conducting Interviews:

The interviews referred here seek to investigate not only the aspirations of elderly for retirement, but also their employment preferences. As it indicates in the Equality and Human Rights Commission Report (Smeaton and Vegeris, 2009), there is a need to extend understanding of the aspirations and experiences of elderly in relation to work and retirement, particularly given the policy push toward longer working lives. As Macnicol (2008) notes the, trends toward earlier retirement may explain, in part, improved life expectancy. Extending working lives and delaying retirement may therefore carry adverse consequences which are likely to vary according to socio-economic group(Refer Appendix 2).

> Do elderly wish to work, and if so, what jobs, terms and conditions do they favour?
> What are their motivations for working or choosing to leave work and what are the ranges of factors that can facilitate or hinder the pursuit of preferences?

The interviews conducted explore seek to the experiences of elderly in the workplace as to how satisfied elderly workers feel about various aspects of their jobs and what would help elderly unemployed people get back into work. There appears to be a growing consensus that early retirement is no longer viable for individuals, employers or national economic performance and that extending working lives is a necessary goal. It is important not to lose sight, however, of the importance of 'choice' and individual preference and to ensure instead that all elderly, regardless of background, have the resources and information necessary to ensure some degree of control over their future. These interviews seek to capture the voices of elderly in order to ensure that their preferences within the workplace, in relation to retirement timing and their aspirations during the retirement years are heard.

In the present study, with a view to providing strong support and validation to the response presented earlier, it is thought appropriate to put to use qualitative data collected from the selected silver workers through the interviews. The qualitative data is discussed below. The findings of the qualitative data are be presented in the following section

The qualitative findings are presented in the following sections:

4.18 Profile of the Selected Silver Workers
4.19 Interviews Conducted with the Selected Silver Workers

4.18 Profile of the Selected Silver Workers

Table 124: Percentage Distribution of the Silver Workers interviewed according to their Background Information

(N=15)

Background Information	Categories	F	%
Age	Young-old	4	26.67
	Old	11	73.33
Sex	Male	14	93.33
	Female	1	6.67
Educational Qualification	Higher Level of Education	9	60.00
	Moderate Level of Education	6	40.00
Type of Organization	Government	1	6.67
	Private	14	93.33
Present Designation	Class I	-	-
	Class II	12	80.00
	Class III	3	20.00
	Class IV	-	-
Type of Work	Full Time	12	80.00
	Part Time	3	20.00

Table 124 focuses on the profile of the silver workers who were interviewed for the purpose of the present study. According to it very high majority (73.33%) of silver workers interviewed belonged to the old age group. Among them little more than twenty five percentages (26.67) belonged to the young –old age group. Further, it was revealed that very high majority (93.33%) of them were male and only one of the silver workers was female. It can be seen from the above table that majority (60%) of the silver workers were highly educated and the remaining forty percent of them were moderately educated. A very high majority of the silver workers (93.33%) were working with private organizations and only one of them (6.67%) was working with a government organization. Further the table reveals that 80 percentages of the silver workers held having class II designations and equal percentages of them (80%) were working full time. A very fewer percent (20%) of them held class III designation and were working part time.

4.19 Interviews Conducted with the Selected Silver Workers

Q-1 Do you think elderly has a right to work after retirement?

Box 1- The Responses quoted below express what the silver workers thought on the issues of working after retirement. They believed that each elderly person who is physically and mentally fit and is willing to work has right to work after retirement.

- There is no question about having a right or not. Do we ask this question to younger generation? Then why raising this question to a retired person? Yes everyone should keep on working if they want to and if they are capable for it. They should be given an opportunity.

- I'm turned 67 and am continuing to work. I like my job and I see no reason to stop. I think I will go on for another couple of years. If there are people who think like me and if they are physically and mentally fit they do have a right to work.

- Though I am 64.I do not feel a day older than 40. Age is all in the mind. There are so many things that I would like to pursue. Right now, there is no rigidity about your age. If you are positive, you hold spirit that is almost age less. Of course elderly persons should be given full freedom to decide about it and they should have right to work if they are willing to.

- A friend of mine who was my colleague and also senior to me in age and designation, retired a year before me. As his retirement was coming closer I was finding him more anxious, worried and disturbed. One fine day I asked him what the matter that was bothering him so much. He replied that he was upset and much worried about retiring. As he could not imagine of life without work, he was worried what kind of changes would take place in his family. He was infact, worried about change in people's behaviour towards him with his retirement. I consoled him, and told him that there are many things he can do even after retirement. Finally the day came and he got retired, after retirement we were unable to meet daily. Almost after six months I got a news morning that he committed a suicide. The news was disturbing and scaring for me too. I was standing on a verge of my retirement and the

news broke my confidence. But gradually I recovered from that shock and made up my mind that I will keep on working. This was possible as my employer thought of giving me an opportunity to work.
- According to me each retired person should have a right to choose when he wants to retire. If he/ she want to work post retirement he should not be forced to retire. If my friend was given a chance to work and if he was given right to continue working post retirement he would not have committed suicide.
- Yes definitely. All the people who are about to retire or on a verge of retirement should be given right to decide whether they would like to continue working or retire. Everyone should have a purpose in life. By working you can actually contribute to what is happening in life .At the end of the day I feel a sense of satisfaction. I do not know how long I will be able to continue working full time, but I will not give up work completely. Work keeps me going. I do not feel like I am disappearing off the planet or isolated from the society. I still want to keep my brain active. So it is very important to have right to work after retirement.
- I think retried people should definitely keep on working, they do have right to work and they can be the role models for others who are going to retire
- Yes, everyone should be given an opportunity to work regardless of gender and age .The only thing that should be taken into consideration is a person's qualities and abilities. I am women and I would love if women decides to continue working after retirement
- *Mere hisab se, ha, retired logo ka haq hai kaam karna aur most importantly ye baat hai ki unka ye haq employers ko samjhna na chahiye.(In my view, yes, retried people have right to work and employers should understand that most importantly it is their right)*

So, it can be inferred from the above responses that the silver workers unanimously felt and agreed on a point that each retired person has the right to work after retirement. The argument posed may be summarized like. One of the silver workers working in a private bank stated that all the people around who are retired or on the edge of retirement should be given the right to decide whether they would like to work or retire. Each elderly or retired person should have a purpose in life. By working you actually contribute to what is happening in life and at an end of a day you get sense of satisfaction. It very important to have right to work after retirement. One of the silver worker working in a corporate stated that "Though I am 64.I do not feel a day older than 40. Age is all in the mind. There are so many things I would like to pursue. Right now, there is no rigidity about your age. If you are positive, you are almost age less. Of course elderly should be given full freedom and they should have right to work if they are willing to." This clearly shows that silver workers hold much positive thinking towards elderly persons those who were working after retirement .They do feel that they have the right to work, so it may be concluded from the above findings that freedom is finally recognized as the basic right of every human being, we are fast approaching the time when society must recognize and ensure the right of every individual for gainful employment. Many stereotypes and prejudices prevail in society concerning employment of elderly persons and employers usually avoid employing them. It has no justification today and it cannot be taken as valid argument. There is an urgent need to formulate an integrated theory of employment to explain a process by which jobs are created and provided to elderly persons. It has roles of political, social, technological and economic factors to contribute to that process."

These responses voiced strongly their feeling of being neglected and discriminated in the society. As a result, there emerged a sharp reaction like 'why raising this question to a retried person? Right implies equality in all matters of life and it is a boon granted by the democracy to all citizens equally. So the reaction given out here is well justified and due attention should be paid to the elderly's aspiring to work after retirement.

Further, it was expressed that right to work makes one physically and mentally fit. In this matter, there should be no rigidity about age and what counts is spirit that makes one ageless. Even at 67 or 64, one may feel younger to 40 even. There prevails a strong feeling that silver workers should be allowe4d freedom to decide to work and if they are willing they should be allowed to work after retirement.

It is important to know just a thought of retirement would affect an elderly persons psychology. In this light one told story of an elderly person who was about to retire. An idea of retirement caused in him anxiety and worry and he felt much disturbed. He was worried about change in people's behaviour to him after retirement. Even if he was consoled and persuaded about options available after retirement he felt so depressed that he committed suicide. Such cases hold an alarm to such shocking effects. The respondent was saved of it because his employer offered him a job after retirement. This aging explains how painful situations can be avoided with sensible handling of the situation with elderly person at an age of retirement. 'What to do next', 'how to fill void', 'how to resolve loneliness and painful passivity' these are big problem that stand opposing them with open teeth to crush them.

In view of this case, there prevails a strong feeling that a person should not be forced to retire. Rather he should have right to decide when to retire. If he wants to continue working he should be allowed as long as his physical and mental health permits. Such free environment would avoid any fatal idea or suicide tendency among elderly persons. It may be noted that in western countries like U.S.A, Canada, the U.K and other European countries there is no age specified for retirement and one is allowed to work as long as he wishes and he can. Of course, after certain age, some options or changes may be suggested and offered to elderly workers as they suit their physical and mental fitness. Positive attitude can save them from any chance of depression and fatal consequences. In this light, if we review the U.S concept of "Bridge Employment" or jobs performed by silver workers in Germany and other European countries. We may notice that there is more of willingness and positive tendency for work to display interest, motivation, openness and commitment to work rather than any kind of compulsion. This tendency enhances efficiency and productive of work and it can be possible only when silver workers enjoy freedom to work and are never bothered and depressed with a thought of retirement.

When the silver workers expressed their feeling for freedom to work their faces gleamed (shine) with sense of satisfaction of contributing something form their side. They do feel that when brain is active they feel life "work keeps me going" and with it they can assert their presence and save them "disappearing from the planet" or isolated in the society. They also shown with confidence that they have something useful to offer and with their knowledge, experience and workaholic attitude they can serve role models to younger workers at workplaces. The only woman respondent expressed that an opportunity to work should be offered "regardless of gender and age" and a person's qualities, calibre and abilities for work should be considered and appreciated in correct spirit.

Further, it was also felt that employers are givers of jobs. They have powers to employ retired persons so they should consider that retired persons have right to work and give thought to it. The overall feeling voiced in the silver workers responses present their reflection on the modern society that demands freedom from stereotypes and biases for elder persons and to recognize an individual right for employment "regardless of age and gender" . Avoiding elderly persons for employment after retirement would be a tendency on employer's part that sees no justification in the modern context. Any argument for it would not sound valid for lack of humanity and equality

It is time to consider how the concept of silver workers 'bridge employment' or in any other forms operate in western markets and an integrated policy of employment should be formulated in India by which jobs are created and offered to elderly persons duly appreciating their long experience, knowledge and skills in light of utility and contribution to the making of modern India. There should be positive mind cultivated among employers and co-workers and of course the policy makers and government agency to recognize utility and value of elderly person to integrate them into labour force with necessary options and changes.

Q-2 What is your opinion about retired elderly persons working after their retirement?

Box 2- The responses quoted below express that the silver workers held positive opinions about elderly persons working after retirement

- There are people who lose energy and enthusiasm as they advance in life by calculating how old they are getting in term of years. If people do not consider their age in just number of years and keep on contributing to the society, I salute them. I would request the government and employers to give them a way to progress and contribute more and more to society.
- It is good and refreshing to see people around of my age who continue to work after retirement. It gives new hopes and I can also see a change that is taking place in a society. It is a change in attitude to accept elderly back in the work sector.
- I feel great to see people like me working. We the "working elderly" are becoming inspiration for the other people and employees who are about to retire or have just retried. We are a source of inspiration to them from us they can learn that life exists beyond retirement like us they too can get an opportunity to work .Life does not end at retirement. They too can work post retirement. They have just "retired and not expired". *Zindgi toh bas abhi shuru hue hai* (Life has just began)
- Retirement is not resignation from life. It is rather an opportunity to live a full dynamic life .I feel encouraged to see people who are active after retirement
- Rather than giving a suggestion I would like to impart a message to people of my age that it is not a time to sit and wait for destiny to decide your future, but to do something valuable that can make your life more meaningful by doing so, you will also enrich your life.
- People who are working after retirement are acting as an eye opener for a society. We are the one who make a society aware that look, we are still capable enough of working even after retirement.
- I do not find many women working after retirement. I wonder why they do not work?? *Jab family ki responsibilities thi tab manage kiya, kaam kiya bachho ko bada kiya ,ghar bhi sambhala, ab kyu nahi? Ab to zimmedariya kam ho gayi hai, ab aap kaam kaijiye apni marzi ka kaam kijiye.(*when you had responsibilities of a

> family, you managed everything, work, reared children, took care of the household. Now why not? Now your responsibilities are reduced and so now do work of your choice.)
>
> - I respect every retired person who is working after retirement. They are one who serve source of inspiration to other people who are afraid of loneliness or feel depressed about retirement.

In the above responses, the silver workers expressed a sense of pride for people who work after retirement. The responses can be summarized like, one of the silver worker working in a corporate mentioned that there are people who lose energy and enthusiasm in life by calculating how old they are getting in term of years. If there are people do not considered their age just in number of years and keep on contributing to a society, I salute them. I would request the government and employers to give them way to progress and contribute more and more to society. Further it can be inferred, that silver workers thinks that people who are work after retirement act as a source of inspiration for other persons who feel depressed and afraid of loneliness about retirement. A silver worker working in finance company stated that Retirement is not resignation from life, but an opportunity to live a full dynamic life .I feel encouraged to see people who are active after retirement. So it can be inferred from the above responses that it is crucial for the silver workers to think about own health and well being .It indicates that they have a strong sense of purpose in life and remain engaged in work of one form or another. Working after retirement can be a very important way to achieve such positive thinking .Working can fill a void in their life and give them a new sense of living.

Silver workers views and opinions reflected sense of pride and confidence that they decide to work after retirement. They show that growing age does not put them off in spirit of life, but shoe their silver heads straight and erect with high spirit. If we review the respondents views we may notice that they truly voice their aspiration to work after retirement on positive mind. They speak of maturity of thinking. It is truly said "life begins at 60" . we interpret it is social context as freedom from family responsibilities. So far you lived for your family and had any time left for you to fulfil your wishes, desires and aspirations. Now since you are free you have time to live for you. The same saying may be applied to what they mean that now they have more meaningful and worthy living with maturity of mind.

We may refer to what they expressed earnestly. They said in their age people may lose energy and enthusiasm to work anymore. But to them an age does not count in years but in deeds. We may call here a verse on Hindi " lamba bhaya to kya bhaya jaise ped-khajur" which mean what's worth if you grow long in years/age like a date tree. The respondents said they believe in contributing something value to society. They rather salute such lofty aspirations and appeal the government and employers to give way to their aspirations through more work and progress.

An idea to continue work after retirement sounds to them good and refreshing that would bring new hope in their later stage of life and affect change in attitude of people to integrate them in labour force at work sectors. The idiom "working elderly" sounds great and fascinating in the sense that silver workers can serve "a source of inspiration" to other people. They can pass a message to them that 'life does not end at retirement' and if they continue to work they do get a feel that 'life exists'. The silver workers feel that have 'just retired and not expired'. They are still feeling that they are living and life for them has just begun.

They further said that in their view "retirement is not resignation from life" but "an opportunity to live a full dynamic life" .when they find someone active after retirement they feel encouragement to involve in activity. They feel like conveying a message that an old age is not a time to sit and wait for destiny to decide your future. If you do something meaningful it will add meaning and worth to your life. By working, you will 'enrich your life' People who work after retirement can act as "an eye opener" to make people aware about their utility to society. The women respondent raised a pertinent question to working women. Before retirement they could manage their jobs with the usual hectic family responsibilities. When they retire in that age their family responsibilities are much reduced and they have good time left for work. So why should they discontinue working? In view of their capabilities, they should look a work of their choice and engage them in work.

One respondent said that he would respect a retried who works after retirement as they serve source of inspiration to other elderly people who fear retirement and are afraid of loneliness and depression at that stage of life. They would serve hem an example to infuse new spirit and hope in life by inspiring them to continue working even after retirement.

Q-3 Should there be a provision made at government organizations for the retired to work after retirement if they wish to?

Box 3- The responses quoted below express that the silver workers do wish that government should make due provisions for the retried to work after retirement if they wish

- I had to search for another job after retirement to boost my occupational pension. The need to search another job aroused because I was thrown out from my first job. The change in legislation will be too late for me. But I do not want that other retired persons who want to continue working suffers similar problems so, I would appeal the government to increase the retirement age in all the sectors and make provisions to create more job opportunities for the retried workers.
- Yes, Promote a good practice to allow provision of flexible working arrangements for people who grow in age.
- Why the government doesn't think about the aged through positive campaign? (sarcastically) *"Beti Bachao"* is doing well, why not *"buddhe bachao"?* We should not be neglected just because we are ageing. Many elderly are committing suicide because of retirement or financial crunch that creep in as one retires. The government should pay due attention to every person who retires the pension would not be enough to survive .If they are willing they should be allowed to work post retirement and for that government should have made some provisions for them
- Yes, government should make provisions for the elderly by which they have right to equal treatment regardless of the age in the matters of recruitment, promotion, retention and training while they work after retirement.
- More opportunities should be created for elderly to work after retirement. There should not be restricted retirement age. Provide websites specially developed to provide information related to elderly who approach retirement.
- We have reserve seats for some of specific castes in the employment sector. Why can't government think of reserving a few seats for the elderly? At least, for those who are educated and capable of working after retirement may be considered for such benefits.

- Most importantly I feel the government should focus on creating work opportunities for women. *Adami toh phir bhi kaam dhund lete hai.Per aurto ke liye kaam dhundhna retirement ke baad thoda zyada mushkil ho jata hai, male dominant society hai,aur meri jaisi aurto ke liye jisne apni aadhi zindgi kaam karte hue nikali ho ghar bethna mushkil hota hai.*(Males, however, manage to find jobs after retirement .But for women it is bit difficult to find out jobs after retirement .The present society is dominated by man and for woman like me who had worked for her life finds it find a difficult to stay at home).
- Provide pre-retirement courses by which older people can be encouraged and supported to engage in work sector.
- Make work possible for elderly after retirement. Provision or opportunities for them to work in a sector or filed where they can contribute their experiences.
- Just providing pension after retirement these days is not enough. People have number of reasons to continue working after retirement .Government should create more workplaces where they can contribute their experiences and knowledge and provide them a chance to work. What if a person has financial crunch? What if a person wants to work to remain physically fit and mentally active? What if person has to work as part of families responsibilities? What if a person wants to work and contribute to a society? Why doesn't the government think and focus on such issues and needs of an elderly worker? Yes the government should make provision for us to work after retirement according to our skills, experience and we should be paid for it.

So, it can be understood from the above responses that the respondents mentioned some hardcore issues in the interest of the desirable provisions that government should make for the silver workers of the Vadodara city .They may be summarized like. One of the silver workers working in an corporate stated that plans to continue working after retirement are associated, among other factors, with feeling of being physically strong enough, being well educated and working in a job described as ideal across a range of dimensions. Silver workers also expressed that they feel that government has failed in abolishing age related discrimination; some of them also raised a question about reservation for the elderly and felt that the government should think and make such provisions. Further, silver workers strongly believed that government should arrange for pre-retirement courses to encourage and support older people to engage in the work sector .Websites should be specially tailored to provide information related to elderly approaching retirement. Silver workers also mentioned about creating more job opportunities for the retired elderly workers and also about increasing the retirement age. Further they expressed that issues related to them are not yet addressed by the government like financial crunch that they face after retirement. They also added that providing pension is not enough for some of them and government should think of creating work opportunities for the elderly so that they can contribute and work according to their skills, experience and knowledge and get duly paid for it.

These responses sounded like strong voices of the silver workers that reflected on an urgent need of attention by the government. The silver workers expect appropriate provisions from the government which can make their life better. These findings support the suggestion of the silver workers that the objective like employment needs and preferences of older people should be duly accommodated by the government in the form of appropriate provisions.

The respondents referred to difficulty many of them faced to find jobs after retirement and appealed the government to raise the age for retirement and crate more job opportunities for people like them. They also requested to promote a practice to provide flexi hours and flexible work arrangement for the silver workers. Retirement and financial constraints with meagre amount of pension cause hard pressing effects on their hearts and a question of how to survive may hurt them in to depression and even drag them to commit a suicide's they urge the government to think out positive campaign like " Buddha bachao" on the patterns of those like " beti bachao". Under such campaign, provision should be made to allow retired persons to work after retirement. They further suggest that a website for elderly workers should be developed and maintained with continuous updates about available job opportunities. The flow of related information should be managed to link needy retried person with jobs at bunnies, government and educational organizations.

Some of the silver workers even demanded reservations of jobs for retire persons to protect their right to work. It may benefit retired persons who have utility and can contribute with their knowledge, experience and capabilities to work in specified filed or area.

Retired elderly women find it more difficult to get jobs. There prevails that in a male dominated society jobs are not so easily made available to retired women. Women who led an active life feel painful to stay at home. So the government should take an initiative to make jobs available to them. There is also suggestion for pre-retirement courses through which proper consultation may be imparted to elderly person on the verge of retirement. It would be a positive step to save them from depression and fatal thinking and encourage and support them to engage in some kind of work after retirement.

If the government provides job opportunities to retired person they can perform productive work by contributing more to a work sector with their knowledge and experience. It has to see that what an elderly person had gained with long term efforts should not be wasted, but utilized in some sense in the benefit of the society and country. There prevails strong feeling among the silver workers that government cannot shake off responsibility to elderly person by realising pension to them after retirement. The government should consider other factors by which elderly retired persons are prompted to work even after retirement and think about possible , provision for work that would suit to retired person's knowledge, skills and experience and of course , capabilities.

In this way the silver workers gave out strong voices to draws attention of the government to an urgent need of work to retired persons. The interviews explain one thing that when no around in family and society is ready to hear retired persons such kind of meeting would provide them a platform to express their anxieties and concern to form collective voice. Only collective voices are heard and inspire people in authority to do something to resolve their problems and their preferences are duly accommodated in the resent conditions.

Q-4 Do you think environment at the workplace is suitable for the retired elderly? (In terms of employer's attitude towards you, your equation with younger colleagues and allocation of work)

Box 4- The responses quoted below express that the silver workers held mixed feelings about work environment and they were not very much satisfied with it. They imparted their view in relation to the employer's attitude towards you, your equation with younger colleagues and allocation of work

- No, as I feel discrimination on the ground of age
- No, being an aged person I always feel under rated, because I am not given an opportunity to work according to my experience and ability.
- No, I feel discriminated in the sense that I do not feel that I am getting the same amount of appreciation for work that younger workers or my young colleagues get.
- I feel that I am forced to do part time work, just because I am aged. In spite of being able to work full time I am not allowed for it.
- I experience complete change in the work environment and in the behaviour of my colleagues. Though I am lucky to get an opportunity to work in the same organization where I used to work before retirement. Some kind of change that I am realising, as I am not allowed to sit at the same table where I used to work before retirement. There is change in behaviour of my colleagues. They used to be kind and nice to me but now they have changed their behaviour drastically. It gives me feeling that they used to respect me for the designation I used to hold and for the person I am. *"chai karta kitli garm* (tea pot is more hotter than tea.) But in regards of my employers I do not have anything to complain. I am getting the similar kind of respect from them.
- I do not found the work environment so friendly to me. I do not feel that I am appreciated for my knowledge and experience .In fact I am capable to contribute as much as a younger employee can do in terms of sharing innovative ideas. But I am never valued for it. I feel neglected by my co workers.

- Work environment is something that one can create. *Aap khud ko low present karoge toh log toh karenge he pareshan kyu hum confidence se kaam na kare? Ha bilkul mujhe mere kaam aur work enivorment se satisfaction hai,* I feel I get the same respect as a human being and as a teacher as other get for their work.
- I feel some kind of isolation while working in the office, I feel neglected because I am working post my retirement age. Some efforts should be made by the employers in order to change the attitude of younger colleagues towards the elderly working after retirement.
- *Ajeeb lage che kaam karvanu, loko nu vartan ajeeb hoy che , hamesha kai pan abhipray aapo hoy toh hestaion thay che, kaik navu karvani eccha. Bas eccha j rahi jay che, kem ke ae tak j nathi madti, dar anubhavu chu, eklta anbhavu chu, badhu bahu kari shakvani eccha che pan loko na vartan thi dar darine kaam karu chu,kyak naukri mathi kadhi na muke.evu lage che ke hu koik alga duniya no manas chu.(*It is strange to work as people behave strangely. If you give your opinion or you want to do something new, your desire is never accepted. I feel lonely and , I do have willing of doing many things. No one appreciate me and I have to work with fear of people around. I always work in the pressure of loosing job and it feels like I am not the part of this world.)
- Some employers look at your age and pass an instant judgement. But when I applied for this job some 2 years ago age simply was not an issue. Its experience and how you do your job that counts. I am the oldest in the office. My colleagues do not see me as an older person, and though all of us work together as a team in these corporate. We get very friendly environment and we all socialise together.
- I had to retire at age of 58 years. I spent two months at home doing nothing. I could not convince myself that I cannot do anything constructive. I decided that the retirement is not meant for me. I am not employed out of sympathy. Age is irrelevant. As long as I can do my job properly, it is not an issue. Do I enjoy working with younger people? Funnily enough, I have never been conscious that I work with people of different age. I suppose it is because we all respect each other and my colleagues never make me feel my age. There's a sense of fulfilment I love my work environment. My workplace become to me like my second home.

So, it can be inferred from the above responses that silver workers expressed dissatisfaction about environment at their workplace. They expressed that, much still needs to be done to change attitude of an employer and especially colleagues towards elderly. Silver workers expressed that they are not given opportunity to work according to their experience and skill; they feel isolated and experience age discrimination at work places. Some of them also reported that they are forced to work part time in spite of having skill and capability to work full time. They also reflected that they feel very awkward to work with younger people. They have many new ideas to carry out the task more successfully, but they cannot express that as they have fear of being terminated from the job. They also added that they are treated so differently at the workplace that they feel as if they are not part of this world. On the other hand there are also silver workers who were happy with the environment at their work places. They expressed satisfaction that they get very friendly work environment and they can socialise with younger colleagues and age had never become an obstacle for them at workplace.

In all, they persistently urged that there is need to bring about a change in the work environment. It should be more work friendly for the retired people to work and they should not be ill treated.

Q-5 Do you think the elderly are exploited by the employers if they want work after their retirement or in retirement period?

Box 5- The responses imparted by the silver workers express that silver workers do feel that elderly are exploited by employers if they want work after retirement.

- Elderly workers are paid lower wages in comparison to what is paid to younger workers in spite of the fact that they were doing same or more amount of work.
- Yes, there is exploitation of the elderly, I work very hard but I am not considered for promotions, just because I am working after retirement.
- I am forced to work for more hours, as there no option of working part time, but I am not paid accordingly
- Flexible work hours are restricted for elderly employees
- Yes, I felt exploited as I am not getting chance to work as per my experience and skills.
- No, I am much happy with my job. I don't feel any kind of exploitation from my employers. I am getting the respect from them and allowed flexibility in the work timings.
- Yes, the employers are exploiting me. I am over burdened with work in comparison to regular employees. I am also paid less.
- It depends on the person working rather than on employers. *Ho sake utna positive thinking rakhna zaruri hai,.*(If possible one should keep positive thinking.)Women have more resistance power than men that is what I feel. I have only one complain *ki women ko kaam milna retirement ke baad kahi na kahi employers he mushkil bana rahe hai, unko bhi muka dijiye (I have one complain that, according to me employers are only making difficult for women to search jobs after retirement. Women's should also be given chance.)*
- I feel that to get an opportunity to work after retirement is a big thing, It becomes possible only because my employer gave me an opportunity. I am happy with my work and also with the pay. In any of the way I do not have any complain nor do I feel any exploitation from employers.

- *Har ek manas khali paisa mate kaam nathi karta, ane jo paisa mate kare pan che , toh shu tame loko paisa mate nathi kaam karta? Toh vadilo sathe aa bhed bhav kem? ame amro atla varsho no anubhav lai ne kaam karva aaviye che kai nai toh thodu adar aapo, Kem amne loko ne hamesha judi najar thi jova ma aave che? Kem amne ae kaam aapva nathi aavta je regular employee ne apva ma aave che? Ek wakhat chance toh aapo? Ek jamana ma ame pan tamari jem j hata ,aaje vadil chiye pan kaam karvani dhagas ane lagan toh ej che , ae haju vadil ke vrudh nathi thai,tame lagan ne kem nathi jota? Aa ek prakar nu shohan j che, mansik shohan.(man does not work just for money. If they do what is wrong about it? Don't you work for money? So why is such attitude shown to the elders? We carry all these years of experience, so would you not give us some respect? Why are we viewed differently? Why don't you give us similar kind of work that you give to regular employee? Just give us an opportunity? Have grown old, but our commitment and enthusiasm for work is not low in any sense. Why don't you look at it? If you do not see it is exploitation ,mental exploitation*

So, it can be inferred from the above responses that silver workers mentioned a number of barriers block the achievement of preferences in relation to hours and flexibility because of which they feel exploited by their employers. It was expressed that they feel exploited as they were not given chance to work according to their experience and skills. They further accused that they were forced to work for more hours, as there was no option of working part time, but they were not paid accordingly. They also perceived that they were treated differently by the employers and they were unrated. They were not given work and responsibilities of the same level that the regular employees were given. They expressed their aggravation towards the employers for not giving them a chance to prove their capabilities

A few of the silver workers could get preferred jobs and were allowed some level of flexibility they expect suitable jobs with better salaries. Some other stated that it is not just money that they were working and they feel exploited by the employers as they were not valued for their experience and treat them in a different way just because they are aged.

The findings reflect the fact that many full-time or flexible hours' opportunities are restricted to a narrow range of jobs and they tend to be lower paid. In another case, jobs were described as incompatible with favoured hours and employers did not allow the silver workers to change their hours as per their need or preferences. There would be problem for those who would like to reduce their hours because a fewer hours are usually associated with lower wages.

The tendency to downshift at older ages, either by means of reduced hours or reduced levels of responsibility, is recognised as important component of exploitation. The silver workers felt dissatisfied as they expected promotion and higher levels of responsibilities. These findings highlight the importance of being avoided and neglected causing to them decline in their 60s. Many of the silver workers continue to perform, both physically and mentally and their level of efficiency and performance cannot be undermined against their younger colleagues. The assumption that the silver workers may decline in work efficiency once they hit their retirement is reflected in discriminatory practices of employees and co-workers.

Exploitation is a burning problem of the present time. It appears to operate on a notion of "survival of the fullest". The strong and powerful dominate over the weal and powerless. It is true about policies, society and also business. When an elderly person decides to work after retirement the biggest problem that troubles him most is exploitation. He feels anxiety with number of doubts and suspicious about a new job like "will I be employed in a similar position?", "will I be given with same level of work and money?", and "will I be treated with same respect and appreciation?"he tends to compare his present employment with his first employment and on finding things on lower scale feels like suffering discrimination and exploitation at the hands of the employers. He feels like suffering injustice. This kind of feeling was expressed by many of the silver workers. Many of them complain about "lower wage for same amount of work as compared to younger workers. "Yes, there is exploitation of the elderly" makes a general feeling. The elderly are not considered for promotions. For there is no option of working part time and they are forced to work for more hours and are not paid accordingly. Flexible hours are not allowed for elderly employees. The work allotted to silver workers is not suitable to his experience and skills. "Over burdened and less money is a complaint received from many of them.

A women respondent said that employers only make things difficult for women to get jobs after retirement. She feels that women possess more power of resistance and they should be considered for jobs after retirement. However, some two silver workers said that they were happy with their jobs and felt no exploitation anywhere. They praise their employers for an opportunity, respect, to allow flexibility in time and work considering their needs and preferences. They perceived that there might be exploitation on with reduce hours of work and lower wages. They did not have to suffer it and so they felt happy about their second employment.

A tendency is noticed among business people to bother more about their profit and ignore any other thing against money. So when they have to employ an elderly person they show a tendency to downshift them with reduced hours of work, reduced responsibilities and reduced rewards. Thinking that these persons are too old to work longer, too weak to work more and carry responsibilities just show pity on them and give them some work and few money for name sake of humanity and earn reputation of being good business man. Against such snobbish tendency, the silver workers reacted sharply that they are still active with physical and mental fitness and maintain similar levels of efficiency and performance and so they should never be understood or undermined in matters of responsibilities and promotions.

Q-6 What would you suggest to the employers as to how they can help the retired elderly?

Box 6- The responses to this question reflect that the silver suggested on the matter that employers can do for retired elderly

- Stop being rude to retired people. Do not even think that we have committed any crime being retired. One of my friends shared his experience with me. He said that when he got retired he received much appreciation for the contribution he made over the years for his tenure in that organization. Everyone treated him very nicely .After a few days when he went to the office once again, he realized a kind of the change in the behaviour of his colleagues. He met and started a conversation with one of his colleagues and to his surprise he found that he seemed not so happy talking to him. Such experience continued at his every visit to the office. One day when he went to the office the peon informed him that the room in which he used to occupy is allotted to someone else. He was not offered a glass of water even and no one even bothered to notice him. Why this kind of change in the behaviour? Just because he was retired? But what about those precious years that he had dedicated to office, his knowledge and experience. Earlier he trained the younger staff .Now they are turning their faces on him without realizing that they grew up and learnt new things under his guidance. *Jene dikro samjhine agad vadvanu prostansah aapyu, dhagas ane atmah vishvas kedvata sikhadayu,aaje aj dikro elto badho atmavishvasi thai gayo ke modhu fervi le che,zidngi no agatya no samay je sanstha ne aapyo ,je jagaya ne biju ghar samjhyu, ae j jagya per thodo samjay vitatvano adhikar pan nathi?*(whom he treated as his son and encouraged to develop enthusiasm and confidence. Today that young guy has become so much confident that now he turns his face on him! He gave the most precious time to this organization, he took the place as his second home and now he is not given right to stay in for short time?
- The elderly should not be discriminated or ignore by the employers at the time of recruitment just because of their age

- Respect and value the experience and knowledge that the retried employees hold.
- Motivate elderly to work after retirement
- Distribute work on fairly ground
- Encourage postponement of retirement
- Allow flexible time schedules for work
- From my experience I would like to suggest that employers should invite retired employees back at least once a year in the organization they seemed to work.
- Develop a post-retirement data with update base recoding of skills and experience a retired person possess.
- Update performance management and reward systems
- *Kaam dijiye, jisse kaam karna hai use mauka dijiye, don't be gender biased and age biased. Aap bhi kabhi na kabhi is duar se guzar ne wale hai ye mat bhuliye.(Give work and give a chance to work. Don't be gender biased and age biased. Do not forget that you will go through such a stage.)*

So, it can be inferred from the above responses that silver workers strongly believed that employers need to begin now to build integrated strategies to encourage employees with valuable skills and experience to stay in the workforce. Employers should provide rewards as a token of appreciation for the work that the silver workers perform. They also expressed that employers should develop a post-retirement data base noting skills and experience that a retired person possesses.

They further suggest that employers should eliminate stereotypes and they should not discriminate or ignore the elderly for their old age at the time of recruitments. They felt stressed that employers should distribute work fairly. Silver workers expressed that employers should invite the retired elderly atleast once in a year in the organization where they served. In all, they persistently urged that knowledge and experience are significant assets for the companies that choose to attract and retain them. These values include commitment and loyalty to the employer, fewer sick days and enhanced length of service. As the workforce ages and contracts, skilled workers will increasingly come to the forefront.

Employers who fail to respond to the threat will put their future growth and profitability at risk, while missing out on the benefits of greater age diversity. To be successful in an increasingly competitive market place, employers need to attract and retain the silver workers for valuable knowledge, skills and experience they possess. They should give due respect to them when they retire

Silver workers always expect some kind of help and support from their employers. Their earnest which that was expressed through their response sums up in one statement "stop being rude to retried people". It implies desire that their spirit is respected in true sense. There is inherent which that with age people also tool at silver hair that indicates maturity and longer experience of work and pay due respect. They should recognize that silver workers still possess utility and efficiency to give better performance. They still can generate innovative ideas, suggest better method of working, and impart valuable lessons to younger workers from their skills and experience. They can still see silver workers in this realistic view and never be carried away with stereotypes, stigmas and biases like "old is gone".

The silver workers also suggest that employers should not view elderly workers different. They should consider them at par with other employers irrespective of age. They should give them an opportunity for similar kind if work and responsibility and consider their enthusiasm and commitment to work to trust them for equal level of performance. If they ignore to see these entire it would amount to mental exploitation that would hurt them to depression.

They added that they understood that at certain age what is important is to continue work preferably in the same organization they would impart more benefits to their past employers. So their employers should find out job options in their organizations. They appeal them to get rid of notion like "the old Vs, useless" and respect their capabilities. They strongly feel that the government should thing of increasing age to retire so that they can work longer and benefit their organization. They may also guide younger workers for better skills and performance using their long experience. The government should form policy to ensure recruitment of the silver workers after retirement.

They further appeal employers to avoid discrimination on the ground of age and pay due consideration value respect silver workers to motivate them by fair distribution of work, postponing retirement, allowing flexible by fair time schedules for work. They may even invite their retired employees once in a year to talk and impart their experiences to workers. They may have something to benefit workers and organizations at large. There is also suggestion to maintain a post retirement data storing information related to knowledge, skills and experience of employees who have retired. The data need to be updated time to time for fresh information. The data may be useful to resolve any problem. The silver workers further felt strongly that if performance management and reward systems are updated time to time on fairground elderly works may be motivated for better and productive performance.

Employers should know that physical exploitation gives rise to grumbling or complaints, but mental exploitation gives out to cause fatal consequences to silver workers to affect more seriously their very spirit of living. So employers should keep in mind the delicacy of this kind and treat elderly workers with positive mind to encourage them for their second employment.

Q-7 What type of opportunities should be created for elderly, who wish to work after retirement? Do you suggest specific work which the elderly can better opt for after retirement?

Box 7- the responses reflect the silver workers feeling that there are many opportunities for them to work after retirement, but the government and employers have to work in that direction

- Teaching related job opportunities should be created for the people from education background providing of tutor/teaching assistants. A person may be employed as an account in any of the chartered accountancy firm if they have experience in banking. In short job where they can apply their knowledge and experience. Job which relate to their past experiences would be appropriate
- *Meri ek khawish hai ki har ek organization, chahe woh government ho ya private, unko ek ya do jitni zarurat ho, unko retired logo ko recruit karna chahiye counsellor ke taur pe, jo un logo ko counsil kar sake guide kar sake, jo aane wale saalo me retired hone wale hai. Taki jo kathnaiya humne sahi hai unko na sehni pade, hum unko samjha paye hamare tajurbe se kuch bata paye.(I have a wish that an organization government or private, should recruit the elders as counsellors, as the requirement goes. They can guide and counsel senior staff who are on the verge of retirement. So that they would not have to suffer that we suffered. They would benefit with our experience.)*
- Employers can use our long experiences by employing us as consultants
- *Mara manva pramane kaam ek umer pachi pan agatya nu hoy che, parvrut rehvu angatya nu hoy che, pachi kaam kai pan hoy. Jaruri ae che ke amne kaam karvani tak aapva ma aave. Ane ae tak madvi tyar j shakaya che jyare employers ane government amri aa jaruarat ne dhyan ma le. (In my opinion, after certain age, activity is important, no matter whatever kind of work one gets. It is necessary that we are given a chance to work and it can happen if employers and the government pay due attention to our needs.)*

- Work opportunities should be created through which retire people gets a chance to continue working after retirement in their own organization.
- Job opportunities should be respectful for which the aged are not treated as old and useless. They should get respect and appreciation for experience and knowledge.
- I think before thinking about job options, it is important for the government that they should allow retired people to work after retirement. Once it is done there will be many fields where we can work .Government may also think of increasing retirement age.
- Clerical job would be better for those who want to work part time .Such opportunities should be made available to retried people.
- Opportunities to work in the same field of experiences should be created as we possess so much of knowledge and experiences of years in the specific field by which the organization will be benefited. We can also get an opportunity to guide the younger employees about matters concerning retirement.
- *Kaam toh bohot hai karne ke liye but employers recruit bhi toh karne chaihye. (There is much work for us to do .Provided employers think of recruiting us.)*

The most important matter mentioned in the above responses that the silver workers expressed an opportunity to work in the same field of experiences. Their knowledge and experiences in that specific field will benefit the organization. It would give them an opportunity to guide younger employees. The silver workers seemed much dissatisfied with the government because they stated that there is an urgent need for government to increase the age of retirement or they allow them to work after retirement. The silver workers also mentioned that clerical work would be more suitable to retired who were willing to work for part time. The silver workers were not happy with the way they are treated at workplaces .They urged to create respectful job opportunities, where they are not treated as old and useless people. They want that they receive due respect and appreciation for their experience and knowledge. It can be concluded from the above findings that the silver workers expected the government to take initiatives in the matter of their re-employment. They feel that there can be good opportunities for them to work, but age limit or lack of opportunities pose huge obstacles.

When silver workers approach for the second employment following the retirement, under force or pressure or out of their own will they exhibit lot of confidence and commitment to work. It is understood that with tit they wish to impress employers so that they may consider for the job. It is required at this stage that an employer should take a positive view and appreciate and encourage them rather than pull them down reminding them about their growing age and declining fitness, both physical and mental. They should not be cruel to them o show pity to them, but appreciating their knowledge, long experience, maturity and skills think about an opportunity of work for them.

Reviewing different job profiles available in their organization, they should short list such job that would suit to their knowledge, skill and experience and to which they can contribute with better efficiency, performance and sharing suggestions. The types of jobs they suggested include teaching jobs, consultancy, accountancy counsellor and the like.

Q-8 What role can civil society play to promote active aging amongst elderly?

Box 8- In the responses quoted below the silver suggested number of roles for civil society to play in prompting active ageing amongst elderly

- Yes there is much that civil society can do. They can support retired people like me to undertake the second careers with which they can combine aspects of work, income and benefits with a desire to make difference in a social activity of value.

- The first thing that civil society including employers can do according to me is to stop sympathising towards elderly or retired people and their families. *Are hum sirf retired hue hai bhai ,mar nahi gaye.Agar itna he pyar hai hamare prati toh hume kam dijiye ,hume aap ki seva karne ka mauka dijiye. Hume sahanubhuti ki zarurat nahi.(we have only retired, we have not expired. If you feel so much for us, give us a chance to serve. We not need your sympathy we want work.*

- Civil society should stop judging people on ground of age. Chronological age would speak about the capabilities of a person. A high active 70 years old person can perform better cognitively than an average person of 35 years. Society should concentrate on the capabilities of a person rather than considering age.

- Misleading perceptions about retirement should be corrected to change attitude of people in a society.

- Stop neglecting the retired people

- Engaging and supporting older people in volunteering and other forms of civic activites would be a welcome step.

- *Agar aap kissi aise sector, ya kisi aise post pe kam kar rahe ho, jaha aap ke liye possible hai , retired logo ko job dena recruit karna toh aap civil society ke bhag hone ka is tarah se bhi farz nibha sakte hai.(If you are working in any sector or post where it is possible for you to recruit retired people you do carry out your duty as a part of a civil society*

> - Respect everyone of all age and work to go hand in hand
> - Do not treat us as useless commodities once we are retired. One day you will be in the same condition. Rather, find ways to use our experienced knowledge, and I am sure, it will help you to achieve success.
> - Bridge a gap perceived between younger and older generation

The respondents expressed that in present context, the civil society should first of all do is stop sympathising the elderly or retired people and their families. They added that they do not need any kind of sympathy from the civil society nor from the employers. They have just retired and if the society is really concerned about them they should create more work opportunities for them. They feel that they have only retired and not expired.

A few of them suggested a the crucial role the civil society can play by engaging and supporting older people in volunteering and other forms of civic activities. Further they demanded that civil society should stop judging people on the basis of their age. Chronological age cannot make known much about the capabilities of a person. A highly active 70 years old person can perform better cognitively than an average person of 35 years. Society should focus more on the capabilities of a person rather than on his/her age. The silver workers also stressed on a need of civil society to support retired people and to consider second career to combine aspects of work, some income and benefits with a desire to make difference in a socially useful activity. Thus it can be concluded from the above findings that the conditions and attitudes of society should be suitable for elderly to contribute productively in workplaces. Society should not treat them as useless commodity. Once they retire they should be helped to live life with new meaning after retirement. Societal sentiments that is prejudiced and at odds with the available evidence should be changed and positive attitude should be cultivated for retired elderly. Work environment and educational provisions need to be improved for the silver workers to be able work with higher productivity. The goal of civil society should be to give retired people an opportunity to work and be productive as long as they wish to do so.

The silver workers were bit emotional when they talked about civic society and how important it is to them. They felt that civic society can do much for them because we are not strangers, but very much its part. People who retire have lived whole life as part of society, born in it, grown up in it, married and led marriage life and now have come to this stage. They have taken much from society in form of care, protection, comfort education , etc. and also given things to society in the form of contribution by work , efficiency, new ideas , new methods to make life more comfortable . They have also given clever and skill full children who now serve the society. They remained busy almost for sixty years doing much for family and society. Now since they have grown in age they had to retire. Retired persons are always read to do adjustment with situation. But if they continue to work after retirement what is wrong with it? On society's part it has to make things convenient and suitable so that they can continue working in their second career.

Silver worker do not prefer to work on number of reasons. They may be health, tiresomeness, some kind of fear of people's indifference and biases like old persons are useless. These reasons prevent them and also discourage them to work. So the civic society has an important role to play here to judge persons by age and correct all false notion misleading perceptions stereotypes and stigma that prevail among younger people that they are "useless and no more of use now". People attitude to the old needs to be corrected so that they stop neglecting them. Silver workers do not want to just be pitted or sympathized. They wish that people sympathy has to be coupled with some kind of support for work.

Silver workers view life after retirement as a new stage in life in which they can shape a second career to combine aspects of work, income and benefits to society. They have earnest desire to earn value in society by word and not to die carrying stigma of being useless and worthless burden on society. So it required that civic society discovers ways to accommodate them in some of work like volunteering and other forms of civic activities. Silver workers would be happy to engage them in any type of work. Some of them are associated with government or private organizations and if they find out a way to accommodate old people in work that would suit their age and capabilities such a support would be a welcome step.

Civic society has to find out way to tap knowledge, skills and experience of old persons an encourage them to contribute and benefit society by sharing and guiding younger people. Younger generation should not treat silver workers as "useless commodity", but take advantage of their knowledge and experience. They should value and respect their elders in society. Silver workers are always eager to share their know-how in the benefit of their own society. Such positive approach on both the sides would work effectively to bridge a gap between the two generations. If people in society keep faith that 'old is gold' and much valuable to them it would resolve number of psychological problems on part of silver workers. It would create more open, frank and healthy society in which all are valued and respected.

What the silver workers expressed sounds very reasonable and practical in the present condition. Because today everything costs and each work earns and in that way the gap between spending and getting is reduced. If silver workers are prompted to work with utility it will enhance their prestige and value in society. The silver workers will get satisfaction of contributing something to society and the society will earn benefits from their knowledge and experience. Thus benefits on mutual ground will pave to healthy atmosphere in which all can live like a happy and integrated family.

CONCLUSION

The qualitative data that was obtained through the interviews schedule with fifteen silver workers prove useful to the present research study. The questions asked to them focused on relevant issues like right to work, opinion about working after retirement, provision made at government organization, work environment, exploitation of the silver workers, employers help to the retired persons , create job opportunity for the elderly and role of civic society to promote the elderly for working after retirement. An attempt was made to obtain responses from the silver workers. Sometimes an interviewer had to encourage and inspire the respondents to share useful and correct information that would be useful for the research

The responses that were imparted at the interviewers reflect first on free and front environment. The silver workers spoke frankly to impart their interviews. Their actual words are quoted verbatim and then the qualitative data that emerge from their responses. Sometimes the silver workers spoke in Gujarati or Hindi and their words were then translated into English to help understanding of what they meant.

It may be noted that while making selection from among the silver worker all different variables for the background information are considered. The idea was to focus on relevant issues from all possible dimensions and to obtain all possible viewpoints from different categories.

The responses imparted by the silver worker who were interviewed project comprehensive picture on each issue. The silver workers being the aged were found a bit sentimental at the prevailing conditions. At time they appeared to be touchy and hurt. But at the same time, they put their point of view with relative confidence about their capability, knowledge and experience. When they make an offer to help and benefit an organization, co-workers, younger workers and society at large their confidence shine on their faces .Considering all such positive aspects of what they expressed, one can say that the silver workers deserve positive attention from employers, government and society. They clearly declared that they do not want to be pitted or sympathised. They expect recognition and respect from all concerned free of bias of age. They expect that they are given a chance to work and contribute more to the relevant fields, organization and society. They offer their experiences to guide younger people and prepare them for possible condition in their later life. Such an offer is quite genuine and it needs serious attention. The present research intends to arouse this kind of positive atmosphere and attitude in employment sectors, organizations and society. So that old retired workers are considered valuable and their knowledge, capabilities and experiences are put to correct use and application by which working sector and society may be benefitted. They may prevail notion in society like "old is gold" to defeat all humiliating notions of the old as worn out, useless and worthless.

The majority of silver workers wish to continue working up to and beyond retirement (some for financial reasons, others for enjoyment or to remain active), and many wish to continue develop their careers. Many silver workers would also appreciate opportunities to change not only their jobs but also their occupations, to try something new. While economic conditions and prohibitive training costs are holding some back, for others a perception of ageism among employers is preventing them from making the changes they desire. Perceptions of self also represent an obstacle, with some silver workers perceiving themselves as too old to initiate change. Cultural change at a societal level alongside the enforcement of age discrimination legislation is likely to improve the employment prospects of silver workers and open up opportunities for occupational change which are likely, in turn, to extend working lives as individuals continue to be motivated and challenged in the workplace. To this end, wider and more affordable training and educational opportunities at older ages are also likely to be beneficial. Although silver workers are broadly content with their jobs, large minorities are, however, dissatisfied with the hours they work and the lack of flexibility they experience in their working schedules. At older ages, adult caring responsibilities and health-related problems become more prevalent. For these groups in particular, flexible and reduced hour's opportunities can become critical for the health and wellbeing of individuals and their dependants. Extending awareness of, and eligibility for, the right to request flexible and reduced hours arrangements is likely therefore to benefit large numbers of silver workers. A range of policies and practices that require auditing and review in the workplace have been highlighted, including recruitment processes, availability of flexible working, workloads and opportunities to continue developing. The considerable progress made by employers over recent years to support silver workers with a range of innovative solutions. Evidence suggests, however, that greater progress has been made in relation to flexible working and the retention of silver workers than on policies and practices directed toward the recruitment of silver workers, job design and work intensification issues.

Finally, a class imbalance of power and control later in life prevails, more advantaged occupational groups better prepared financially to exercise choice. The policy impetus towards extended working lives and delayed retirement may therefore be associated with quite distinct consequences for different socio-economic groups. Trends towards earlier retirement may explain, in part, improved life expectancy. Any moves to prolong employment must therefore be accompanied by a consideration of working conditions and individual scope for choice must be supported.

This change might best be realised through dual processes comprising engaging with and appraising these workers' worth. That is, through a process that supports employment opportunities. All of this takes time and requires considerable and sustained commitment from government, industry bodies and industry sector councils. In the meantime, but also to support and sustain the change in employer attitude, silver workers or collectively may increasingly be required to rely more on their own organization in maintaining their workplace competence than younger workers. It seems that to bring about desired changes, the focus for policy and practice considerations needs to simultaneously engage employers of silver workers and include a process whereby the contributions of these workers can be appraised and used to transform employers' perspectives. That will mean, change beyond the introduction of regulations or subsidies for the employment or re-employment of silver workers. There also needs to be interlinked or entwined processes that press employers to reflect upon the contributions of these workers and thereby challenge their biases and prepared causes of action. Some associated initiatives might be to: de-emphasise the term 'silver workers' to engage with a more helpful and positive titling of workers beyond retirement , a realignment of the existing classification of 'silver workers' which more helpfully accommodate the scope of needs for workers who are aged or retried and consideration of how best workplace environments and government policies, as well as practices by workers themselves might be enacted to secure longer and more productive working lives for those working after retirement. In short, current deficit discourses used to describe silver workers to be transformed through a process by which perceptions of and decision about silver workers are more informed by evidence from practice.

Part -2 Employers

A coin had two sides. Likewise, an issue or a problem has two sides. When there is discussion two ideas need to be considered in the interest of a whole view and correct understanding. The present discussion has dealt with the first side of the silver workers who are the target group of the issue on discussion. This side has the target group of employers who have employed the silver workers in their organization. They made the second side of the issue. The second part of the present discussion seeks to review the findings and their analytical outcome with a view to balance the study still further.

The silver workers as employees occupy the central focus of the present study and so major part of the study is devote to matters related to them. But the employers who employ them in their organization cannot be ignored. In the first part initiative, courage and concern they have shown to silver workers to grant jobs allow to work again after retirement, that positive attitude in the matter can encourage more of elderly to think of working after retirement. It is commendable that they have not fallen under influence of stereotypes negative perceptions and biases about elderly persons prevailing in society and resorted to bold action of employing elderly. We can say such generous employers can create a new history for silver workers in the midst of so much of negativity about them.

The discussion now of negativity draws on the collected data relate to the employers. It seeks to review the context that prompted them to employ silver workers in view of day to day systems and processes at their organizations. It plays special focus on how flexible working is accommodated in these already existing processing without affecting efficiency and productivity of business. Employers always talk about "the demands of the jobs"

It means that a particular set of constraints are necessitated by particular jobs or roles and they may highlight a range of practices that may operate in a single workplace. These practices may go in relation to workers in different occupation. The discussion would aim at understanding how the employers structure a working day. It provides an important context of whether they can offer flexibility to the silver workers, up to what extent and how it help them growing business. The flexibility that can be allowed to the silver workers may be defined in view of the employer, his business and the characteristics of his organization, such as size, sector, and retirement age. Hence, first the profile of the employers was reviewed.

The previous sections considered the reasons, problem, and perceptions about retirement, satisfaction and influencing factors that have made the concerns of silver worker participation in the labour market more prominent. It also explored the problems faced by silver workers who re-enter the labour market. Secondly it was explored about what conditions of work and employment need to be considered in order to develop comprehensive policies from national to local level. Such policies are intended to ensure equitable circumstances for silver workers in the workplace, as well as the opportunity at some point to retire with dignity. Now the employer's part will be taken into consideration

This part of the chapter draws on the quantitative data obtained from the employers. It seeks to explain the context of what the employer's practice in employing the silver workers. It examines the day-to-day systems and processes of the employers with a specific focus on the ways in which flexible forms of working were or were not embedded in these practices.

Examining what the employers define as 'the demands of the job', the particular sets of constraints necessitated by particular jobs or roles may highlight a range of practices that may operate within a single workplace, in relation to the staff engaged in different occupations. Although the silver workers would not form the specific focus in this part, understanding the way which the employers would structure a working day provides an important context to understanding what they were able or unable to offer the silver workers in a form of flexibility. The employer and their characteristics of the organization such as, size, retirement age, sector and organization would define different forms of flexibility the employers can offer and the constraints would affect on flexibility adversely. The tables below would present the related data in the manner like.

4.19 Profile of the Employers

4.20 Details about the Employees

As per the plan of the chapter, the data obtained through the responses of the selected silver workers should project a triangular perspective on the silver workers decision to work after retirement. The part I of the chapter presents two dimensions of the perspective viz. quantitative perspective on the basis of the data and the qualitative perspective on the basis of the responses of the silver workers. It projects objective and subjective perspective on the subject under the study. The part II seeks to project the third dimension of the perspective through the views expressed by the counterparts of the silver workers. They are the employers who employ the silver workers in their organizations

4.20 Profile of the Employers

Table 125: Percentage Distribution of the Employers According to their Designations

(N=50)

Designation	F	%
Manager	14	28.00
Department Head	12	24.00
Branch Head	9	18.00
Director	8	16.00
Development Officer	7	14.00

All (100%) the employers interviewed were males. The table 125 reveals that designations on which employers of the silver workers were engaged included manager (28%), department head were (24%) branch head (18%), director were (16%) and development officer were (14%). This person held higher position in the respective organizations at which the silver workers were employed after retirement. This table shows that all employers were having higher position at their work place

As the data reflect, all the fifty employers, held higher position at the organizations at which the silver workers were employed. They appeared to hold key positions like manager, department head, branch head, director and development officers, from these positions they would be able to plead a case for elderly candidate and influence decision of recruitment with their recommendations. But among them, those holding the positions of director and branch head would prove more influential in the matter of employing silver workers.

Table 126: Percentage Distribution of the Employers According to their Age

(N=50)

Age	F	%
Middle Aged	25	50.00
Aged	25	50.00

Table 126 reflects on the age shows that equal percentages (50%) of the employers belonged to middle aged and aged group and all (100%) of them were males. This table reveals both middle aged and aged were working on the higher positions, but it was important to notice that they were all males.

In view of age, all the employers were evenly divided in to middle age group and aged group. Majority of them were more experienced in business and some of them were still young and less experienced in business. It indicated that their age and experience may speak about their open attitude and positive mind about silver workers.

Table 127: Percentage Distribution of the Employers According to their Experience in the organisation/company/institution/ corporate/firm

(N=50)

Experience (In Years)	F	%
More experienced	30	60.00
Less experienced	20	40.00

Table 127 shows that 60 percent of the employers possessed work experience of 24 years and more in the organisation/company /institution/corporate/firm and 40 percent of them had less than 24 years of experience. This table shows that higher percentages of employers possessed more years of experience.

Table 128: Percentage Distribution of the Employers According to the Type of Organizations

(N=50)

Type of Organization	F	%
Private Organizations	20	40.00
Corporate	9	18.00
Firms	8	16.00
Agencies	7	14.00
Business houses	6	12.00

Table 128 shows that 40 percentages of employers were working in private organizations. Little less than one fifth percentages (18%) of them were working were working in corporate, little more than fifteen percent (16%) were working in firms and 14 percent were working in agencies and the remaining 12 percent of them were working in business houses.

Many of the organization at which the silver workers were employed were private organizations. Some were corporate houses, some business firms, some agencies and some were business houses. No government organization and public sector company seemed to employ elderly persons. It shows that since private companies enjoy more flexibility of decisions they would think of employing aged people. In the government and public set up, age of retirement is fixed by rule and so it allows no flexibility about considering aged persons. Further, in view of huge problem of unemployment and other restrictions they usually express inability for it. Further, as unemployment prevails on large scale supply of unemployment youths always exceed a demand of workers. So the procedure of recruitment is further tightened with eligibility tests, personal interviews, site interviews etc. in view of very high competition among youths aspiring jobs, a chance of elder persons for jobs at government and public sector organization id further minimised

Table 129: Percentage Distribution of the Employers According to the Finance Resource that they Resort for the Organizations

(N=50)

Finance Resources	F	%
Business savings	38	76.00
Operating profits	32	64.00
Bank loans	18	36.00
Introducing new partners	11	22.00
Private loans	10	20.00
Private savings	3	6.00

Table 129 reveals that high percentages (76%) of employers were utilizing the business savings as the finance resources for the organizations. Whereas 64 percent of them were using operating profits for the purpose. 36 percent of the employers obtained bank loans and 22 percentages managed to introducing new partners in their business. Almost equal percent of them (20%) used private loans and very less (6%) were using private savings as the finance resources for their organizations. When a question of employing elderly person arises one naturally thinks about financial arrangements. Some owners of business may project as a pretext for their inability to employ elderly persons, as they always weigh productivity and profit against the amount of work that elderly persons would be able to put. Keeping this possibility in mind, finance resources were reviewed at the employers organization resorted to.

The data revealed that good majority of the employing organization resorted to their own business savings that they raised from their earning or profit. A majority of them arranged the finance from their operating profit. Some of the organizations preferred into new partnership with a view to raising the finance. Some even relied on private loans from private money lenders and on their own private savings. Employing persons in organization is usually perceived as risk in business and so reliability of finance comes to be deciding factor.

Table 130: Percentage Distribution According to the Age of Retirement Prescribed at the organizations

(N=50)

Retirement Age	F	%
58 years	36	72.00
60 years	14	28.00

Table 130 shows that high majority (72%) of the organizations had prescribed retirement age of 58 years. While only 28 percent organizations had prescribed retirement age of 60 years. This shows that majority of the organizations still prefer to retire their employees at an age of 58 years

Another point for which employers would feel resentful to employ elderly person's persons is age of retirement at all the organization ranged from 58 to 60 years. The employers as such preferred to retire employees at 58 or at the most, at 60 years of age. Yet to is really appreciable about the employers that they have accommodated e4lerly persons in their workplace. It would be interesting to review how an on which ground they have taken such a so –called risky decisions in business and what calculations goes with it. This kind of curiosity takes us to the point of reviewing the status of silver workers at those organizations.

4.21 Details about the Employees

Table 131: Percentage Distribution of the Employers According to Number of the Silver Workers working in their Organisations

(N=50)

Silver Workers	F	%
1-5	47	94.00
6-20	2	4.00
21-100	1	2.00

Table 131 reflects that very high majority (94%) of organization employed 1 to 5 silver workers in organizations. Whereas only two of the organizations employed 6 to 20 silver workers in organization. Only at one organization a good number of 21 to 100 silver workers were employed. This table reveals that at very less number of organizations more number of silver workers were recruited after retirement.

The data related to the silver workers employed at the employer's organization reflected that out of fifty organization almost 47 organization employed upto five silver workers. Some two of them had employed six to twenty silver workers and only one organization had employed more than twenty silver workers.

Table 132: Percentage Distribution of the Employers According to Increase in Number of Elderly Workers in the Organizations

(N=50)

Number of Employees	F	%
Same	36	72.00
Less	11	22.00
Not Sure	3	6.00

Table 132 shows that at high majority (72%) of the organization the number of silver workers remained the same as compared to the number of last year. While at 22 percent of the organizations the number of silver workers decreased. A very less six percent of the employers were not sure about the difference in numbers of silver workers at the organizations

The data also shows that in comparison of the last year the number of silver workers remained same at good majority of the organization and at some their number decreased. Just three organizations were unable to report surely about the status of the silver workers employed with them. It was a relief that majority of the employers retained the silver workers. Yet it sounds discourage that the status of the silver worker did not improve over a year which means that no progress was reported in the matter.

Table 133: Percentage Distribution of the Employers Opinion Regarding Employing Female Silver Workers in the Organisations

(N=50)

Employing Elderly Females	F	%
No not Sure	38	76.00
No reply	7	14.00
Have employed	5	10.00

Table 133 reflects on the opinion of the employers about employing elderly females. High majority of employers (76%) said they were not sure about employing female silver workers in their organizations. Whereas 14 percent of them refused to answer and only five of them were positive about employing female silver workers in their organizations. This indicates that organizations were not favourable to employ female silver workers.

Employing female silver workers is an issue that operates on different consideration as there prevail number of reservations about female silver workers. This projection seemed to be reflected in the related data (table 131) which present that almost three fourth of the organization, were unable to report anything with surety. From seven organizations, no reply was received and five organizations admitted that they did not employ any female silver worker. The data thus project that no organization had taken a clear and positive view on the matter or so to say, were not favourable to employ female silver workers. Probably the employers were influenced with misleading negative dominated perceptions or stereotypes that prevail in male dominated society.

Table 134: Percentage Distribution of the Employers According to their Roles in the Organisations

(N=50)

Roles in the Organizations	F	%
Responsible to manage the actual recruitment processes	24	48.00
Specifying requirements for employees but do not conduct interviews for the recruitment	15	30.00
Specifying both requirements for employees and conduct interviews for the recruitment	11	22.00

Table 134 focuses on the roles that the employers play in the organisations. As identified almost half percent (48%) of the employers were responsible to manage the actual recruitment processes. Whereas little less than the one third (30%) percent of them were involved to specify the requirements for employees to be recruited. But they do not conduct interviews for the actual recruitment. Only 22 percent of them were involved in specifying both requirements for the employees and also conducting the interviews for actual recruitment

Roles and responsibilities assume lot of significance in work sector. An employee value is attached to the facts related the roles and responsibilities that he/she is assigned in an organization. It would be encouraging to note that almost fifty percent of the silver workers were involved in the recruitment procedure and some thirty percent of them were assigned a work of specifying requirement for newly employed. Some of them were involved in both the role. It means that the employers appeared to value and respect their knowledge and long term experience in an area of work and sought for their opinion in the matter of new recruitment. It can be surely understood at such positive treatment the silver workers would be highly pleased and satisfied

Table 135: Percentage Distribution of the Employers According to Reasons Organisations for not Retaining retired Silver Workers after Retirement

(N=50)

Reasons	F	%
Government regulations/policies get in way	47	94.00
Elder workers are more expensive	25	50.00
Elder workers are not valuable as young workers	17	34.00
Not an urgent or pressing issue	12	24.00
Work is too physical to employ people beyond a certain age	11	22.00

Table 135 specifies the reasons for not retaining silver workers after retirement. When asked about why organizations do not retain elderly very high majority (94%) of the employers gave the reason of government regulations/policies. Whereas 50 percent of the employers said that elder workers are more expensive and 34 percentages explained that elder workers are not valuable as younger workers. 24 percent of the employers said that it's not an urgent or pressing issue for them and the remaining 22 percent of them said that work is too physical to employ people beyond a certain age. The table reveals that high percent organizations were facing more difficulty in employing silver workers as government rules and regulations do not allow it. This indicates that even if they are willing to recruit silver workers they cannot do it. Such a condition highlights that government policies need to be revised in the benefit of the elderly who want to work after retirement.

The employers expressed their inability to retain elderly or silver workers at their organization beyond an age of retirement. They gave variety of reasons for it. A very high majority of them gave valid reason of the government regulations that restrict an age of retirement at 58 or 60 years and would not approve of employment exceeding it. About half of them gave an economic reason, like "elderly workers are more expensive" in the sense that calculation about them would not fit with productivity and profit. Some one third of them posed reasons of age when they expressed "elder workers not valuable as young workers" they perhaps meant efficiency of man hours and machine hours to ensure high productivity. In addition, they lack technical skills to operate computers and manage computerized operations which are a reality of the day at workplaces. About one fourth of the employers put forth reasons like "no urgency" or "no pressing issue" for them to employ elderly persons and about same number of them said that it was not feasible for them to employ persons beyond a certain age. The former group indicate that unless the employers are insisted they would not think about employing elderly persons. Someone or government has to exert pressure on them to consider the issue in positive light. The latter group indicated of demands like feasibility of work and time, special concession and assistance in view of the age and the like. So these two groups showed a kind of resentment to employ silver workers at their organization.

Table 136: Percentage Distribution of the Employers According to the Best Age to Contribute to the Organizations

(N=50)

Age (In Years)	F	%
Under 30 years	7	14.00
30-44 years	12	24.00
45-54 years	2	4.00
55 years and Above	6	12.00
At any Age	23	46.00

Table 136 reveals what employers thought about best age to contribute to their organizations. 14 percent of them stated that age below 30 years would be best suited to contribute. While 24 percent of them opined that age group of 30 to 44 years would be best suited to contribute. Very less (4%) of them believed that age between 45 to 54 years would be better of age to contribute, while 12 percent of them were in favour of the age of 55 years and above. While 46 percent of them did not specify any age for the purpose and believe that an employee can contribute best to the organization at any age if he/she keeps that sentiment. The table shows that higher percentages of employers did not believe in any age as a factor to contribute to work sector. Rather than insisting on an age an employee they believe that can contribute best to the organizations provided he/she possess efficiency and willingness for it.

There arises a question of efficiency in view of a workers age. So the data concerning the employers view about an age at which one can contribute at his/her best. On reviewing the data, some of them believed that one can contribute at his/her best under age of 30 years. They perhaps referred to freshness of human energy and modern knowledge and skills. About half of them viewed that a worker can contribute at best in an age from 30 to 44 years. A few of them mentioned the nest age to contribute from 45 years to 54 years. Some of them believed that an age of 55 years and above would be the best age to contribute. Against all these varied views, half of the employers believed that a worker can contribute best at any age. They probably thought that age cannot be mark or yardstick to measure one's contribution. One's performance speaks for his efficiency innovativeness and commitment to work and contribution can be measured with these three yardsticks. Thus, the last view sounds realistic, reasonable and appreciable.

Table 137: Percentage Distribution of the Employers According to their Opinions regarding Formal Policies/Programmes for Recruitment of Employees who are Approaching Retirement Age

(N=50)

Formal Policies/ Programmes	F	%
No formal policies	31	62.00
There are formal policies	11	22.00
Planning to develop a policy	8	16.00

Table 137 shows that 62 percent of the employers reported that there is no formal policies/programmes to encourage employees who are approaching the retirement age to continue working in the company/organization. Whereas 22 percent of them informed that that they do have such policies and programmes in their organizations and 16 percent of them regretted that they do not have such policies or programmes but they are planning to develop such policies and programmes to encourage. Employee approaching the retirement age to continue working in the organizations. The above table reveals that that there is an urgent need to frame formal policies to encourage silver workers to work after retirement. Higher percentages of the organizations were unable to employ silver workers in absence of suitable policies and regulations

Another important point raised with the employers about whether there was a need of formal policy or programme to employ silver workers' good majority of them held an opinion that no formal policy was rewired in the matter of employing silver workers. Employers should first apply their practical business sense to work out their feasibility to accommodate silver workers in their workforce. It has to go with human considerations to see how best they can work in its favour and pay positive considerations to offer options and adjustments and assistance in work and time in view of their senior age.

Some one fourth of the employers admitted that there are formal policies, but they did not clarify how much they adhere to them and give positive mind to employing silver workers. Several of them admitted about no policy and that they are planning to develop a policy. It means they are ready to pay positive consideration to employing silver workers. This projection indicated that majority of the employer's appeared serious and positive about employing silver workers and some appeared to be strikers putting out this or that pretext to not employing silver workers.

Table 138: Percentage Distribution of the Employers Concerned about Loss of Valuable Knowledge faced by the Company/Organization

(N=50)

Loss of Valuable Knowledge	F	%
Very concerned	41	82.00
Somewhat concerned	9	18.00

In view of the impact of retirement of employers to an organization, the employers' were asked a pertinent question. When an employer retired and leave an organization, do you perceive its adverse effect like' loss of valuable knowledge' to an organization? How much would you be said that they were 'somewhat concerned'? They explained the loss like as employee is recruited in an organization he carries with it knowledge and skill. Both enhance and consolidated further, as he gains experience. An organization too is benefitted with his/her improved knowledge and skill in the form of efficiency and productivity through its useful application in business. Table 138 shows that the very high majority (82%) of employers were much concerned that retirement of elderly employees would cause loss of valuable knowledge to their organizations. Only 18 percent of them were somewhat concerned about loss of valuable knowledge. This table show that higher percentages of employers were aware about loss of valuable knowledge as the elder employees would retire from a job with long tenure.

Thus, in their sense knowledge became valuable when it proves utility through productivity application in business. Any employers grumble about young candidate who appear at interviews for jobs that they possessed knowledge by qualifications or degrees, but they are unable to explain its utility by application in business. So knowledge is important, but more important is its utility and that is where its value lies. The employers perception related to their employers reaching an age of retirement was further confirmed with an analysis of intensity index. For the purpose, some 10 items were short listed derived from the related matters and the intensity index was calculated for each of them. The items focus on influential factors in the employers even after retirement. These workers were approaching an age of retirement soon and wish to work after they retire on certain considerations.

Knowledge is treasure that grows bit by bit as a person grows in years. More knowledge is held by an older person. This is a traditional notion which seems be defeated in the light of an age of computers and internet. Today we find that at young age of early or mid twenties youth come out of universities holding PhD's, M.B.A's and the like and employed in higher positions with handsome salaries. It sounds very attractive and encouraging to younger generation and they may be bit arrogant about it. There may be no wrong about it. In fact it is a right picture of literacy in human society. But the knowledge we mean here is not just information or rich data bank of information built up with computers and the internet. We mean knowledge as information converted into one understanding and enhance his/her level of maturity. It required years to go by during which a person gives his mind to the information he/she has obtained from the websites and books with relevant knowledge. When we say "loss of valuable knowledge" we mean this knowledge and it built up in age. As a person reaches an age of retirement his knowledge operates with his/her practical experience to generate real understanding and maturity about it.

4.22 Item Wise Findings Regarding the Influential Factors in deciding the time to Retire

The employers perceptions related to their employees reaching an age of retirement were further confirmed with an analysis of intensity index. For the purpose the items were short listed derived for the related matters and the intensity index was calculated for each of them. The items focus on influential factors in the employers view even after retirement.

The scale to judge the influential factors included 10 items, and under each item three options were specified. It indicated three intensity indices related to the influential factors in deciding time to retire. The items, for which more number of employers had marked, are reported below:

Table 139: Overall Intensity Indices Showing the Influential Factors in Deciding Time to Retire

(N=50)

Items	Intensity Indices
Desire to be productive and helpful	2.54
Desire for income	2.44
Recognition received for work	2.36
Desire for health benefits0	2.06
Enjoyment derived from work	2.01
Sense of fulfilment derived from work	1.96
Social interaction with co-workers	1.72
Opportunity to continue to learn	1.62
Sense of responsibility to help co-workers	1.46
Opportunity to work a reduced hours for period of time prior to retiring completely	1.09

Table 139 shows that the overall intensity indices regarding influential factors that the employers considered for employees in organisation approaching the retirement who want to continue working after the expected retirement age. They ranged from 2.54 to

1.09. It means that there prevailed great to less extent of agreement on the above mentioned items about the influencing factors

According to the influencing factors, great extent of agreement was held by the employers in the following items.

- Desire to be productive and helpful
- Desire for income
- Recognition received for work

The table further reveals that employers showed some extent of agreement on the following factors which can prompt silver workers to work after retirement.

- Desire for health benefits
- Enjoyment derived from work
- Sense of fulfilment derived from work
- Social interaction with co-workers
- Opportunity to continue to learn

Table 139 also revealed that less extent of agreement was shown by the employers related to the following factors.

- Sense of responsibility to help co-workers
- Opportunity to work a reduced Schedule for a period of time before retiring completely

4.23 Item Wise Findings Regarding the Qualities Considered by Employer while Employing Silver Workers

The scale to judge the qualities that employers expect while employing silver workers included 22 items. Under each item three options were specified which indicated the three intensity indices related to the qualities. The items, on which more number of employers had marked, are specified below:

Table 140: Overall Intensity Indices Showing the Qualities Considered by Employer Expect while Employing Silver Workers

(N=50)

Items	Intensity Indices
Reliable	2.76
Trustworthy	2.76
Listens carefully and follows instructions	2.68
High physical strength and stamina	2.58
Energetic and enthusiastic	2.58
Work full-time and willing to work longer hours if required	2.44
Lot of experience	2.34
Having Similar background	2.22
Works peacefully	2.18
Willing to be flexible and work varied hours (including shorter hours) if required	2.14
Innovative	2.14
Mentally very sharp	2.12
Specialist skills	2.06
Adapts well to change	2.05
Over-qualified for the job	2.04
Enjoys challenges	2.04
Works effectively as part of a team	2.04
Ambitious	2.03
Able take the initiative	2.03
Ability to work in different areas of the business as needed	2.01
Work independently	1.96
Promising employee with recent training	1.84

Table 140 indicates the overall intensity wise qualities considered by employer while employing silver workers. They ranged from 2.76 to 1.84. It means that there was great extent to some extent of agreement. It can be seen from the above table that the employers showed greater extent of agreement about the qualities that they would expect while employing silver workers with regards to the following items.

- Reliable
- Trustworthy
- Listens carefully and follows instructions
- High physical strength and stamina
- Energetic and enthusiastic

Further it can be seen from the above table that employers showed some extent of agreement a regards to following qualities as an advantage to recruit silver workers.

- Work full-time and willing to work longer hours if required
- Lot of experience
- Having Similar background
- Works peacefully
- Willing to be flexible and work varied hours (including shorter hours) if required
- Innovative
- Mentally very sharp
- Specialist skills
- Adapts well to change
- Over-qualified for the job
- Enjoys challenges
- Works effectively as part of a team
- Ambitious
- Able take the initiative
- Ability to work in different areas of the business as needed
- Work independently
- Promising employee with recent training

4.24 Item Wise Findings Regarding the Advantages of the Employer while recruting Silver Workers

The scale to judge the advantages considers by employer while employing silver workers included 18 items. Under each item three options were indicated which indicated the three intensity indices related to the advantages. The items, for which more number of employers agreed are specified below:

Table 141: Overall Intensity Indices showing the Advantages of the Employers while recruiting Silver Workers

(N=50)

Items	Intensity Indices
Established network of contacts and clients	2.68
Helped in crisis	2.52
Dedication would render significant business advantage	2.46
Loyal to the organizations	2.46
Lower propensity to quit or change a job	2.34
Ability to guide other workers	2.28
High level of engagement in work	2.24
Strong work ethics	2.18
Do not need guidance	2.12
Highly skilled	2.08
Valuable experience	2.07
Hard working	2.06
Highly productive	2.04
Positive attitude	2.04
Valuable insights into customers and business needs	2.03
More dependable	2.01
Diversity of thoughts and new approaches to teamwork	2.01
More readily available to start work	1.64

Table 141 shows that overall intensity wise advantages that an employer would consider by recruiting silver workers. They ranged from 2.68 to 1.64. It means that there prevailed greater to some extent of agreement on the advantages among the employers.
It can be seen from the above table that employers showed greater extent of agreement on the advantages of recruiting silver workers with regards to following items.

- Established network of contacts and clients
- Helped in crisis

It can be further revealed from the above table that employers agreed to some extent for the following item as the advantages of recruiting silver workers

- Dedication would render significant business advantage
- Remained loyal to the organization/ company
- Lower propensity to quit or change job
- Ability to guide other workers
- High level of engagement in their work
- Strong work ethics
- Do not need guidance
- Highly skilled
- Valuable experience
- Hard working
- Highly productive
- Positive attitude
- Valuable insights into customers or business needs
- More dependable
- Diversity of thoughts and new approaches to teamwork
- More readily available to start work

4.25 Item Wise Findings Regarding the Disadvantages of the Employer in Recruting Silver Workers

The scale to judge the disadvantages that employer would consider by recruiting silver workers included 17 items. Under each item three options were mentioned which indicated the three intensity indices related to the disadvantages. The items, for which more number of employers agreed, are reported below:

Table 142: Overall Intensity Indices showing the Disadvantages if the Employers in Recruiting Silver Workers

(N=50)

Items	Intensity Indices
Lower productivity	2.76
Less receptive to training and skills	2.74
High wage expectation	2.72
Fear changes in work place	2.64
Do not keep updated with latest technology	2.54
Prefer to work on own tasks and methods	2.44
Integrating diverse generations of workers and accommodating part time and flexible schedules	2.32
Reculant to travel	2.06
Reculant to learn new technologies	2.06
Less flexible compared to younger workers	1.98
Negative attitude towards organizational change	1.98
High rate of absenteeism	1.86
Unable to meet physical demands of the job	1.64
Lack of innovative thinking	1.58
Source of greater health security and health expense	1.38
Persistent health problems hampering jobs	1.28
Lack Poise and Confidence	1.22

Table 142 represents the overall intensity wise disadvantages that an employer considers by recruiting silver workers. They ranged from 2.76 to 1.22. It means that there prevailed greater to less extent of agreement among the employers.

It can be seen from the above table that employers showed greater extent of agreement on the disadvantages of recruiting silver workers with regards to following items.

- Lower productivity
- Less receptive to training and skills
- High wage expectation
- Fear changes in work place
- Do not keep updated with latest technology

It can be further revealed from the above table that employers agreed to some extent for the following item as the disadvantages of recruiting silver workers

- Prefer to work on own tasks and methods
- Integrating diverse generations of workers and accommodating part time and flexible schedules
- Reculant to travel
- Reculant to learn new technologies
- Less flexible compared to younger workers
- Negative attitude towards organizational change
- High rate of absenteeism
- Unable to meet physical demands of the job
- Lack of innovative thinking

Further it can be revealed that employers agreed to lesser extent for the following items as disadvantages of recruiting silver workers

- Source of greater health security and health expense
- Persistent health problems hampering jobs
- Lack Poise and Confidence

It may be understood from the above discussion on the employers' perspective on the silver workers that searching qualified elderly would be a challenge to them. They would find it a big puzzle to confuse with doubts about what they would gain or lose.

Some kind of fear would make them bit reculant to employ silver workers in their organizations

It can be revealed from the findings that professional efficiency was highly perceived by the employers and there cannot be compromise on them. The second group of disadvantage relate to job relate requirements and they were perceived as disadvantage, but some kind of concession or adjustment may be allowed to the silver workers. The third group indicates disadvantage causing appear to have less agreement to call them as disadvantages, but rather natural unavoidable conditions that may need different kind of considerations. From this, it may be a big challenge to the employers and unlike recruiting younger candidate they have to be more careful, while recruiting silver workers and apply precise, positive and versatile thinking to their limitations in view of prospects of their business.

In view of the disadvantages discussed about, the employers would be facing a bug challenge about employing silver workers. Against so much of positive dimensions of silver workers as viewed as advantages , the disadvantages sound more puzzling and unavoidable in moral work changes, a adjustments and inadmissible concession, which may not be so feasible with normal work schedules and special arrangements for it may not be economically viable in the present business status.

The employers reported about the challenges that they faced in searching qualified elderly workers. Although they were able to locate an elderly candidate with good qualifications all sorts of attitude problems coming up would spoil prospects to employ him. They were like unwilling to work on lower salaries, rigidity of mind, inflexibility to work on lower salaries, lacking technical knowhow and confidence to cope with advance technologies, unwilling to work full time , lacking experience, suitable to the requirements of a job, lacking enthusiasm to work, unwilling to work on lower designations and expecting higher monetary rewards for work. These challenging traits in silver workers are drawn on the ground on general experiences with them reported or shared by several people. They project problem areas that pose challenges to the employer in their view to recruit silver workers in their organizations so against all good talks about the silver workers reasonable and legitimate claim for ' right to work' and all good appeals and pleading in their favour, these problem areas demand adequate attention and efforts on the part of elderly workers. So that way may be given to their claim 'right to work' with active support from all concerned in business, industry professional fields , educational fields, social work field and of course in the government.

In this manner, the present discussion seeks to review all relevant matters concerning silver workers decision to work after retirement with all angels and dimensions emerging from the data collected for the study and their analysis through different technical test and methods. It also considers the objective and subjective implication of the responses obtained from the respondents. To go still further, it considered the employers pints of view as counterpart of the employed silver workers perception to weigh the validity and project balanced overview on the silver workers decision to work after retirement.

Silver workers exist all over the globe and form a sizeable component of the population and society of all countries. They can be ignored neither their wishes, desires, aspirations can be undermined, neglected and rejected. Since they have stopped working after and rejected. Since they have stopped working after retiring from their first employment they on the large form inactive or passive and idle human component of society. According to the proverb "an idle mind is devils workshop", idle elderly persons may divert to damaging and unproductive activities causing number of ill to spoil healthy environment. Before the conditions go to dogs' to affects human society adversely some constructive thinking is required paving way to constructive efforts. There is an urgent need to engage human minds in one or other kind of work suiting to a person's capacity and capability.

Western societies have worked out some kind of arrangements of work for retired elderly persons. In the U.S.A , it is floated in the name of "bridge employment" .there may be similar programmes operated in many countries. In fact, it is mandatory for any sensible society to arrange for such a programme to avail opportunity of work or job to elderly persons. Elderly persons should be given due attention by which they may be integrate in current workforce. They offer to contribute with their knowledge and experience. They will be motivated to work to provide relevant competencies with which organizations will certainly be benefitted. In this light, a observation served at different times by Olesch (2005); Reinberg and Hummer (2004) and Wagner (2000) is worth considering. It coveys that the predicted lack of specialised staff might promte post retirement activity, as silver workers accumulated work experience and knowledge will be valuable for filling the gap in the workforce.

Since in different countries and societies the conditions and situation would vary with geographical and climatic and also cultural diversities. Yet an issue and problems concerning elderly persons remain radically alike. In that condition, a model of silver works employment after retirement may be adapted to the prevailing conditions with necessary changes. The western model of bridge employment; can be adopted to suit the Indian context and conditions in view of variable and influential factors that promote elderly persons to work after retirement. Unlike the considerations in India are motivated by socio-economic pressures. So keeping this in mind, a suitable model of silver workers post retirement employment may be evolved for India to save elders from depression and fatal suicidal predicament. By engaging elders in to suitable work after retirement would allow them to feel satisfaction and motivation with utility of their knowledge and experience. It would prove a great boon to them.

While working on such models, expectations of employers and job requirement too should be granted due consideration so that silver workers are accepting in the present workforce without sacrificing business interest and prospects. Silver workers do need self introspection to know their limitation that might hamper or damage business interest. They need to work to improve or correct them in the interest of their better adaptability to the business world in India. Their sincere efforts will certainly earn them appreciation for being valuable addition to workforce.

Silver workers have many attributes that are of benefit to the labour market. They bring a myriad of skills and experience developed throughout their careers, both at and away from work. Many have highly developed judgment, problem-solving abilities, and interpersonal skills, have forged valuable relationships with customers or clients, and are willing to help employers out on a part time or seasonal basis. Silver workers are typically strongly committed to their jobs and tend to remain in jobs longer than younger workers. In a recent survey of its members in Alberta and B.C., the Canadian Federation of Independent Business (CFIB) found that over three quarters of those who responded feel elderly bring a strong work ethic, experience, qualifications and loyalty to the workplace. However, misconceptions about silver workers still abound. Employers may be reluctant to look at initiatives to attract or retain silver workers because of unfounded concerns about the willingness of silver workers to learn new skills and new technologies and practices. The reality is that many silver workers are keen and capable of learning new skills, but may be overlooked for training. Employers may also be concerned that declines in physical and mental abilities among silver workers will

In many fields, knowledge and skill requirements for existing jobs are increasing. Some silver workers may feel they do not have the knowledge and skills they need to be comfortable and productive in today's workplaces. For many, this may be because they have not been provided with–or taken advantage of–opportunities to continue to increase their knowledge and skills and become comfortable with new technologies throughout their careers. Training opportunities in many companies continue to focus on younger employees, despite research which shows on-the-job training and "the opportunity to learn something new" is something silver workers seek in a job. Again, Silver workers are not a homogeneous group, and employers need to think carefully about the kinds of training and opportunities needed. Promoting a culture of life-long learning may be the best approach to ensuring all employees have the skills and developmental opportunities they need, both to be competent at their jobs and to remain engaged in the workforce.

CONCLUSION and SUGGESTIONS

"Rest is a good thing, but boredom is its brother."
Voltaire

This study represents an attempt to investigate the determinants of labour force participation among silver workers in Vadodara city. This study has explored the experiences of older people in the workplace, how satisfied elderly are with various aspects of their jobs. There appears to be a growing consensus that early retirement is no longer viable for individuals, employers or national economic performance and that extending working lives is a necessary goal. It is important not to lose sight, however, of the importance of 'choice' and individual preference and to ensure instead that all older people, regardless of background, have the resources and information necessary to ensure some degree of control over their future.

The results of this study revealed that silver workers are very much motivated to work after retirement the reasons behind it is not only the financial need but many other factors like to remain active, to share knowledge expertise with the younger generation, to remain healthy were the reason for them to work post retirement. Although most silver workers were not that content with their jobs, as they dissatisfied with the hours they work and the lack of flexibility they experience in their working schedules. For these groups in particular, flexible and reduced hour's opportunities should be designed. Perceptions of self also represent an obstacle, with some elderly perceiving themselves as too old to initiate change. Cultural change at a societal level alongside the enforcement of age discrimination legislation is likely to improve the employment prospects of elderly and open up opportunities for occupational change which are likely, in turn, to extend working lives as individuals continue to be motivated and challenged in the workplace. To this end, wider and more affordable training and educational opportunities at older ages are also likely to be beneficial.

The culture and values of the silver workers are significant assets for the companies that choose to attract and retain them. These values include commitment and loyalty to the employer, fewer sick days, reduced injuries, and enhanced length of service. As the workforce ages and contracts, skilled workers will increasingly come at a premium.

Managers who fail to respond to the threat will put their future growth and profitability at risk, while missing out on the benefits of greater age diversity. To be successful in an increasingly competitive market place, managers need to attract and retain silver workers and, yes, love them when they are 62.

Employers need to begin now to build integrated strategies to encourage employees with valuable skills and experience to stay in the workforce while the organization transfers their expertise or develops/recruits the talent needed to replace them. Like any commodity, silver workers are getting more valuable as they get scarcer. A few things managers can do to retain their silver workers include:

- Eliminate stereotypes
- Motivate silver workers
- Distribute work fairly
- Encourage postponement of retirement
- Allow flexible work timings
- Invite retired employees back at least once a year for a company gathering.
- Develop a post-retirement data base noting skills and experience of each retiree.
- Update performance management and reward systems

Based on the results, some policy recommendations that can help to increase the labour force participation of silver workers can be outlined in bid to promote active ageing. This can include steps to raise the mandatory retirement age, develop and open more employment opportunities for silver workers, develop geriatric training centres to equip the elderly with knowledge and skills needed by employers, provide financial incentives to encourage employers to hire and retain silver workers. A range of policies and practices that require auditing and review in the workplace have been highlighted, including recruitment processes, availability of flexible working, workloads and opportunities to continue developing.

Through this study an attempt has been made to capture the voices of older people in order to ensure that their preferences within the workplace, in relation to retirement timing and their aspirations during the retirement years, are heard.

Messages of the Employers

Challenges faced by the employers in searching qualified elder workers

- Retired people are not willing to work on lower salaries, so it would be bit difficult to find such employees
- They have rigid mind and less flexible to adjust to prevailing set-up ,that is the major problem in recruiting them
- Lacking of knowledge and confidence about the advance technologies
- Lack of people willing to work full time
- Finding an employee having experience from the same filed
- Facing difficulty in searching employee's possessing enthusiasm for work that they used to display before retirement.
- Not finding an employee who is ready to take up training sessions.
- Not finding an employee who is flexible in term of work timings
- E difficult to find an employee with less family responsibilities
- Scarcity of workers having suitable resume for the jobs on the job sites
- They are not ready to work on lower designations
- They expect higher salaries

Important Message for people who are planning to do productive work in retirement

- Keep your resume update and readily posted on the job site so that recruiters can approach you easily.
- Be active and productive as long as your health permits
- There is no age for learning. Learn and keep yourself active. Do not let your ego to spoil your career
- Always remember that you are trunk of knowledge to others. Be ready to share knowledge with younger workers to enhance their as capability and know how about a job on hand
- Live your life king size, be helpful to other people at a workplace and be cheerful

- Forget your post/designation that you had before retirement and accept what is being offered to you in this new innings
- Be open and readily adaptive to the changes in the work sector.
- Do not demand for the respect, earn it by your won virtue of a good worker.
- Be receptive towards the change and learning new technologies
- Do not demand for the same salary that you were getting before you retired. Give priority to the work rather than to money
- Just be what you are and be confident about it. Don't try to act wise, raise your voice against wrongs and odds in the working situations.
- Stop sympathizing yourself as being a retired. Be an employee and start gearing up yourself to work with the younger people. Never think that you are inferior to them that in any sense.
- Stop being stiff minded. If you want to work you need to learn you need to adjust with the situation.
- Do not compare your present with your previous job.
- Don't feel that you are not capable to work with younger colleagues do not lose your confidence
- Keep yourself active and just share your experience with others to enrich the younger employees
- Learn new technologies, and try to be technology friendly. It is the only way you can sustain in the employment sector after retirement.
- No work cab be less important until and unless you enjoy doing it. Enjoy the work that you are doing.
- Try not to impose your thoughts and methods of working on other employees because with the chaining time methods also changes.
- Consider the work opportunities that come in your way rather than sitting and waiting for the ideal one. It is just work that ultimately matters
- If you want to work, give importance to work and ignore the amount paid to you.
- It is good to work on the basis of your past experiences. But every time you're past experiences may not work well for the present job. So better try to think about some new techniques and innovative methods that can be more advantageous for task given to you

RECOMMENDATIONS FOR FURTHER STUDIES

- Similar studies can be conducted in relation to variables other than those taken in the present study such as marital staus, gender, family pressure, social isolation , fear and anxiety due to retirment

- Similar study can be conducted to know the reasons ,difficulties and problems faced by by elderly who are self employed

- A comparative study cab ne conducted involving the elderly who are working after retirement and those who are not working

- A longitudinal study of this topic could effectively examine how occupation, health, and socioeconomic status earlier in life help determine one's retirement decisions and behaviours. Such longitudinal research could also help identify how spousal characteristics, marital circumstances, and family circumstances more broadly influence important decisions that are made in later life.

CHAPTER – 5

SUMMARY

5.1 Introduction

India has largest population in the world. On average, an elderly person is expected to live between 18 and 20 years beyond 60.The number of older persons in India is projected to increase from 90 million in 2008 to 298 million in 2051 and 505 in 2001.the portion of the elderly would reach 20 percent in 2051, from 8 percent in 2008 about 75 percent of the elderly are in rural areas.

The ageing of populations is one of the successful outcomes of demographic transition, in particular, mortality transition. The developed countries of the world have already experienced the process of ageing and its consequences and have developed policies and programmes to avert crisis in not only providing economic and social security but also promoting economic growth. Developing economies such as the countries of South Asia are also well on their way to having a similar ageing population. However, they are either prepared to face the consequences or to manage the growing numbers of the elderly through appropriate policies of welfare and social protection. Although the proportion of the elderly who are 60 years of age and above would seem to be relatively low in the biggest populous giants of the world such as China and India, in terms of absolute numbers, they have much more elderly persons than many other regions (countries) of the world because of their huge population bases. The recent spurt in empirical studies related to the elderly in the developing world is attributed not only to increasing numbers but also to deteriorating living conditions of the elderly accentuated in part by rapid modernisation and urbanisation as well as internal and international migration. The projected increase of the elderly populations in both absolute and relative terms is, in many developing countries, a subject of growing concern for demographers, planners, policymakers, actuarial experts and pension economists. It has been, indeed, a matter of grave concern for countries such as India, Sri Lanka and Bangladesh, Pakistan and Nepal. (Treas and Logue, 1986; World Bank, 1994, 2000; 2001; Government of India, 1999, 2001; Alam, 2006; Irudaya Rajan, Mishra, and Sarma, 1999; Irudaya Rajan, 2008; Leibig and Irudaya Rajan, 2003; Irudaya Rajan, Risseeuw and Perera, 2008).

India has largest population in the world. On average, an elderly person is expected to live between 18 and 20 years beyond 60.The number of older persons in India is projected to increase from 90 million in 2008 to 298 million in 2051 and 505 in 2001.the portion of the elderly would reach 20 percent in 2051, from 8 percent in 2008 about 75 percent of the elderly are in rural areas.

The twentieth century and the beginning of this one have seen an unprecedented demographic transition in the form of population ageing. Globally, life expectancy at birth increased from around 47 years in the 1950s to 67 in 2008, an increase of 20 years in the space of half a century. The gain has been impressive among less developed regions, i.e. 24 years compared to 10 in developed regions (UN, 2007). In India, the gain has been 21 years (Irudaya Rajan, 2008). India has the second largest number of older persons1 in the world. On average, an older person is expected to live 18-20 years upon reaching 60. When people live longer, what mechanisms are available to them to remain active and productive in employment and other gainful activities? How much unemployment and poverty are there among older persons? Are they covered under existing social security schemes and/or do they own financial assets and property? Are they assured of income through pension and retirement benefits? Are widowed women dispossessed? Is there any special social security provision for older women and widows? What are the policy responses? This paper aims to address these issues in the Indian context.

The reduction in fertility level, reinforced by steady increase in the life expectancy has produced fundamental changes in the age structure of the population, which in turn leads to the aging population. India had the second largest number of elderly (60+) in the world as of 2001. The analysis of historical patterns of mortality and fertility decline in India indicates that the process of population aging intensified only in the 1990's. The older population of India, which was 56.7 million in 1991, is 76 million in 2001 and is expected to grow to 137 million by 2021.

The current problem of the policy makers to extend socio economic security for the poor is the demographic ageing and increased number of aged in the country.s population. The growth of the aged population which is either dependant on the young or unemployed or working for food during the evening yeas of their life is a challenge to the social security systems in the country. As there is no correct definition to the aged, we consider , that the population above the age of sixty as aged. This can be safely taken as the retirement age in the organized employment in the country is between 58 years to 60 years on majority. According to the data available from the decennial census the number of aged has increased from about 19.6 million in 1951 to 75.93 million in 2001 or by 287 percent over 50 years period. Their share of population increased from 5.5 to 6.8 percent. However in effect, nearly 72 percent of the increase in the number of the aged has to be attributed to population growth, where as the balance 28 percent has been due to the aging of the population.

More than 100 million populations (8% of total population) in India are elderly, higher than the combined population of UK and Canada. In India according to living arrangement by analysing 39,694 elderly data from NFHS-2. Overall 3% of total elderly are living alone in India, 1.7% men and 4.5% women. Significant variations in morbidity among the elderly exist with respect to living arrangement and gender.

Today India is home to one out of every ten senior citizens of the world. Both the absolute and relative size of the population of the elderly in India will gain in strength in future. Among the total elderly population, those who live in rural areas constitute 78 percent. Sex ratio in elderly population, which was 928 as compared to 927 in total population in the year 1996, is projected to become 1031 by the year 2016 as compared to 935 in the total population. The data on old age dependency ratio is slowly increasing in both rural and urban areas. Both for men and women, this figure is quite higher in rural areas when compared with that of urban areas. More than half of the elderly populations were married and among those who were widowed, 64 percent were women as compared to 19 percent of men. Among the old-old (70 years and above), 80 percent were widows compared to 27percent widowers. Men compared to women are found to be economically more active. In 1991, 60 percent of the males were main workers whereas only 11 percent of the females were main workers. Out of the main workers in the 60+ age group, 78 percent of the males and 84 percent of the females were in the agricultural sector. Since women's economic position depends largely on marital status, women who are widowed and living alone are found to be the worst among the poor and vulnerable.

Given the trend of population aging in the country, the older population faces a number of problems and adjusts to them in varying degrees. These problems range from absence of ensured and sufficient income to support themselves and their dependents to ill health, absence of social security, loss of social role and recognition and to the non-availability of opportunities for creative use of free time. The needs and problems of the elderly vary significantly according to their age, socio-economic status, health, living status and other such background characteristics. The prospect of loneliness often accompanies the process of aging. In fact, many old people, unable to bear this loneliness, commit suicide, and many are clamouring for the right to die rather than be forced to live with the indignities and hopelessness of old age(commit aging suicide). Aging also hardens the likes and dislikes of a person— his or her prejudices, perceptions, and value judgments that refuse to acknowledge the reality of aging.

Among the several problems of the elderly in our society, economic problems occupy an important position. Mass poverty is the Indian reality and the vast majority of the families have income far below the level, which would ensure a reasonable standard of living. As people live longer and into much advanced age (say 75 years and over), they need more intensive and long term care, which in turn may increase financial stress in the family. Inadequate income is a major problem of elderly in India (Siva Raju, 2002). Nearly half of the elderly are fully dependent on others, while another 20 percent are partially so (NSSO, 1998). For elders living with their families-still the dominant living arrangement their economic security and well being are largely contingent on the economic capacity of the family unit. Particularly in rural areas, families suffer from economic crisis, as their occupations do not produce income throughout the year. Nearly 90 percent of the total workforces are employed in the unorganised sector. They retire from their gainful employment without any financial security like pension and other post retirement benefits

5.2 Objectives of the Study
(A) Objectives related to Silver Workers

1. To study the profiles of silver workers working in Vadodara city.
2. To study the reasons of silver workers to work after retirement with respect to
   a. Personal reasons
   b. Familial reasons
   c. Financial reasons
   d. Work related reasons

3. To study the differences in the reasons of silver workers to work after retirement in relation to the selected variables:
   a. Age
   b. Educational qualification
   c. Last Designation
   d. Present salary
   e. Health status
   f. Type of family

4. To study the influence of work on silver workers

5. To study the differences in influence of work on silver workers in relation to the selected variables:
   a. Age
   b. Type of work (Present)
   c. Present designation
   d. Health status

6. To study the problems faced by silver workers at their workplace

7. To study the difference in the problems faced by silver workers at their workplace in relation to the selected variables:
   a. Age
   b. Educational qualification
   c. Present salary
   d. Health status
   e. Present designation
   f. Perceptions about old age

8. To study the satisfaction of silver workers in relation to their work status

9. To study the differences in satisfaction amongst silver workers in relation to the selected variables:
   a. Type of work (present)
   b. Present salary
   c. Present designation

(B) Objectives Related to Employers

10. To study the profiles of organizations employing silver workers

11. To study the reasons of employers for recruiting silver workers in their organizations/companies/institutions/firms/business houses/corporate.

12. To study benefits of employing silver workers in their organizations/companies/institutions/firms/business houses/corporate.

13. To study the problems faced by employers by employing silver workers in their organizations/companies/institutions/firms/business houses/corporate.

5.3 Null Hypotheses of the Study

1. There will be no significant differences in the reason of silver workers to work after retirement in relation to the selected variables:

    a. Age
    b. Educational qualification
    c. Last designation
    d. Present salary
    e. Health status
    f. Type of Family

2. There will be no significant differences in influence of work on silver workers in relation to the selected variables:

    a. Age
    b. Type of work (Present)
    c. Present designation
    d. Health status

3. There will be no significant difference in the problems faced by silver workers at their workplace in relation to the selected variables:

    a. Age
    b. Educational qualification
    c. Present Salary

    d. Health status

    e. Present designation

    f. Perceptions about old age

4. There will be no significant differences in satisfaction amongst silver workers in relation to the selected variables:

    a. Type of work (Present)

    b. Present salary

    c. Present designation

5.4 Methodology

5.4.1 POPULATION OF THE STUDY

The population of the present study comprised of silver workers those who are officially retired (58 and above) working for productive purpose/still working and earning after their retirement. The other group of sample consisted of employers from Vadodara city who have recruited those silver workers in their offices/institution/firms and Business houses residing in Vadodara city of Gujarat State.

5.4.2 SAMPLE SIZE AND SELECTION PROCEDURE OF THE SAMPLE (SILVER WORKERS AND EMPLOYERS

The sample of the present study comprised of two types of respondents one were the silver workers and other were the employers who employed silver workers. In total there were three hundred and fifty respondents from which three hundred were silver workers who were working post retirement and fifty were the employers who recruit those retired silver workers in their organizations, corporate, banks, companies, firms and colleges from Vadodara city of Gujarat State.

In order to indentify an employer which is the second sample of the study, the researcher approached the same organization where the silver workers were found working during their retirement. The size of the organisation (i.e number of employees) was one important factor in shaping the experience, ethos and practice of employers.

A purposive sampling method was used to draw the sample. Researcher identified banks/corporate/organizations/companies/firms functioning actively and recruiting silver workers and the organization recruiting those silver workers after retirement in Vadodara city. Researcher visited those banks/corporate/organizations/companies/firms and asked about silver workers who were recruited there after retirement. Almost fifty silver workers were identified initially those who were working after their retirement.

Those silver workers provided the names and addresses of the other silver workers whom they knew. The names and addresses of silver workers were also collected from colleagues, friends, relatives, neighbours, who knew silver workers those who were working after retirement. Same organizations were approached by the researcher in order to identify the employers .The snowball sampling technique was used to identify the sample.

5.4.3 CONSTRUCTION OF RESEARCH TOOLS

The present study was an exploratory research. Therefore, survey method was preferred for studying the reasons of silver workers and for the employers who recruit them. The questionnaire, perception scale and rating scales were the tools used for data collection. In addition to obtain a picture of ideal working situation during retirement open ended question were incorporated. The main aim to incorporate open ended questions was to attract unfiltered impressions of the silver workers descriptions of their circumstances and experiences. The tools were constructed keeping in mind various purposes after reviewing related literature desired from books, journals and other literatures. As a first step, main topics for survey were defined such as former professional career, motivation for working during retirement, changing profession when entering retirement, and type of work in retirement. The pilot study helped the researcher to frame the questionnaire. The tools were prepared in English and then translated into Gujarati for better comprehension of the silver workers and to ensure ease in communication

5.4.4 DESCRIPTION OF RESEARCH TOOL USED FOR SILVER WORKERS
A questionnaire consisting of six sections was prepared to study the reasons, perceptions, problems, their work related satisfaction and factors that influence silver

workers, to work after retirement. The sections, content and response system used in the research tool of silver workers are detailed in the table1

Table: Description of Research Tools of the Silver Workers

Sections		Content	Response System
Section-1	Part-A	Background Information of the Silver Workers	Check list cum Questionnaire
	Part-B	Family Background	Check list cum Questionnaire
	Part –C	Present Occupational Status	Check list cum Questionnaire
	Part-D	Work History	Check list cum Questionnaire
	Part –E	Health Status	Checklist
Section-2	Part-A	Reasons of Working after Retirement	4-Point Rating Scale
	Part-B	Perceptions about Retirement	3-Point Rating Scale
Section -3		Influence of Work on Silver Workers	3-Point Rating Scale
Section -4		Problems Faced by Elder Workers at Workplace	4-Point Rating Scale
Section -5		Satisfaction at Workplace	3-Point Rating Scale
Section -6		Suggestions	Open Ended Questions and checklist

5.5 Validity of the Research Tools

To check the validity of the research tools, the questionnaires were sent for review by experts from the following institutions:

- Dean, Faculty of Family and Community Sciences, The Maharaja Sayajirao University of Vadodara , Vadodara
- Head, Faculty of Family and Community Sciences, The Maharaja Sayajirao University of Vadodara , Vadodara
- Associate Professor, Department of Extension and Communication, Faculty of Faculty of Family and Community Sciences , The Maharaja Sayajirao University of Vadodara, Vadodara
- Associate Professor, Department of Psychology, Faculty of Education and Psychology, The Maharaja Sayajirao University of Vadodara, Vadodara

- Associate Professor, Department of English, Faculty of Arts, The Maharaja Sayajirao University of Vadodara, Vadodara
- Associate Professor, Department of Statistics, Faculty of Science, The Maharaja Sayajirao University of Vadodara, Vadodara
- Associate Professor, Faculty of Masters in Social Work, The Maharaja Sayajirao University of Vadodara, Vadodara

The experts were requested to check the questionnaire for:
- Content validity
- Nature of the Statements
- Clarity of language and ideas
- Appropriateness of the response system

The suggestions given by experts were incorporated in the tools

5.6 Reliability of the Research Tools

The test-retest method was used for measuring the reliability of the questionnaire. The tool was administered on five silver workers and five employers in Vadodara City. To measure the reliability of the tool, it was administered again on the same persons after a gap of fifteens days. The coefficient of correlation between the two sets of scores was calculated to find out the reliability of the tool by using the following formula:

$$r = \frac{\sum xy}{\sqrt{\sum x^2 \sum y^2}}$$

Where, r = Coefficient of correlation
X = Score of First test
Y = Score of Second test
The tool reliability was found 0.92

5.7 Pre-testing of the Research Tools

The prepared questionnaires were pre-tested on ten silver workers and ten employers in the Vadodara city. The researcher simplified some terms that respondents could not follow. Silver workers and employers selected for pre-testing of the tool took about thirty to thirty five minutes to fill the questionnaire.

5.8 Procedure of Data Collection

The data were collected from 300 silver workers and 50 employers who recruit those retired silver workers in their organizations, firms, corporate, business houses, from different areas of Vadodara city during December 2012 to May 2013. With regards to acquisition of respondents, large organisations were systematically contacted who supposedly maintained contacts with their retirees. Some respondents were acquired using personal contacts known to the researcher or from respondents in a snow ball process. Thus making the study's sample a cumulative sample. A large number of silver workers were identified through companies/organizations/Corporate/institutes/firms/colleges who were recruiting retired silver workers. A permission to collect data from silver workers as well as employers was sought from the various authorities of the concerned organizations. The silver workers and employers were contacted and the data was collected by meeting them according to their convenience of time and place. The questionnaires were distributed to silver workers. They were collected back after a week or fifteen days.

Many a times, silver workers took more than 30 to 35 minutes to fill the questionnaire as it required them to do some thinking on the items and relating it to their working practise and experiences. Interview method was used to collect data from those silver workers, who faced difficulty in reading or were not used to filling questionnaire. Six to seven hundred questionnaires were distributed amongst the silver workers as well as employers out of which 378 in total were returned.

- Various reasons were found for not returning the questionnaire such as:
- Losing the questionnaire
- Unwilling or uninterested in the study/in filling questionnaire
- Not filling the questionnaire after many reminders
- Few silver found the questionnaire too lengthy and some information which about they were hesitant to answer

Interview schedule was prepared as tool for the employers and interview method was used to collect the data. Tools were prepared in English language. Employers took around 15 to twenty minutes to answer the questions.

No major difficulties were faced during the data collection and it completed peacefully. Majority of the silver workers and employers were interested in the study as it was related to them.

5.9 Scoring and Categorization of the Data of Silver Workers

Different types of scoring procedures were use for giving weightage to various items of all the parts of the tools used to collect information regarding the variables of the study. The scoring pattern and categorization of the silver workers and employer are discussed separately in the following lines:

5.9.1 CATEGORIZATION OF VARIABLES

The tool contains questions regarding profile of the silver workers. The categorization of the **Independent and Dependent variables** for a silver worker was done as follows

Table : Categorization of Independent Variables for Silver Workers

Variables	Basis	Categories
Age	58-66 years	Young-Old
	67-74 years	Old
Educational Qualification	Graduate to Doctorate	Higher Level of Education
	Diploma to Higher Secondary	Moderate Level of Education
	Primary to Secondary	Low Level of Education
Designation	Class I	Higher order Designation
	Class II	
	Class III	Middle order Designation
	Class IV	Low order Designation
Present Salary	Less than 17,000 Rupees	Low Income Group
	17,000 Rupees	Middle Income Group
	More than 17,000 Rupees	High Income Group
Health Status	0-1 Health Problems	Healthy
	2-4 Health Problems	Somewhat Healthy
	More than 4 Health Problems	Less Healthy
Type of Family	Living Alone	Living Alone
	Living with Partner	Living with Spouse
	Living with Children	Living with Family
Type of Work	8 hours	Full Time
	Less than 8 hours	Part Time
Perceptions about Old Age	Above Mean	Most Favourable
	Mean and Below Mean	Favourable and less favourable

Table : Categorization of Dependent Variables for Silver Workers

Variables	Basis	Categories
Reasons of Working	Above Mean	More Number of Reasons
	Mean	Moderate Number of Reasons
	Below Mean	Less Number of Reasons
Influence of Work	Above Mean	High Level of Influence
	Mean	Moderate Level of Influence
	Below Mean	Low Level of Influence
Problems at Workplace	Above Mean	More number of problems
	Mean	Moderate number of Problems
	Below Mean	Less number of Problems
Satisfaction at Workplace	Above Mean	High satisfaction
	Mean	Moderate Satisfaction
	Below Mean	Less Satisfaction

5.9.2 REASONS TO WORK AFTER RETIREMENT

To measure the reasons of silver workers to work after retirement, the scores were given to the silver workers as shown in the (Appendix 1, Section 2-A). The minimum and maximum possible ranged from 1 to 36. However, the scores achieved by the respondents ranged from 1 to 36 and they were categorized as follows:

Aspect Wise total Obtainable Scores:

Aspects	Number of Statements	Maximum Obtainable Scores	Minimum Obtainable Scores
Financial	10	30	10
Familial	11	33	11
Work	7	21	7
Personal	8	24	8
Total	36	108	36

The range of intensity indices were calculated overall and aspect wise to measure the extent of reasons of the silver workers to work after retirement. To describe the extents of reasons, the range of intensity indices were decided as follows:

The range of intensity indices were decided as follows:

Extent of Reasons	Scores	Range of Intensity Indices
Great Extent	3	2.51-3.00
Some Extent	2	1.51-2.50
Less Extent	1	1.00-1.50

Range of the scores for describing the reasons of silver workers to work after retirement was decided as follows:

Type of Reasons	Score
Less Number of Reasons	36-60
Moderate Number of Reasons	61-85
More Number of Reasons	86-108

Range of mean scores for describing the reasons of silver workers to work after retirement were decided as follows:

Range of Mean Scores	Categories
Less Number of Reasons	Below Mean
Moderate Number of Reasons	Mean
More Number of Reasons	Above Mean

5.9.3 PERCEPTIONS ABOUT RETIREMENT

The perception scale was developed to measure the intensity of the perceptions of silver workers about retirement. It was a 3 point scale. The scoring of the responses on a scale was done as follows:

Scoring pattern according to the nature of statements in the perception scale regarding silver worker's perception about retirement

Nature of Statement	Agree to Great Extent	Agree to Some Extent	Agree to Less Extent
Positive	3	2	1
Negative	1	2	3

The total numbers of statements were 46. The minimum and maximum obtainable scores ranged from 46-138. Range of scores describing the perceptions of silver workers regarding retirement was decided as follows:

Type of Perceptions	Score
Less Favourable	46-76
Favourable	77-107
Most Favourable	108-138

Aspect Wise Obtainable Scores were as follows

Perceptions about Retirement	Number of Statements	Maximum Obtainable Scores	Minimum Obtainable Scores
Favourable	17	51	17
Unfavourable	29	87	29

The range of intensity indices were calculated overall and aspect wise to measure the extent of perceptions about retirement of the silver workers. To describe the extents of perceptions, the range of intensity indices were decided as follows:

Range of Intensity Indices:

Extent of Perceptions	Scores	Range of Intensity Indices
Great Extent	3	2.51-3.50
Some Extent	2	1.51-2.50
Less Extent	1	1.00-1.50

Categories for describing the perceptions of silver workers regarding retirement was decided as follows:

Range of Mean Scores	Categories
Less Favourable and Favourable	Mean and Below Mean
Most Favourable	Above Mean

5.9.4 INFLUENCE OF WORK ON SILVER WORKERS

To measure the influence of work on silver workers, a three point scale was developed. The overall intensity indices were calculated to measure the extent of influence of work on silver workers. The total number of statements in the scale was 24 and the possible obtainable score ranged from 24-72.

Obtainable Scores were as follows

Content	Number of Statements	Maximum Obtainable Scores	Minimum Obtainable Scores
Influence of work	24	72	24

To describe the extent of work, the obtainable scores and range of intensity indices were decided as follows:

Range of Intensity Indices:

Extent of Influence	Scores	Range of Intensity Indices
Great Extent	3	2.51-3.00
Some Extent	2	1.51-2.50
Less Extent	1	1.00-1.50

Range of the scores for describing the intensity of influence of work was decided as follows:

Extent of Influence	Score
Low Level of Influence	24-40
Moderate Level of Influence	41-57
High Level of Influence	58-72

To find out overall and item wise influence of work intensity indices were calculated. Range of mean scores for describing the intensity of influence of work was decided as follows:

Categories	Basis
Low Level of Influence	Below Mean
Moderate Level of Influence	Mean
High Level of Influence	Above Mean

5.9.5 PROBLEMS FACED BY SILVER WORKERS AT WORKPLACE

To measure the extent of problems faced by silver workers at workplace a four point rating scale was prepared which included twenty five statements. The maximum obtainable score was hundred and minimum obtainable score was twenty five. The scoring of the statements in the scale was done as follows:

Obtainable Scores were as follows:

Content	Number of Statements	Maximum Obtainable Scores	Minimum Obtainable Scores
Problems faced by silver workers at their workplace	25	75	25

The intensity indices were found out overall and item wise to measure the extent of problems faced by silver workers at workplace. The categorization of intensity indices was as follows

The range of intensity indices were decided as follows:

Extent of Problems	Score	Range of Intensity Indices
Great Extent	3	2.51-3.00
Some Extent	2	1.51-2.50
Less Extent	1	1.00-1.50

Range of the scores for describing the intensity of problems at workplace was decided as follows:

Categories	Basis
Less Problems	Below Mean
Moderate Problems	Mean
More Problems	Above Mean

5.9.6 SATISFACTION AT WORKPLACE

To measure the extent of satisfaction of silver workers at workplace a three point rating scale was prepared which included twelve statements. The maximum obtainable score was thirty six and minimum obtainable score was twelve. The scoring of the statements in the scale was done as follows:

Obtainable Scores were as follows:

Content	Number of Statements	Maximum Obtainable Scores	Minimum Obtainable Scores
Satisfaction of Work	12	36	12

The intensity indices were found out overall and item wise to measure the extent of satisfaction of silver workers at workplace. The range of intensity indices was as follows:

The range of intensity indices were decided as follows:

Extent of Influence	Scores	Range of Intensity Indices
Great Extent	3	2.51-3.00
Some Extent	2	1.51-2.50
Less Extent	1	1.00-1.50

Range of the scores for describing the intensity of satisfaction of silver workers at workplace was decided as follows:

Type of Satisfaction	Score
Less Satisfaction	12-20
Moderate Satisfaction	21-29
High Satisfaction	30- 36

To find out overall and item wise satisfaction of silver workers at workplace intensity indices were calculated. Range of the mean scores for describing the intensity of satisfaction of silver workers at workplace was decided as follows:

Categories	Basis
Less Satisfaction	Below Mean
Moderate Satisfaction	Mean
High Satisfaction	Above Mean

5.10 Scoring and Categorization of Data of Employers

5.10.1 QUALITIES OF RECRUITING SILVER WORKERS

To measure qualities that employers considered while recruiting silver worker, a three point scale was developed. The overall intensity indices were calculated to measure the extent. To describe the qualities, the obtainable scores and range of intensity indices were decided as follows:

Obtainable Scores were as follows

Content	Number of Statements	Maximum Obtainable Scores	Minimum Obtainable Scores
Qualities of the Employees	22	66	22

The intensity indices were found out overall and item wise to measure the extent of qualities of an employee. The categorization of intensity indices was as follows:

Range of Intensity Indices:

Extent	Scores	Range of Intensity Indices
Great Extent	3	2.51-3.00
Some Extent	2	1.51-2.50
Less Extent	1	1.00-1.50

Range of scores for describing the qualities of the employees was decided as follows:

Extent	Scores
Great	22-36
Some	37-51
Less	52-66

5.10.2 ADVANTAGES OF RECRUITING SILVER WORKERS

To measure advantages that employers takes into consideration while recruiting silver worker, a three point scale was developed. The overall intensity indices were calculated to measure the extent. To describe the Advantages, the obtainable scores and range of intensity indices were decided as follows:

Obtainable Scores were as follows

Content	Number of Statements	Maximum Obtainable Scores	Minimum Obtainable Scores
Advantages	18	54	18

Range of Intensity Indices:

Extent	Scores	Range of Intensity Indices
Great Extent	3	2.51-3.00
Some Extent	2	1.51-2.50
Less Extent	1	1.00-1.50

Range of scores for describing the advantages of employing silver workers was decided as follows:

Extent	Scores
Great	18-30
Some	31-43
Less	44-56

5.10.3 DISADVANTAGES OF RECRUITING SILVER WORKERS

To measure disadvantages that employers takes into consideration while recruiting silver worker, a three point scale was developed. The overall intensity indices were calculated to measure the extent. To describe the disadvantages, the obtainable scores and range of intensity indices were decided as follows

Obtainable Scores were as follows

Content	Number of Statements	Maximum Obtainable Scores	Minimum Obtainable Scores
Disadvantages	17	51	17

Range of Intensity Indices:

Extent	Scores	Range of Intensity Indices
Great Extent	3	2.51-3.00
Some Extent	2	1.51-2.50
Less Extent	1	1.00-1.50

Range of scores for describing the disadvantages of employing silver workers was decided as follows:

Extent	Scores
Great	17-28
Some	29-40
Less	41-52

5.10.4 INFLUENTIAL FACTORS IN RECRUITING SILVER WORKERS

To measure the factors that influence the employers takes while recruiting silver worker, a three point scale was developed. The overall intensity indices were calculated to measure the extent. To describe the influential factors, the obtainable scores and range of intensity indices were decided as follows:

Obtainable Scores were as follows

Content	Number of Statements	Maximum Obtainable Scores	Minimum Obtainable Scores
Influential Factors	10	30	10

Range of Intensity Indices:

Extent	Scores	Range of Intensity Indices
Great Extent	3	2.51-3.00
Some Extent	2	1.51-2.50
Less Extent	1	1.00-1.50

Range of scores for describing the influential factors in employing silver workers was decided as follows:

Extent	Scores
Great	10-16
Some	17-23
Less	24-30

5.11 Statistical Analysis of the Data

A statistical package for social sciences (SPSS) was used to analyze the data. Different statistical measures for various purposes used were as follows:

Table : Plan for Statistical Analysis of the Data of Silver Workers

No.	Purpose	Statistical Measure
1	Background Information of the Silver Workers	Frequencies, Percentage and Intensity Indices
2	Reasons and Perceptions of Silver Workers to work After Retirement	T-Test, ANOVA (F-test) Intensity Indices
3	Influence of work on Silver Workers	T-Test, ANOVA (F-test) Intensity Indices
4	Problems faced by Silver workers at work place	T-Test, ANOVA (F-test) Intensity Indices
5	Satisfaction at Workplace	T-Test, ANOVA (F-test) Intensity Indices
6	Suggestions	Intensity Indices

5.12 Major Findings of the Study

5.12.1 SILVER WORKERS

- Sample of the study were silver workers working after retirement and residing in Vadodara city.
- High majority of them belonged to old age group
- Very high majority of them were males
- Very high majority of silver workers had high level of educational qualification
- 55 percentages of them had pension as their main source of income
- Very high majority of them were married and they were living with family
- Nearly half percentages of them joined the job within small gap (within 1 to 3 years) of their retirement.
- High majority of (76%) of them were not working in same organizations
- Nearly forty percentages (39.67%) of them were working on temporary basis. Whereas 96.33 were working on permanent basis before they retired.
- Except three silver workers (1%) all (99%) were working in private organizations after retirement.
- Majority (61.33%) of them were working for full time after retirement
- 63.33 were having class III designations on present job. Whereas before retirement 45.33% of them were working on class I designation.
- Nearly half percentages (48.33%) were having less salary in their present jobs. Whereas 55.67 percentages had moderate salary before retirement.
- 63 percentages of **silver workers faced problems in searching jobs due to lack of** :
    - job advertisements
    - jobs according to their abilities and skills
    - Jobs with same designation that they had before retirement
    - Jobs in city they live
    - Jobs according to past experiences
    - Jobs paying salary as earlier

- Almost 74 percentages of the silver workers faced difficulties in procuring present job.
- 85 percentages of them were prepared to work even before they retired

- When asked about age of re-retirement almost 35 percentages of silver workers believed that they want to continue working till heath permits as to kill time it's important to remain active.
- 52 percentages of them had worked for almost 32 years before retirement (average duration)
- Nearly 65 percentages of the silver workers were healthy
- Social and familial reason were found as the main reasons for silver workers to work after retirement
- **Major reasons to work were:**
    - To get attention and respect from the family
    - Become financially independent
    - To stay physically and mentally active
    - Cannot imagine life without work
- 37.67 percentages of silver workers had less favourable perceptions about retirement
- Majority of silver workers started to plan about retirement much before they actually retired
- Little more than half (51%) of them started to plan for finance at 51 years and below age
- 67 percentages of them reported that they enjoyed Brahmacharya (student stage of life) the most
- Half percentages of the silver workers were likely to retire after achieving certain amount of retirement money
- Nearly forty percentages of silver workers believed that employers, government and co-workers were primarily responsible for preparing the workers for retirement.
- 61.33 percentages of silver workers had **high level of influence in terms of** :
    - Getting respect and attention from family
    - Recognition in society
    - Being able to face people with confidence
- Almost forty percentages of silver **workers faced more number of problems related to work and workplace like:**
    - Fear and anxiety of losing job
    - Working on new technology
    - Working with younger generation

- 45.33 percentages of silver workers had moderate level of satisfaction related to their work and workplace.
- High majority of the silver workers reported that there is need for specific personnel polices for elder employees.
- Silver workers suggested that employers can provide opportunity to:
  - Guide and teach young workers
  - Work few hours
  - Enjoying stimulating workplace

5.12.2 EMPLOYERS

- All (100%) employers were males. Designations on which employers of the silver workers were engaged included manager 28 percentages, department head were 24 percentages branch head were 18 percentages, director were 16 percentages and development officer were 14 percentages.

- Equal percentages (50%) of the employers belonged to middle aged and aged/silver workers group and all (100%) of them were males. This table reveals both middle aged and aged were working on the higher positions, but it was important to notice that they were all males.

- Majority 60 percentages employers had work experience of 24 years and more than 24 years in the organisation/company /institution/corporate/firm and 40 percentages of them had less than 24 years of experience. This table shows that high percentages of employers were having more years of experience.

- Very high majority (94%) of organizations/companies had employed 1 to 5 silver workers in their organization. Whereas only 4 percent of organization/companies had 6 to 20 silver workers and only 2 percent of organizations companies were had 21 to 100 silver workers in their organizations/companies.
- High majority (72%) of the organization/company had same number of silver workers as compared to last year. While 22 of them had less number of silver workers and very less six percentages of the employers were not sure about the difference in numbers of silver workers in the organization company as compared to last year

- High majority of employers (76%) were not sure about employing female silver workers in their organization/companies. Whereas 14 percentages of employers refused to answer and only 10 percent of the employers had employed five female silver workers in their organization/company.
- Reliability, trustworthy, listens carefully and follows instructions were the main **qualities** that employers prefer while employing silver workers
- Established network of contacts and clients, helps in crisis, dedication provides significant business advantage, remain loyal to the organization were considered as the **advantages** for employers in recruiting silver workers
- Lower productivity, less receptive to training and skills. High wage expectation, fear change in workplace, do not keep updated with technology were considered as **drawback's** by employers in recruiting silver workers

CITED LITERATURE

1. Agewell Research and Advocacy Centre (2008) Impact of Economic Slowdown on Older Persons of India Agewell Economic Study Assessment of the Impact of Economic Slowdown on Older Persons of India_December Agewell Foundation M-8A, Lajpat Nagar-II, New Delhi-110024 Ph.: 011-29836486, 29840484 Website: www.agewellfoundation.org

2. American Association of Retired Persons (AARP) (2002) Staying Ahead of the Curve. The AARP Work and Career Study. Retrieved from AARP website: http://assets.aarp.org/rgcenter/econ/d17773_multiwork_1.pdf

3. American Association of Retired Persons (AARP) (2007) *Staying Ahead of the Curve 2007. The* AARP Work and Career Study. Full Report, September 2008. A National Survey Conducted for AARP by Synovate Inc.

4. Aboulafia, M. (2001) The cosmopolitan self: George Herbert Mead and continental philosophy. Champaign, Ill: the University of Illinois Press.

5. Amornsirisomboon, P. (1992) Factors Related to Employment Status of Elderly in Thailand. M.A. in Population and Social Research, Mahidol University. (in Thai).

6. Bansal, K.K. and Sharma, N. (2006) Retirement: An Emerging Challenge for 264-272 the Planners ,Indian Journal of Gerontology a quarterly Journal devoted to Research on Ageing VOL. 20, NO. 3

7. Brown, S. K. (2003) Staying ahead of the curve 2003: The AARP working in retirement study. Washington, D.C.: AARP Knowledge Management. Retrieved November 26, 2007 from http://assets.aarp.org/rgcenter/econ/multiwork_2003.pdf

8. Bird, C. (1994) Second Careers. New Ways to Work After 50. Boston: Little, Brown and Company

9. Barnes, H., Smeaton, D. and Taylor, R. (2009) *An ageing workforce: The employers perspective*. Institute for Employment Studies Research Report No. 468. London: Institute for Employment Studies.

10. Becker, G.S. (2009) Human capital: A theoretical and Empirical Analysis, with Special reference to Education, Chigaco: University of Chicago Press

11. Boonnak, A. (1994) The Study of Needs to Seek for Job and Social Welfare for the Establishment of a Placement Service Center of the Elderly in Bangkok Metropolis. Bangkok: Institute of Population Studies, Chulalongkorn University.(in Thai).

12. Bailey, L., and Hansson, R. (1995) "Psychological Obstacles to Job or Career Change in Late Life." Journal of Gerontology 50: 280-293.

13. Brown, S. K. (2003) Staying ahead of the curve 2003: The AARP working in retirement study. Washington, DC: AARP.

14. Boonyanupong, K., Boonyanupong, S., and Chanta, S. (1990) Elderly's Life in Chiangmai. Institute of Social Research, Chaiangmai University. (in Thai).

15. Bal, P. M. and Kooij, D. (2011). The relations between work centrality, psychological contracts, and job attitudes: The influence of age. European Journal of Work and Organizational Psychology. 20(4): 497-523.

16. Calvo, E. (2006) Does working longer make people healthier and happier? *Work Opportunities for Older Americans,* series 2. Retrieved January 19, 2007, from the Center for Retirement Research at Boston College's web site: http://www.bc.edu/centers/crr/issues/wob_2.pdf.

17. Cameron, M.P. and Waldegrave, C. (2009) 'Work, retirement and wellbeing among older New Zealanders', in P. Koopman-Boyden and C. Waldegrave (eds), Enhancing Wellbeing in an Ageing Society: 65–84 year old New Zealanders in 2007, Hamilton: Family Centre Social Policy Research Unit and Population Studies Centre, University of Waikato

18. Calo, T. J. (2005) The generativity track: A transitional approach to retirement. Public Personnel Management, 34, 301-312

19. Chariyaratpaisarn, M. (2000) Nakhonpathom: Elderly's Health. Faculty of Technical Science, Rajabhat Kampangsean. (in Thai).

20. Chayovan, N. (1995) Tendency, Demographic and Social characteristics, and Health of Elderly in Thailand. Seminar of Elderly in Thailand. May 3-4, Pattaya: Regent Marina. (in Thai).

21. Dhillon, P. and ladusingh, L. (2011) Economic activity in post retirement life in India. Asia-Pacific Population Journal. Vol. 26 issue 3, page 55-71. 17page.

22. Dorbitz, J., and Micheel, F. (2010) Continued employment after retirement - potential, settings, and conditions. Population Research Currently, S. 2-7.

23. Dittrich, Dennis A. V., Büsch,V. and Micheel, F. (2011) Working beyond retirement age in Germany: The employee's perspective Chapter in Book "Older workers in a sustainable society"

24. Deborah, S. Sandra, V. and Melahat Sahin-Dikmen (2009) Older workers: employment preferences, barriers and solutions Equality and Human Rights Commission, Policy Studies Institute, First published Winter 2009 ISBN 978 1 84206 230 2

25. Elezua, C. C. (1998). Counselling for retirement. *The Counsellor*, 16, 1, 6-10. Industrial Training Fund (ITF, 2004). *Life in retirement*. Jos: Center for Excellence Press.

26. Feldman, (1994) The Decision to Retire Early: A review and Conceptualisation. In: The Academy of Management Review 19,2: 285-311 (DOI:10.2307/258706).

27. Farr, J. Tesluk, L., P. E., and Klein, S. R. (1998) Organizational structure of the workplace and the older worker. In K. Schaie and C. Schooler (Eds.), Impact of work on older adults (pp. 143-185). New York, NY: Springer Publishing Company.

28. Gobeski, K. Beehr, T. (2009) How retirees work: predictors of different types of bridge employment. In: Journal of Organizational Behavior 30,3: 401-425 (doi: 10.1002/job.547).

29. Goldman, D. and Smith, J (2011) "The Increasing Value of Education to Health." Social Science and Medicine 72(10):1728-1737.

30. Government of India National Policy on Older Persons (1999) Ministry of social justice and empowerment, New Delhi.

31. Gordon, M. Johnson, R. and Toder ,E. (2008) Will Employers Want Aging Boomers? The Retirement Policy Program Discussion Paper 08-04 July ,The Urban Institute 21 00 M Street, N.W. / Washington D.C. 20037 / www.retirementpolicy.org

32. Grube, A. Hertel , G. (2008) Age-related differences in work motivation , job satisfaction and emotional experience while working . In : Economic Psychology 10.3 : 18-29

33. Irudaya Rajan, S. (2000) Financial and social security in old age, in Murli Desai and Siva Raju,S.(eds.) Gerontological Social Work in India: Some Issues and Perspectives,B.R.Publishing,Delhi

34. Irudaya Rajan, S. (2005) Chronic Poverty among the Indian Elderly. Chapter 5. Pp.168197 in Aasha Kapur Mehta and Andrew Shepherd (eds). Chronic Poverty and Development Policy in India. Sage Publications, New Delhi

35. James, J., Jennifer E. Swanberg ,J. and Sharon P. McKechnie ,J. (2007) Generational Differences in Perceptions of Older Workers' Capabilities Issue Brief 12 November in the Center on Aging and Work/Workplace Flexibility at Boston College, funded by the Alfred P. Sloan Foundation, is a unique research center established in 2005.

36. Khotrakul, S. (1993) Problems of the Elderly. Bangkok: National Social Welfare. (in Thai).

37. Keukulnurak, S. (1997) A Comparative Study on Economics Activities of Never Married and Married Aged in Thailand. M.A. in Population and social Research, Mahidol University. (in Thai).

38. Lord, R. and Farringdon, P (2006) Age-related differences in the Motivation of Knowledge Workers. Engineering Management Journal, , September. 18(3), 20-26.

39. Lord, R. (2002) Traditional Motivation Theories and older Engineers, In: Engineering Management Journal 14,3: 3-7.

40. Loretto, W., Vickerstaff, S. and White, P. (2005) Older Workers and Options for Flexible Work. Equal Opportunities Commission Working Paper Series No. 31. Manchester: EOC.

41. Loi, J. L. P, and Shultz, K. S. (2007) Why older adults seek employment: Differing motivations among subgroups. Journal of Applied Gerontology, 26, 274-289.

42. Macnicol, J. (2008) 'Older Men and Work in the Twenty-First Century: What can the History of Retirement Tell Us?' Journal of Social Policy, 37, 4: 575–95.

43. Munnell, A. H., Sass, S., and Soto, M. (2006) Employer attitudes towards older workers: Survey results. Chestnut Hill, MA: Center for Retirement Research at Boston College. Retrieved November 26, 2007 from http://www.bc.edu/centers/crr/issues/wob_3.pdf 3

44. Marsh, A. and Sahin-Dikmen, M. (2002) Discrimination in Europe (London, Policy Studies Institute, November) (2003): Discrimination in Europe (Brussels, European Commission, May), available at http://europe.eu.int/comm/employment_social/publications/2003/cev403001_en.pdf (at June 2005).

45. Maykut, P. and Morehouse R. (1994) Beginning Qualitative Research: A Philosophic and Practical Guide. London: The Falmer Press.

46. Maestas, N. (2010) "Back to Work: Expectations and Realizations of Work after Retirement." The Journal of Human Resources 45(3):718-748.

47. Mermin, G. B. T., Johnson, R. W., and Murphy, D. P. (2007). Why do boomers plan to work longer? Journal of Gerontology: Social Sciences 62B S286 – S294

48. Mermin, G. B. T., Johnson, R. W., and Toder, E. (2008). Will employers want aging boomers? Urban Institute Retirement Policy Discussion Paper 08-04. Retrieved September 15, 2009, from http :// www . urban . org / UploadedPDF / 411705_aging_boomers . pdf ? RSSFeed = Urban . xml

49. National Sample Survey Organisation (1998) Morbidity and Treatment of Ailments (NSS 52nd round) report no. 441, New Delhi, government of India.

50. National Policy on Older Persons (1999) Ministry of social justice and empowerment ,Government of India Shastri Bhavan,New Delhi

51. National Institute of Social Defence (2001). A Solution To The Problems Of Older Persons, Newsletter, 2(3),Delhi

52. National Sample Survey Organization (2005) Employment and Unemployment Situation in India NSS 61st round ,(July 2004 – June 2004-05 Report No. 515(61/10/1) (Part – I)

53. National Statistical Office, (2001) A Study on the Impact of the Economic Crisis on Households. Bangkok: National Statistical Office, Office of the Prime Minister. (in Thai).

54. National Statics office (1998) Status of the Elderly. Bangkok: National Statistical Office, Office of the Prime Minister. (in Thai).

55. Odin, S. (1996). The social self in Zen and American pragmatism. Albany; State University of New York Press.

56. Patrickson, M. and Ranzijn, R. (2004) 'Bounded choices in work and retirement in Australia', Employee Relations, Vol. 26 No 4, pp. 422-43

57. Parnes, Herbert S. and David G. Sommers. (1994) "Shunning Retirement: Work Experiences of Men in Their Seventies and Early Eighties." Journal of Gerontology: Social Sciences 49: S117-S124.

58. Pitt-Catsouphes, M., and Smyer, M. A. (2007) The 21st century multi-generational workplace (Issue Brief No. 09). Chestnut Hill, MA: Boston College Center on Aging and Work/Workplace Flexibility. Retrieved November 1, 2007 from http://agingandwork.bc.edu/documents/IB09_ MultiGenWorkplace_001.pdf

59. Pittayanon. S., (1992) Labour Economics. Bangkok: Chulalongkorn University Printing. (in Thai).

60. Quinn, J., "Has the Early Retirement Trend Reversed?" (unpublished paper), accessed online at http://fmwww.bc.edu/ec-p/wp424.pdf; and Joseph F. Quinn and Gary Burtless, "Is Working Longer the Answer for an Aging Workforce?" *Issues in Brief* 11 (December 2002), Center for Retirement Research, Boston College University, accessed online at www.bc.edu/centers/crr/ib_11.shtml, on Feb. 13, 2006. For annual LFPR from 1963 to 2003 for men and women ages 55-61, 62-64, 65-69, and 70 and over, see Federal Interagency Forum on Aging Related Statistics, *Older Americans 2004: Key Indicators of Well-Being* (Washington, DC: Federal Interagency Forum on Aging Related Statistics, 2004), accessed online at www.agingstats.gov, on Feb. 13, 2006.

61. Ruttanavijit, P. (1995) Labour Force Particiration of the Elderly in the Central and the Northeastern Regions of Thailand. M.A in Population and Social Research, Mahidol University. (in Thai).

62. Rix, S. E. (1990) "Older Workers." In Choices and Challenges: An Older Adult Reference Series, edited by E. Vierck. Santa Barbara, CA: ABC-CLIO, Inc..

63. Ruhm, C.J. (1990) 'Bridge jobs and partial retirement', Journal of Labor Economics, 8, 482501.

64. Rabl, Tanja (2010) Age, discrimination, and achievement motives – A study of German Employees. In: Personnel Review 39,4: 448-467 (doi: 10.1108/00483481011045416).

65. Reynolds, S., Ridley, N., and Van Horn, C. (2005) A work-filled retirement: Workers' changing views on employment and leisure (Work Trends Survey No. 8.1). New Brunswick, NJ: John J. Heldrich Center for Workforce Development, Rutgers University. Retrieved October 30, 2007 from http://www.heldrich.rutgers.edu/uploadedFiles/Publications/WT16.pdf

66. Sharanjit U., and Sisira S. (2007) World Health and Population, 9(4) .doi:10.12927/whp.2007.19516 Aging, Health and Labour Market Activity: The Case of India

67. S. Spencer and S. Fredman (2003) Age equality comes of age: Delivering change for older people, London, Institute of Public Policy Research.

68. Stein, D.; Rocco, T. S.; and Goldenetz, K. A. (2000) "Age and the University Workplace. A Case Study of Remaining, Retiring, or Returning Older Workers." Human Resource Development Quarterly 11, no. 1 (Spring 61-80).

69. Shultz, Kenneth S. (2003) Bridge employment: Work after retirement. In: Adams, Gary A.; Beehr, Terry A. (Eds.): Retirement: Reasons, processes, and results. New York: Springer. 215-241.

70. Siva Raju, S. (2002) "Meeting the Needs of the Poor and Excluded In India", Situation and Voices, the Older Poor and Excluded in South Africa and India, UNFPA, Population and Development Strategies, No. 2, 93-110.

71. Statistics Canada. (2006) "Continuous Learning, Work and Participation in Society." A Portrait of seniors in Canada Catalogue no. 89-519:107-136.

72. Szinovacz, M.E. (2003) 'Contexts and pathways: Retirement as institution, process, and experience', pp. 6-52 in G.A. Adams and T.A. Beehr (eds) *Retirement: Reasons, Processes, and Results*. New York: Springer Publishing Company.
73. Towers, P. (2005)The Business Case for Workers Age 50+: Planning for Tomorrow's Talent Needs in Today's Competitive Environment, , Washington DC: AARP
74. Towers, P . (2008) Investing in training 50+ workers: A talent management strategy. Retrieved from American Association of Retired Persons website: http://www.aarp.org/work/work-life/info04_2008/_investing_in_training_50_workers_a_talent_management_strategy.html
75. United Nations (UN), (2002), International Plan of Action on Ageing, Second world assembly on ageing, 8 to 12 April 2002, Madrid.
76. University of Indianapolis. (2005) Gray matters : Opportunities and Challenges for Indiana's Aging Workforce : Phase 1--the Aging Matrix Publisher: Indianapolis : University of Indianapolis Center for Aging and Community,
77. United Nations (2007) World population ageing (New York).
78. United Nations Population Fund (UNFPA) (2002) Population ageing and development: Social, Health and Gender Issues, No. 3: 21.
79. Vijay Kumar, S. (2002) Economic Issue of Elderly in India
80. Vaidyanathan, R. (2003) "Pension Products for the Self Employed in India," Asia Pacific Risk and Insurance Association, 7th Annual Conference, Bangkok
81. World Health Organization (2002) "Active Aging: A Policy Framework," Second United Nations World Assembly on Aging, Madrid, Spain, April
82. Waldman, D. A., and Avolio, B. J. (1993) "Aging and Work Performance in Perspective: Contextual and Development Considerations." Research in Personnel and Human Resource Management 11: 133-162.
83. Wang, Mo; Shultz, Kenneth (2010) Employee Retirement: A Review and Recommendations for Future Investigations. In: Journal of Management 36,1: 172-206 (doi: 10.1177/0149206309347957).
84. Yesudian, C.A.K. (1998) "Socioeconomic Implications of Aging," WHO Symposium Aging and Health: A Global Challenge for the 21st Century, Kobe, Japan, and November 10-13,.

BIBLIOGRAPHY

1. Central Statistical Organization (2000) A Report: Programme for the Elderly, Government of India, New Delhi.

2. Eschtruth, A., Sass, S., and Aubry, J. (2007). Employers lukewarm about retaining older works (Issue in Brief WOB No. 10) Chestnut Hill, MA : Center for Retirement Research . Federal Interagency Forum on Aging-Related Statistics . (2008). Older Americans 2008: Key indicators of well-being . Washington, DC : U.S. Government Printing Office .

3. Ferraro, K.F. (2009). Editing in the rearview mirror . Journal of Gerontology: Social Sciences

4. Ferraro, K. F., Shippee, T. P., and Schafer, M. H. (2009). Cumulative inequality theory for research on aging and the life course . In V. Bengtson,

5. Freedman, M. (2007). Encore: Finding work that matters in the second half of life . New York : Public Affairs .

6. Friedberg, L., and Owyang, M. (2002). Not your father's pension plan: The rise of 401(k) and other defi ned contribution plans . Review/Federal Reserve Bank of St. Louis

7. Fronstin, P. (2005). The impact of the erosion of retiree health benefi ts on workers and retirees (EBRI Issue Brief No. 279) Washington, DC : Employee Benefi t Research Institute .

8. Ghilarducci, T. (2008). When I'm sixty-four: The plot against pensions and the plan to save them Princeton, NJ : Princeton University Press .

9. Gilleard, C., and Higgs, P. (2000). Cultures of ageing: Self, citizen, and the body New York : Prentice Hall .

10. Gilleard, C., and Higgs, P. (2005). Contexts of ageing: Class, cohort and community

11. George (Eds.), Handbook of aging and the social sciences (5th ed., pp. 255 – 272). San Diego, CA : Academic Press .

12. Hardy, M. A., and Hazelrigg, L. (2007). Pension puzzles: Social Security and the great debate New York : Russell Sage .

13. Henretta, J. C. (2001). Work and retirement. In R. H. Binstock and L. K.

14. Hershey, D. A., Jacobs-Lawson, J. M., McArdle, J. J., and Hamagami, A. (2007). Psychological foundations of financial planning for retire- ment. Journal of Adult Development

15. Helpage International (1999) In Judith Randel, Tony German and Deborah Ewing (Eds) The Ageing and Development Report: Poverty, Independence and the World's Older People, Earths can Publications Ltd, London.

16. Irudaya Rajan, S. (2001). "Social assistance for poor elderly: How effective?" in Economic and Political Weekly, Vol. 36, No. 8, pp. 613-17.

17. Irudaya Rajan, S.; Sarma, P.S.; Mishra, U.S. (2003). "Demography of Indian aging, 2001-2051", in Journal of Aging and Social Policy, Vol. 15, Nos. 2 and 3, pp. 11-30

18. Irudaya Rajan, S, Myrtle Perera and Sharifa Begum. (2005). The Economics of Pensions and Social Security in South Asia. Chapter 5, Pp.196-257 in Mohsin Khan (ed). Economic Development in South Asia. Tata McGraw Hill, New Delhi.

19. Irudaya Rajan, S. (2006). Population Ageing and Health in India. Background Paper Series 1, Cente for Enquiry into Health and Allied Themes. Mumbai. www.cehat.org

20. Irudaya Rajan, S., U. Mishra and P. Sankara Sarma (1999).*India's Elderly: Burden or Challenge?* Sage Publications, New Delhi,

21. Irudaya Rajan, S. and S. Kumar (2003) "Living Arrangements among Indian Elderly: New Evidence from National Family Health Survey". In *Economic and Political Weekly*, 38 (1): 75-80,.

22. Irudaya Rajan, S. and K. Zachariah (eds.) (1997)*Kerala's Demographic Transition: Determinants and Consequences*. Sage Publications, New Delhi,.

23. Johnson, R. W. (2002). The puzzle of later male retirement. Economic Review/Federal Reserve Bank of Kansas City

24. Johnson, R. W. (2004). Trends in job demands among older workers, 1992- 2002 .Monthly Labor Review

25. Johnson, R. W. (2009). Managers' attitudes toward older workers: A re- view of the evidence. In S. J. Czaja and J. Sharit (Eds.)

26. Joint Committee on Taxation. (2008). Estimates of federal tax expenditures for fiscal years 2008 – 2012 Washington, DC: U.S. Government Printing Office.

27. Lahey, J. (2005). Do older workers face discrimination? (Issue in Brief No. 33) Chestnut Hill, MA : Center for Retirement Research.
28. Lippmann, S. (2008). Rethinking risk in the new economy: Age and cohort effects on unemployment and re-employment. Human Relations
29. Lowenstein, R. (2005). The end of pensions. New York Times Magazine pp. 56 – 63, 70, 82, 90.
30. Lumsdaine, R., and Mitchell, O. (1999). New developments in the economic analysis of retirement. In O. Ashenfelter and R. Layard (Eds.), Handbook of labor economics (vol. 3, pp. 3261 – 3308). New York : North-Holland. Luo, M. (2009). Longer unemployment for those 45 and older. New York Times, p. A11.
31. Lusardi, A., and Mitchell, O. (2007). Financial literacy and retirement pre-paredness: Evidence and implications for financial education. Busi- ness Economics
32. Moore, E. (1946). Preparation for retirement. Journal of Gerontology 1 202 – 211.
33. Muldoon, D., and Kopcke, R. (2008). Are people claiming social security benefits later? (Issue in Brief No. 8-7). Chestnut Hill, MA : Center for Retirement Research.
34. Munnell, A., Webb, A., and Golub-Sass, F. (2007). Is there really a retirement savings crisis? An NRRI analysis (Issue in Brief No. 7-11) Chestnut Hill, MA : Center for Retirement Research.
35. Munnell, A. H., and Sass, S. A. (2008). Working longer: The solution to the retirement income challeng Washington, DC : Brookings Institution Press. Oliver, C. (2008).
36. NSSO (1988) *The Aged in India : A socioeconomic profile NSS* 52nd Round (July 1995- June 1996), Government of India.
37. National Sample Survey Organization. (2006). Morbidity, health care and the condition of the aged. NSS 60th round, (January-June 2004), Report No. 507 (New Delhi, India, Ministry of Statistics and Programme Implementation).
38. Polivka, L., and Longino, C. F., Jr (2006). The emerging postmodern culture of aging and retirement security. In J. Baars, D. Dannefer

39. Quinn, and Joseph F. 1999. "Has the Early Retirement Trend Reversed?" Paper presented at the First Annual Joint conference for the Retirement Research consortium, Washington, DC, May 20-21
40. Rao, K.V. (1995) Rural Elderly in Andhra Pradesh: A Study of Their Socio Demographic Profile, unpublished doctoral dissertation, Andhra University, Visakhapatnam (mimeo).
41. Retirement migration: Paradoxes of ageing New York : Routledge .
42. Rix , S. (2008). Age and work in the United States of America . In P. Taylor (Ed.),
43. Roscigno , V. , Mong , S. , Byron , R. , and Tester , G. (2007). Age discrimination, social closure and employment . Social Forces 86 313 .
44. Siva Raju, S.(1991) Health care system in India: need for comprehensive evaluation, in Primary Health Care, C.A.K. Yesudian (ed.) Tata Institute of Social Sciences, Bombay.
45. Siva Raju, S.(1997) Medico-Social Study on the Assessment of Health Status of the Urban Elderly, Tata Institute of Social Sciences, Bombay,(mimeo).
46. Siva. S. (2000) Ageing in India : An overview in, *Gerontological Social Work in India: Some Issues and Perspectives*. (eds) Murli Desai and Siva Raju, Delhi.
47. Savishinsky , J. S. (2000). Breaking the watch: The meanings of retirement in America Ithaca, NY : Cornell University Press .
48. Schafer , M. , and Ferraro , K. (2009). Data sources for studying aging . In P. Uhlenberg (Ed.), International handbook of population aging (pp. 19 – 36). New York : Springer .
49. Schulz , J. H. , and Binstock , J. H. (2006). Aging nation: The economics and politics of growing older in America
50. United Nations (1999) Population Ageing 1999, United Nations Population Division, Department of Economic and Social Affairs, New York.
51. United Nations. (2003). Announcement of theme for International Day for Older Persons, 2003 (http://www.un.org/esa/socdev/ageing/stmntid03.htm)
52. United Nations. (2002). World Population Ageing, 1950-2050, Department of Economic and Social Affairs, Population Division, New York
53. World Bank (2000) Attacking poverty, World DevelopmentReport,2000/2001, Oxford University Press, New York.

54. Why Population Aging Matters Global Perspective. 2007. National Institute on Aging National Institute of Health U.S. Department of Health and Human Services U.S. Department of State, pp.6-7.

55. Westport, CT : Praeger . Sennett, R. (1998). The corrosion of character: The personal consequences of work in the new capitalism New York : Norton

WEBLIOGRAPHY

- Gorman M.(2000) Development and the rights of older people. In: Randel J, et al., eds. The ageing and development report: poverty, independence and the world's older people. London, Earthscan Publications Ltd.,1999:3-21.
- Thane P. The muddled history of retiring at 60 and 65. New Society. 1978;45(826):234-236.
- http://ssmrae.com/admin/images/4d42135670d9d65349c0013b55f0bff6.pdf
- ("Sathy Gaya"-Gone crazy after age 60 years? Jan 17, 2007)
- 'Satya gaya' ---- Gone crazy after age 60 years? By aht42002 Jan 17, 2007
- http://www.indianexpress.com/res/web/pIe/ie/daily/19990408/ige08107.html
- http://in.rediff.com/money/2005/aug/25spec1.htm
- http://www.retirement-abc.com/The-Ups-and-Downs-of-Retirement.html
- **http://www.aifs.gov.au/institute/pubs/WP14.html**
- www.me-jaa.com/mejaa4/sso.pdf
- http://www.retirementplanblog.com/WT16-Retirement.pdf
- http://assets.aarp.org/rgcenter/econ/d17772_multiwork.pdf
- http://group.aomonline.org/cms/Meetings/Atlanta/Workshop06/Streams/Aging/CMS%20AgingWorkforcePaper-DeLong-FINAL6-21-06.pdf
- http://www.metlife.com/assets/cao/mmi/publications/studies/mmi-studies-living-longer.pdf
- http://assets.aarp.org/rgcenter/econ/aging_workforce.pdf
- http://assets.aarp.org/rgcenter/econ/mw_employers.pdf
- http://cac.uindy.edu/media/GrayMattersI.pdf
- http://www.urban.org/uploadedPDF/411705_aging_boomers.pdf
- http://www.globalresearch.com.my/proceeding/icber2010_proceeding/PAPER_138_LaborForce
- http://economicscience.net/files/Working%20beyond-retirement-age-in-Germany_20-10-10.pdf
- http://group.aomonline.org/cms/Meetings/Atlanta/Workshop06/Streams/Aging/CMS%20AgingWorkforcePaper-DeLong-FINAL6-21-06.pdf
- http://www.aegon.co.uk/downloads/pdf/pdf20080813.pdf

- http://ipsr.healthrepository.org/bitstream/123456789/307/3/THCT2004_Yukolnee%20Kangsasitiam_eng.pdf
- http://www.google.co.in/url?q=http://www.hrmguide.com/career/workinglonger.htmandsa=Uandei=d57jTKiSBMXzcamhlfMLandved=0CCEQFjAEandusg=AFQjCNEKnc1rML5E08Y6QCQacNm9Veq8XQ
- http://www.metlife.com/assets/cao/mmi/publications/studies/mmi-studies-living-longer.pdf
- http://assets.aarp.org/rgcenter/econ/aging_workforce.pdf
- http://assets.aarp.org/rgcenter/econ/mw_employers.pdf
- http://cac.uindy.edu/media/GrayMattersI.pdf
- http://www.urban.org/uploadedPDF/411705_aging_boomers.pdf
- http://www.globalresearch.com.my/proceeding/icber2010_proceeding/PAPER_138_LaborForce
- http://economicscience.net/files/Working%20beyond-retirement-age-in-Germany_20-10-10.pdf
- http://group.aomonline.org/cms/Meetings/Atlanta/Workshop06/Streams/Aging/CMS%20AgingWorkforcePaper-DeLong-FINAL6-21-06.pdf
- http://www.retirementplanblog.com/WT16-Retirement.pdf
- http://assets.aarp.org/rgcenter/econ/d17772_multiwork.pdf
- http://group.aomonline.org/cms/Meetings/Atlanta/Workshop06/Streams/Aging/CMS%20AgingWorkforcePaper-DeLong-FINAL6-21-06.pdf
- http://www.metlife.com/assets/cao/mmi/publications/studies/mmi-studies-living-longer.pdf
- http://assets.aarp.org/rgcenter/econ/aging_workforce.pdf
- http://assets.aarp.org/rgcenter/econ/mw_employers.pdf
- http://cac.uindy.edu/media/GrayMattersI.pdf
- http://www.urban.org/uploadedPDF/411705_aging_boomers.pdf
- http://www.globalresearch.com.my/proceeding/icber2010_proceeding/PAPER_138_LaborForce
- http://economicscience.net/files/Working%20beyond-retirement-age-in-Germany_20-10-10.pdf
- http://group.aomonline.org/cms/Meetings/Atlanta/Workshop06/Streams/Aging/CMS%20AgingWorkforcePaper-DeLong-FINAL6-21-06.pdf

- http://www.aegon.co.uk/downloads/pdf/pdf20080813.pdf
- http://ipsr.healthrepository.org/bitstream/123456789/307/3/THCT2004_Yukolnee%20Kangsasitiam_eng.pdf
- http://www.google.co.in/url?q=http://www.hrmguide.com/career/workinglonger.htmandsa=Uandei=d57jTKiSBMXzcamhlfMLandved=0CCEQFjAEandusg=AFQjCNEKnc1rML5E08Y6QCQacNm9Veq8XQ

Appendix 1: Tool for Elderly

Section-I

A. Background Information

Direction: Following are the items related to your personal information, please tick mark (✓) against appropriate options and give details wherever specified

1. Name : _____

2. Mailing Address : _____
   _____

3. Contact no : **(M)** _____ **(R)** _____

4. E-mail I.d : _____

5. Educational Qualification :

   Doctorate _____
   Post Graduate _____
   Graduate _____
   Diploma Holder _____
   Upto higher secondary school _____
   Upto Secondary school _____
   Upto primary school _____

6. Age (in years) : _____

7. Sex : Male _____ Female _____

8. Marital status : Married _____ Single _____
   Divorced _____ Widowed _____
   Separated _____ Live in relationship _____
   Any other specify _____

9. Religion : Hindu _____

   Muslim _____

   Christian _____

   Parsi _____

   Sikh _____

   Jain _____

   Any other _____

10. Caste : _____

11. Native Place : _____

12. Do you have your own house?

    Yes_____ No _____

Kindly give the details about your house:

Sr. no.	Type of House	Own	Rented	Companies Accommodation	Son's / daughters house, relatives house
a.	Flat				
b.	Bungalow/Tenement				
c.	Row house				
d.	Any other				

13. Do you have your own vehicle?

    Yes_____ No _____

    If yes please specify:

    i. Two wheeler _____

    ii. Four wheeler _____

a) Do you drive?

   Yes_____ No _____

b) If yes please specify which vehicle you drive

  i. Two wheeler _____
  ii. Four wheeler _____
 c) When do you drive?

  While going for:
  i. Work/job   _____
  ii. Social purposes   _____
  iii. For household related task (shopping, banking, paying bills, _____
   booking tickets)
  iv. To visit a doctor   _____
  v. Any other specify   _____

14. What do you do in your leisure time?

 a) Read
- Newspaper _____
- Magazine _____
- Books _____

 b) Listen to
- Bhajans _____
- Music _____
- Religious Lectures _____
- Political Lectures _____
- Social Lectures _____
- Educational Lectures _____
- Health Lectures _____

 c) Visit
- Temple _____
- Garden _____
- Relatives _____
- Neighbours _____
- Restaurants _____

- Theater/Cinema house_____
- Club/Mahila Mandal _____
- Any other _____

d) Play games
- Indoor _____
- Outdoor _____

e) Sleep _____

f) Do creative work(embroidery, stitching, painting) _____

g) Chintan/Yoga/Mediation _____

h) Go for walk _____

i) Learn/use computers _____

j) Help in household work _____

k) Play/take care of grandchildren _____

l) Any other _____

B. About Family

Direction: Following are the questions related to your family, please tick mark (✓) against appropriate options and give details wherever specified.

1. Type of family:

    a) Living alone   _____

    b) Living with spouse   _____

    c) Living with family   _____

    d) Any other   _____

2. Total Number of family members: _____

    Given below is the table, please fill in the details about your family members:

Names	Your Relationship with them	Age	Educational Qualification	Marital Status	Occupational Status			Disabilities	
					Working	Not Working	Physical	Mental	

3. Sources of your family's income per month

Sr. No.	Sources of Income	Income/ Amount
a.	Pension	
b.	Interest of fixed deposits	
c.	Rental income	
d.	Interest from investment	

C. About your Occupation

Direction: Following are the questions related to your **present occupation** (after retirement), please tick mark (✓) against appropriate options and give details wherever specified

1. Date of Retirement : _____

2. Date of joining present job after retirement : _____

3. Name of the organization/company/industry/ Firm/corporate you are presently working in
   _____

4. Is it the same organization where you used to work before retirement?

   Yes _____   No_____

5. Employment status

   a) Temporary   _____
   b) Permanent   _____
   c) Contract basis   _____
   d) Consultancy   _____

6. Type of organization:

   a) Government   _____
   b) Non-government   _____
   c) Corporate   _____
   d) Business house , _____
   e) Agency   _____
   f) Firm   _____

7. Type of work

   a) Part time   _____
   b) Full time   _____

8. Designation : _____

a) Is it the same designation you were having before retirement?

Yes_____ No _____

If <u>no</u> please specify the designation you were having before retirement

_____

_____

9. Salary/ Income : _____
   a) Fixed   _____
   b) Consolidated   _____
   c) On the basis of work I do   _____

10. What type of duties do you perform as part of your job?

_____

_____

   a) Are these the same duties as you used to perform before retirement?

   Yes _____ No _____

   If <u>no</u> please specify the duties in your job you performed before you retired.

   _____

   _____

11. Working hours
   a) Per day   _____
   b) Per week   _____

12. Distance of work place from your residence (in Kms) _____

13. After retirement is the present job your first?

   Yes _____ No _____

If no than please provide the details of your work <u>you did after retirement</u>:

Jobs	Designation	Date of Joining	Date of Leaving	Salary	Employment Status				Type of organization	Type of Work	
					Temporary	Permanent	Contract Basis	Consultancy		Part Time	Full Time
1st				a. Weekly ☐ b. Monthly ☐ c. Amount: _____					Government ☐ Non-government ☐ Agency ☐ Firm ☐ Business house ☐ Corporate ☐		
2nd				a. Weekly ☐ b. Monthly ☐ c. Amount: _____					Government ☐ Non-government ☐ Agency ☐ Firm ☐ Business house ☐ Corporate ☐		
3rd				a. Weekly ☐ b. Monthly ☐ c. Amount: _____					Government ☐ Non-government ☐ Agency ☐ Firm ☐ Business house ☐ Corporate ☐		

14. Who helped you to get the present job?

    a) My Family   _____

    b) My friend   _____

    c) My relatives   _____

    d) My colleague   _____

    e) My own initiative/active search(Newspaper advertisement _____
/website like 2nd Innings/ internet browsing)

15. What problems did you faced while searching a job after retirement?

    Kindly tick mark (✓) on the problems you faced while searching job.

    a) **GE**: If you faced problems to "Great Extent"
    b) **SE**: If you faced problems to "Some Extent"
    c) **LE**: If you faced problems to "Less Extent"

Sr.No.	Statements	GE	SE	LE
	Problems faced in searching job			
a.	Lack of job advertisements			
b.	Lack of many organizations /companies who recruit elderlies			
c.	Lack of job according to my qualification			
d.	Lack of job according to my abilities/expertise			
e.	Lack of job in the city I live in			
f.	Lack of job matching to my past experience			
g.	Lack of jobs of same designation (referring designation before retirement)			
h.	Lack of job with the pay/salary I used to get before retirement			

16. Did you get the present job easily or you had to work hard to get this job?

    a) Easy_____ b) Worked hard_____

17. Do you receive any social security benefits from your current job?

    Yes _____ No _____

    If <u>yes</u> please specify the benefits you receive _____
    _____

18. Why are you working on the present job?

    This job gives me

    a) Money   _____
    b) Opportunity to learn new skills   _____
    c) Good health benefits   _____
    d) Self-respect   _____

e) Respect in my family   _____
f) Respect from co- workers   _____
g) Freedom to share my views   _____
h) Flexibility in work timings   _____
i) Opportunity to use of my education _____
j) Friendly work environment   _____
k) Opportunity to do quality work _____
l) Good reputation in society   _____
m) Good pension plan   _____

19. Before you retired, did you expect or think of working after retirement?

Yes _____   No _____

20. Are you currently doing the type of work that you expected to do after retirement?

Yes _____   No _____

If no please specify the kind of work you would like to do_____

_____

21. What do you miss in your present job?

_____

_____

22. In comparison to the past how intense (passionate) is your work today?

_____

_____

23. What are the current retirement benefits that you are receiving?

a) Pension   _____
b) Health benefits   _____
c) Security benefits _____

D. Work History

Direction: Following are the questions related to your **last occupation** (before retirement), please tick mark (✓) against appropriate options and give details wherever specified

Kindly give details about your last job before retirement:

1. Name of the organization : _____
2. Designation : _____
3. Date of Joining : _____
4. Date of leaving : _____
5. Salary/ Income : _____
   a) Fixed   _____
   b) Consolidated   _____
   c) On the basis of work I do _____

6. Employment status
   a) Temporary   _____
   b) Permanent   _____
   c) On contract basis   _____
   d) Consultant   _____

7. Type of work
   a) Part time   _____
   b) Full time   _____

8. Type of organization:
   a) Government   _____
   b) Non-government   _____
   c) Corporate   _____
   d) Business house   _____
   e) Agency   _____
   f) Firm   _____

E. Health Proforma

Direction: Following is the list of health related problems, please tick mark (✓) against specific health problem if you are facing it.

Type of Problems:

a) Problems related to _____
Digestive system
(Gastric troubles, acidity, constipation, dysentery, diarrhea, indigestion, gastritis, vomiting nausea)

b) Problem of oral cavity _____
(Ulcers, inflammation of tongue, excessive salivation, lack of salivation, missing/ broken teeth, full/partial denture, caries/toothache, swollen gums)

c) Problems related to _____
respiratory system
(Recurrent cold, running nose, recurrent tonsillitis, pneumonia, aasthma, lung cancer)

d) Problems related to _____
cardiovascular system
(Blood pressure, pain in chest, enlargement of heart, pneumatic heart disease, hypertension)

e) Problems related to _____
genitourinary system
(Urinary tract infection,

      kidney stone, oedema,
      renal failure, dialysis, prostitis)

f)   Problems pertaining to   _____
    locomotors system
    (Osteomalacia, osteoporosis,
     osteosderosis, rheumatoid,
     arthritis, spondlitis, low backache
     after sleep, fever, frozen shoulders)
      Muscle (inflammation of muscle
     hard swellings)

g)   Problems related to   _____
    central nervous system
    (Tension, headaches
     migraine, sleep disturbances,
     Sudden/gradual dimness
     of vision, double vision (squint)
    convulsive attacks

h)   Problems related to   _____
     Endocrine system
     (Hypoglycemia, diabetes,
     hypothyroidism)

I)   Miscellaneous problem   _____
    (Aanemia, skin disorders,
    allergies, hearing aid,
    artificial limbs, calipers)

Section-II

A. Reasons of Working after Retirement

Direction: Listed below are the reasons of working after retirement, please tick mark (✓) against the statement in the column which describes the extent of your reason for working after retirement.

    a) **GE**: If you agree with the statement to "Great Extent"
    b) **SE**: Represents "Some Extent"
    c) **LE**: Represents "Less Extent"
    d) **NA**: Represents " Not Applicable"

1. What are the major reasons of your working after retirement?

Sr. No	Statements	GE	SE	LE	NA
1.	**I am working after retirement because**				
a.	I could be financially independent				
b.	I can spend money according to my own wish				
c.	I do not receive pension				
d.	I am not getting sufficient pension				
e.	I ran out of my savings				
f.	I want to build additional retirement savings				
g.	I want to pay off my mortgage				
h.	I incur heavy expenditure on my medicines				
i.	I want to reinvest for capital growth				
j.	I want to support my children financially				
k.	I am alone in my family				
l.	I can maintain my lifestyle				
m.	I can get attention and respect from family				
n.	I have important financial responsibility towards family				
o.	I want to buy another property				
p.	I want to renovate my house				
q.	I am sole bread earner of the family				

r.	I have responsibility of my children's education					
s.	I and my spouse need additional income for health care					
t.	I got the opportunity to work which is not too stressful					
u.	I got the opportunity to work on my dream job					
v.	I got an opportunity to learn new job skills					
w.	I got chance to do work that is not too physically demanding					
x.	I cannot imagine my life without work					
y.	I would be bored sitting idle					
z.	I find this job interesting					
aa.	I could stay physically active					
bb.	I could stay mentally active					
cc.	I could be productive, useful and helpful					
dd.	I could be around people					
ee.	I want to enjoy social interaction with colleagues					
ff.	The pay offered to me was too good to refuse					
gg.	Income from other sources is not enough					
hh.	There is desire in me to learn new things					
ii.	Long term care of my dependents					
jj.	My family is pressuring me to work					

B. Perceptions about Retirement

Part of every human being's self-image is based on their age, whether it is their chronological or their "subjective age", or how old they feel. Accordingly, when people reach retirement age, these two perceptions can widely differ. Society may view an individual of 65 as "ready to be put out to pasture", while that same individual still views himself as an active, energetic and productive member of the community. Consequently the negative stereotypes perpetuated by society often cause people to behave differently towards the elderly than they would had such harmful biases not been so deeply ingrained. : It's worth analyzing this concept a little closer, before we arrive there, to make sure it's a place we want to go. What is the purpose and meaning of "retirement" to you? Below listed are the perceptions about retirement, please tick mark (✓) against appropriate options and give details wherever specified:

1. Since when did you started planning related to finance for your retirement? **(Please mention age)** _____

    a) After retirement _____
    b) At the time of retirement _____
    c) Much before retirement _____

2. Which stage of your life did you enjoy?
    a) **GE**: If you agree with the statement to "Great Extent"
    b) **SE**: Represents "Some Extent"
    c) **LE**: Represents "Less Extent"

Sr. No.	Statements	GE	SE	LE
a.	Brahmacharya (Student stage of life)			
b.	Grahasta (Family stage of life)			
c.	Vanprastha (Indicates departure from material possession)			
d.	Sanyasa or renunciation(The person leaves society to spend the remaining part of his life in meditation and contemplation of God solitude			

3. How would you perceive retirement period as?
   a) **GE**: If you agree with the statement to "Great Extent"
   b) **SE**: Represents "Some Extent"
   c) **LE**: Represents "Less Extent

Sr. No	Statements	GE	SE	LE
1.	**According to me retirement means**			
a.	A stage to relax			
b.	A stage to have fun			
c.	A stage to fulfill dreams and aspirations which could not be fulfilled earlier			
d.	A stage to travel			
e.	A stage of more maturity			
f.	A stage to get involved in religious activities			
g.	A stage to serve family			
h.	A stage with more control over personal time			
i.	A stage to enjoy with grandchildren			
j.	A stage with less family responsibilities			
k.	A stage with less financial responsibility			
l.	A stage of freedom from work pressures			
m.	An opportunity to contribute to the society			
n.	An opportunity to share knowledge and experience			
o.	More respect in society			
p.	Getting more attention from the family			
q.	Working after retirement because I enjoy working			
r.	Establishing new routine			
s.	Feeling too young to retire			
t.	Worrying about retiring			
u.	Working in order to get by financially			
v.	unable to face people with confidence			
w.	Feeling unwanted in society			

x.	Having the fear of being dejected or left out by family members			
y.	Accommodating in post-retirement lifestyle is difficult			
z.	Learning a new survival skill for postretirement life			
aa.	Managing new and low social status			
bb.	Managing irregular or non-payment of retirement benefit			
cc.	Managing surplus time at my disposal			
dd.	Coping with long hours with my partner without our children			
ee.	Developing of feelings of inferiority complex			
ff.	Starting of old age			
gg.	Sense of worthlessness			
hh.	Decline in social life			
ii.	Loss of interest in life			
jj.	Less fun in life			
kk.	Health deterioration			
ll.	Cursed stage of life			
mm.	Physically unable to do household work			
nn.	A period of misery			
oo.	A slide to dependency			
pp.	Fear of isolation			
qq.	Feeling of insecurity			
rr.	Loosing charm of looks			
ss.	Prone to disease			
tt.	Problems of ageing and imminent death			

4. Do you think during retirement age you need more money?

    Yes _____ No _____

    If **Yes**, then on which aspects
    a) Health emergencies   _____
    b) House maintenance   _____
    c) Domestic services   _____
    d) Leisure and entertainment   _____
    e) Tour and travels   _____
    f) Old age homes   _____

5. For which of the following reasons are you prepared to spend more money in retirement?
   a) Deterioration in health _____
   b) Death of Partner _____
   c) Not being able to take care of self _____
   d) Being a burden on children _____
   e) Running out of money _____
   f) Being able to leave some money for children/grandchildren _____

6. Which are important factors in deciding the time to retire?
   a) When I achieve certain amount of money for retirement _____
   b) When I am eligible for retire health benefits _____
   c) When I accomplish certain career or job related goals _____
   d) When my children start earning _____

7. How have you prepared yourself for retirement?
   a) By reading books of renowned authors _____
   b) By attending lectures of religious guru _____
   c) By discussing with friends who have already retired _____

8. Who do you think should be primarily responsible for helping workers prepare for retirement? (Here worker is referred to the people who are working and not yet retired from their job)
   a) Co-workers _____
   b) Employers _____
   c) Government _____
   d) All of three _____

9. Which one of these do you think probably caused some retirees to have inadequate income or savings?
   a) They did not plan well for retirement _____
   b) They believed other would look out financially for them _____
   c) Medical bills used up their savings _____

Section- III

Influence of Work on Elder Workers

Sr. No.	Statements	GE	SE	LE
	Due to Working			
a.	I am able to receive health benefits and wellness supports			
b.	I get respect and attention from my family			
c.	I am able to get recognition in society			
d.	I am able to contribute my experience to the society			
e.	I am able to support my children financially			
f.	I am able to face people with confidence			
g.	I am able to work on new technologies such as computer, mobile, i-pad			
h.	I am overburdened with responsibilities			
i.	I am able to be physically active			
j.	I am able to be mentally active			
k.	I am able to have interaction with people			
l.	I am able to accomplish certain career or job related goals			
m.	I am facing more health problems			
n.	I feel more stressed after working for the whole week			
o.	I am able to save money			
p.	I am not able to spend time with my family			
q.	I am not able to take care of my spouse			
r.	I m able to spend more for my health needs			
s.	I am able to spend for my leisure/entertainment activities			
t.	I feel insulted to work under younger generation			
u.	I do not have to depend on my children for financial requirements			
v.	I do not get enough leisure time			
w.	My health is not permitting me to work for long hours			
x.	My economic status has improved			

Section IV

Problems Faced by Elder Workers at Workplace

Since there is prescribed retirement age in organizations/companies/business houses/firms/agencies, when you are working beyond that age, you may be facing some problems. Enlisted below are the problems which you may be facing at your workplace. Kindly tick mark (✓) on the problems you face and give details wherever specified.

a) **GE**: If you face problems to "Great Extent"
b) **SE**: If you face problems to "Some Extent"
c) **LE**: If you face problems to "Less Extent"
d) **N.A** If it is not applicable

Sr. No	Statements	GE	SE	LE	NA
	Problems Faced at Work Place				
a.	I am discriminated due to age				
b.	Working on new technologies like computers ,laptops, fax, E-mails				
c.	Not feeling comfortable working with young generation				
d.	Over burdened with work				
e.	Not being able to face people with confidence				
f.	Facing difficulty in traveling to work place				
g.	Always having fear and anxiety of losing job/work				
h.	Finding office hours very long				
i.	My nature of comparing my present and previous work/job				
j.	My job is physically demanding				
k.	My opinions and experience are not valued				
l.	Work environment is not suitable				
m.	Work is not interesting				
n.	Co-workers are not giving respect				
o.	Co-workers are not willing to work with me				
p.	Co-workers are neglecting me				
q.	Lack of necessary skills or education				
r.	Lack of appreciation from boss				

s.	Lack of independence in terms of taking decision related to work			
t.	Lack of flexibility related to working hours			
u.	Lack of clearly defined roles and responsibilities			
v.	Remuneration is not sufficient			
w.	Work place is very far from my residence			
x.	Designation given to me is not appreciating my experience			
y.	Not able to concentrate while working			

24. Do you think elder workers are treated unfairly when employers are:
a) Making hiring decision   _____
b) Assigning desirable work   _____
c) Determining salary increase   _____
d) Laying off employees   _____

Section V

Satisfaction at Work Place

Direction: Following are the statements related to the satisfaction at work place. Please tick mark (✓) against appropriate options and give details wherever specified.

a) **GE**: If you agree with the statement to "Great Extent"
b) **SE**: Represents "Some Extent"
c) **LE**: Represents "Less Extent"

Sr. No	Statements	GE	SE	LE
a.	I have good opportunities for learning new job skills			
b.	People are very friendly			
c.	Welfare facilities are good			
d.	I find my work offer challenges to advance my skills			
e.	I have full freedom to do my own work			
f.	Salary i get for nature of my work is enough			
g.	My boss shoulder some of my worries about work			
h.	I believe in the principles by which my employer operates			
i.	I feel satisfied with work's value system			
j.	I get encouragement from employers to take my own decisions in day to day work			
k.	There is good arrangement for settlement of disputes and readdressal of our grievances			
l.	Employees co operate with each other and there are no quarrels			

1. To what extent do you feel appreciated today?

   _____

   _____

2. How far do you feel you meet the demands of <u>work today</u>?

3. How important or meaningful was your <u>work in past</u>?

4. How important or meaningful is your work today?

5. At what age do you think you will be <u>able financially to retire</u> from full/part time work for pay?

6. Regardless of when do you think you will be able to retire from full/part time job/work for pay, <u>at what age, ideally, would you like to retire</u>?

Section VI
Suggestions

Direction: Following are the items related to suggestions, please tick mark (✓) against appropriate options and give details wherever specified

1. Do you think there should be specific personnel policy for elder employees in organization?

   Yes_____ No_____

   If yes what should these specific personnel policies contain?

   _____

   _____

2. Where do you see the greatest need for action by the employers concerning engagement of elder employees?

   a) Support transfer of knowledge and experience _____
   b) Interchange between young and old _____
   c) Make work of older people possible _____
   d) Change of attitude/ valuation/ appreciation _____
   e) Observance of demands in everyday work life _____
   f) Make further development possible _____
   g) Change public policies _____
   h) Payment regulations _____
   i) Concentrate on younger people _____
   j) No need for action _____

3. Which services for elder employees do you think are especially important?

   a) Heath care services _____
   b) Reduced/flexible working hours _____
   c) Adapted demands and workplace design _____
   d) Counseling/support _____
   e) Integration into company _____

f) Further education   _____
g) Contact   _____
h) Company pension scheme   _____
i) Domestic supply   _____

4. Which of the following could an employer provide that would make working in later life more attractive?

   a) Ability to guide and teach young workers   _____
   b) Opportunity to work fewer hours   _____
   c) Opportunity to learn new skills   _____
   d) Ability to undertake less physically demanding work   _____
   e) New kinds of work   _____
   f) Ability to continue earning an income   _____
   g) Enjoyable and stimulating work place   _____
   h) Nothing   _____

5. What important message do you want to give to the people who are planning to do productive work in retirement?

   _____

   _____

Appendix 2: Tool for Employers

Section-I

Background Information

Direction: Following are the items related to the organization/ company, please tick mark (✓) against appropriate options and give details wherever specified

1. Name : _____

2. Designation : _____

3. Age : _____

4. Sex : Male _____ Female _____

5. Your Experience in this : _____
   Company/Institution/Firm (in years)

6. Name of the organization/company : _____
   _____

7. Address : _____
   _____

8. Email : _____

9. Contact no : (M) _____

   (o) _____

10. Year of Establishment : _____

11. Vacancies in the organization/company : _____
    (in present year)

12. Type of organization:

    a) Government   _____
    b) Non-government   _____
    c) Corporate   _____
    d) Business house   _____
    e) Agency   _____
    f) Firm   _____

13. What are objectives/mission of your organization/ company?

_____

_____

14. Annual turnover of the organization/company _____

15. Paid staff(in numbers) :

    a) Full time   _____

    b) Part time   _____

    c) Consultancy basis   _____

16. What are the financing resources you resort to for your organization/company?

    a) Operating profits   _____

    b) Business savings   _____

    c) Private savings   _____

    d) Bank loans   _____

    e) Private loans   _____

    f) Introducing new partners   _____

    g) Not sure/refused   _____

17. What is the retirement age in your organization/company?

_____

18. What is the organization /company's policy for retirement?

_____

_____

19. What is organization/company's policy in terms of voluntary retirement?

_____

_____

20. What are the retirement benefits provided by your organization/ company?

_____

_____

Section-II

Information related to Elder Workers

Direction: Give information of Elder workers working in your organization/ company, please tick mark (✓) against appropriate options and give details wherever specified

1. What makes it challenging to find qualified elder workers with the experience and skills that your organization/company needs?

   _____

   _____

2. Currently, how many elder workers are working in the organization/company?
   a) 1– 5   _____
   b) 6 – 20   _____
   c) 21 – 100   _____
   d) More than 100 _____
   e) Not sure/refused _____

3. Compared to last year, the present number of elder workers you currently have are more, few, the same, or are you not sure?

   _____

4. At what levels are elder workers employed?

   _____

   _____

5. Do you employ elderly females in your company?
   a) Yes   _____
   b) No not sure _____
   c) Refused   _____

6. As regards to recruitment in organization/company, which of the following best describes your role?
   a) I am responsible for managing the actual recruitment process _____
   b) I generally specify requirements for employees but do not   _____
      conduct the actual recruitment

c) I specify both requirements for employees and_____ conduct the actual recruitment

d) Other (specify)_____

7. What would you say are the main reasons your organization/company does not do more to attract or retain elder workers?

   a) Not an urgent or pressing issue   _____
   b) Work is too physical to employ people past a certain age _____
   c) Elder workers are more expensive   _____
   d) Government regulations/policies get in way   _____
   e) Elder workers are not as capable as young workers   _____
   f) Elder workers are not valuable as young workers   _____

8. Thinking about the type of person you recruit most often, choose the quality that best describes that person from the following qualities:

Sr. No	Statements	GE	SE	LE
a.	An employee who can work full-time and is willing to work longer hours if required			
b.	An employee who is willing to be flexible and work varied hours (including shorter hours) if required			
c.	An employee with a lot of experience			
d.	A promising employee with recent training			
e.	An employee who works calmly			
f.	An employee who is trustworthy			
g.	An employee who is reliable			
h.	An employee who enjoys challenges			
i.	An employee who listens carefully and follows instructions			
j.	An employee who is able take the initiative			
k.	An employee who adapts well to change			
l.	An employee who is mentally very sharp			
m.	An employee with physical strength and stamina			
n.	An employee who is over-qualified for the job			
o.	An employee with similar background			
p.	An employee with specialist skills			

q.	An employee with the ability to work in different areas of the business as needed			
r.	An employee who works effectively as part of a team			
s.	An employee who can work independently			
t.	An employee who is energetic and enthusiastic			
u.	An employee who is innovative			
v.	An employee who is ambitious			

9. Throughout a person's working life, there are times when they are able to make a larger or smaller contribution to the workplace. In your experience, at what age do people make the best contribution to the business?

   a) Under 30 years of age   _____
   b) 30-44 years of age   _____
   c) 45-54 years of age   _____
   d) 55 or over years of age   _____
   e) At any age   _____

10. Compared to all other workers in your organization which of the following do you consider being advantages/reasons of employing elder workers in your organization /company?

    a) **GE**: If you agree with the statement to "Great Extent"
    b) **SE**: Represents "Some Extent"
    c) **LE**: Represents "Less Extent"

Sr. No.	Statements	GE	SE	LE
a.	They have high level of engagement in their work			
b.	They have ability to mentor other workers			
c.	They have valuable insights into customers or business needs			
d.	They are highly productive			
e.	They have invaluable experience			
f.	They have strong work ethics			
g.	They have established network of contacts and clients			
h.	They are more dependable			
i.	Their dedication provide significant business advantage			

j.	They are hard working			
k.	They have positive attitude			
l.	They are highly skilled			
m.	They remain loyal to the organization/ company			
n.	They do not need guidance			
o.	They can be count in crisis			
p.	They have diversity of thoughts and new approaches to teamwork			
q.	They are more readily available to start work			
r.	They have lower propensity to quit or change job			

11. Compared to all other workers in your organization which of the following do you consider to be disadvantages/problems of elder workers in your organization/ company?

   a) **GE**: If you agree with the statement to "Great Extent"
   b) **SE**: Represents "Some Extent"
   c) **LE**: Represents "Less Extent"

Sr. No.	Statements	GE	SE	LE
a.	They are not flexible compared to young workers			
b.	They are not receptive to training & skills			
c.	They are unable to meet the physical demands of the job			
d.	They have persistent health problems			
e.	They have lower productivity			
f.	Integrating multiple generations of workers and accommodating part time and flexible schedules			
g.	They prefer to work on own tasks and methods			
h.	They fear changes in work place			
i.	They are reculant to learn new technologies			
j.	They have negative attitude towards organizational change			
k.	They have lack of innovative thinking			
l.	They lack Poise & Confidence			
m.	They are source of greater health security and health expense			

n.	They have high rate of absenteeism			
o.	They do not keep up with technology			
p.	They are reculant to travel			
q.	They have high wage expectation			

12. Does your organization have any formal policies or programs to encourage employees who are approaching retirement to <u>continue working</u>?

   a) Yes　　　　　　　　　　　　　_____

   b) No, but we plan to develop a policy _____
   and/or program with this objective

   c) No　　　　　　　　　　　　　_____

13. How concerned are you, if at all, that your organization may lose valuable knowledge related to your business and/or hard to- replace skills over the next ten years as employees retire?

   a) Very concerned　　　　_____
   b) Somewhat concerned　　_____
   c) Not too concerned　　　_____
   d) Not at all concerned　　_____

14. How influential do you think each of the following factors would be in causing employees in your organization who are approaching retirement and want to continue working beyond their expected retirement age?

   a) **GE**: If you agree with the statement to "Great Extent"
   b) **SE**: Represents "Some Extent"
   c) **LE**: Represents "Less Extent"

Sr. No.	Statements	GE	SE	LE
a.	Desire for income			
b.	Enjoyment derived from work			
c.	Sense of fulfillment derived from work			
d.	Desire to be productive and feel useful			
e.	Sense of responsibility to help co-workers			
f.	Social interaction with co-workers			

g.	Desire for health benefits			
h.	Opportunity to continue to learn			
i.	Recognition received for work			
j.	Opportunity to work a reduced schedule for a period of time before retiring completely			